T0192535

Pharmacoeconomics

Pharmacoeconomics
From Theory to Practice

Second Edition

Edited by
Renée J.G. Arnold, PharmD, RPh

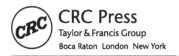

CRC Press
Taylor & Francis Group
Boca Raton London New York

CRC Press is an imprint of the
Taylor & Francis Group, an **informa** business

Second edition published 2021
by CRC Press
4 Park Square, Milton Park, Abingdon, Oxon, OX14 4RN

and by CRC Press
6000 Broken Sound Parkway NW, Suite 300, Boca Raton, FL 33487-2742

© 2021 selection and editorial matter Renée J.G. Arnold individual chapters,
the contributors
CRC Press is an imprint of Taylor & Francis Group, an Informa business

First edition published by CRC Press 2009

International Standard Book Number-13: 978-1-138-58983-4 (Hardback)
International Standard Book Number-13: 978-0-367-52136-3 (Paperback)

Library of Congress Cataloging-in-Publication Data

Names: Arnold, Renee J. G., editor.
Title: Pharmacoeconomics : from theory to practice / edited by Renée J.G. Arnold.
Description: Second edition. | Milton Park, Abingdon, Oxon ; Boca Raton, FL : CRC Press, [2020] | Includes bibliographical references and index.
Identifiers: LCCN 2020013270 | ISBN 9781138589834 (hardback) |
ISBN 9780367521363 (paperback) | ISBN 9780429491368 (ebook)
Subjects: LCSH: Drugs–Cost effectiveness. | Pharmacy–Economic aspects. | Decision making.
Classification: LCC RS100 .P433 2020 | DDC 615.1–dc23
LC record available at https://lccn.loc.gov/2020013270

Contents

Preface

The genesis of this book was the pharmacoeconomics research and other outcomes projects that my colleagues and I have completed for our pharmaceutical company and government clients over the years. The chapters' ideas came specifically from the Introduction to Pharmacoeconomics course that I developed and currently teach for the Icahn School of Medicine at Mount Sinai Master of Public Health Program. I have extensively collaborated with many of the colleagues who have written chapters for this book and I am truly grateful to them who, despite being extremely busy, have contributed their valuable time and collective wisdom to make this book useful and practical. This book is meant to introduce the major concepts and principles of pharmacoeconomics, with particular emphasis on modeling, methodologies, and data sources and applications to real-world dilemmas. Readers will learn about the use of pharmacoeconomics in drug reimbursement and pricing internationally. Examples of pharmacoeconomic models used to support these purposes in government, the pharmaceutical industry, and healthcare settings are also given.

The first edition of this book focused on pharmacoeconomic analyses of a public health vaccination program and collaboration among members of the pharmaceutical industry, academia, and government in the development of the human papillomavirus vaccine. In this second edition, we broaden the focus to include more recent examples of published analyses and/or current thinking about relevant issues, such as new chapters on multicriteria decision analysis (MCDA), discretely integrated condition event (DICE) simulation, global implementation of value frameworks, international experience in use of pharmacoeconomics in drug reimbursement, and anticipated future developments in the field. In addition to cost, the book examines a full range of ethical and moral issues, as well as overall public health and commercial concerns that are often involved in decisions entailing pharmacoeconomic decision-making. Unfortunately, this book was already in galleys when the novel severe acute respiratory syndrome (SARS-CoV-2, also referred to as Covid-19) became a global pandemic in 2020, so has been addressed only in a few instances here and in a final small chapter. Suffice it to say, however, that a multitude of issues described in the book are extremely relevant to the public health and economic consequences being faced currently and for years to come.

Lest the reader think these issues esoteric or untimely, the reader is referred to multiple articles both in the scientific literature and lay press (e.g., *The New York Times* and *Wall Street Journal*) on comparative cost-effectiveness of medications for pandemic diseases, such as the novel coronavirus-19, prevalent diseases, such as hepatitis C and atopic eczema, and also for rare diseases such as spinal muscular atrophy.

These principles are being embodied, for example, in the much-discussed US Institute for Clinical and Economic Review (interestingly, the same acronym as an oft-used concept in pharmacoeconomics – the incremental cost-effectiveness ratio, or ICER) evaluations and in guidances rendered by the UK's National Institute for Health and Care Excellence (NICE). Pharmacogenomics, or the use of personalized medicine, will be combined with cost-effectiveness analyses, to inform and improve healthcare decision-making. Thus, improved and cost-effective decisions, using the best available, evidence-based medicine, will require that both clinical and economic expertise, as epitomized in this book, be used.

Renée J. G. Arnold, PharmD, RPh

Acknowledgments

I gratefully acknowledge my colleague and friend, Dr. Sean Ekins, who prompted me to write the first edition of this book and also contributed a chapter to both the first and second editions. I also acknowledge all of my illustrious coauthors (according to chapter number) Drs. William F. McGhan, Mark Roberts, Ken Smith, J. Robert Beck (who included updated examples and created a new figure!), Sanjeev Balu, Alan Haycox (who took on an additional chapter besides his own), Lieven Annemans, Jo Mauskopf (who was so kind as to update Dr. Annemans' chapter with incredibly helpful text, examples, and illustrations), Kevin Marsh (who provided a new chapter on MCDA), Sumitra Sri Bhashyam (new chapter coauthor), Jaime Caro (with his wit and insight about what the future may hold in our field and who has kindly provided me with professional guidance), Stuart Birks, Gordon Guyatt, Dianne Bryant, Andrew Firth, Maarten Postma, Chris Sampson, Neil X. Hawkins (who provided the international counterpoint to our new value-based pricing chapter), and Ryung Suh. Lastly, in terms of this second edition, I gratefully thank Ms. Hilary Lafoe and Ms. Jessica Poile who encouraged me to be thorough and unrelenting in pursuing excellence and to my excellent editors, Subathra Manogaran and Sunantha Ramamoorthy.

Although not included in this newest edition, I would also like to thank Dr. Michael Drummond for his support initially in my health economics and outcomes research career (I recruited him as the keynote speaker for the first International Society for Pharmacoeconomics and Outcomes Research [ISPOR] meeting) and throughout my career in the field; he always responded in a forthright and helpful manner. Speaking of ISPOR, I also gratefully acknowledge the late Dr. Marilyn Dix Smith and Dr. Alan Bakst, who approached me after a CEPOR meeting in North Carolina to help cofound ISPOR, originally founded as the Association for Pharmacoeconomics and Outcomes Research (APOR), in 1995. Marilyn was my true mentor in the organization. I would also like to thank my parents, Jack and Betty Goldberg; Jack was a true clinical pharmacist whom everyone who went to his pharmacies called "Doc" and who was my inspiration to enter the field. Betty continues to be an inspiration in my scientific and personal endeavors. Both have been an inspiration about the power of persistence. Lastly, I would be remiss if I do not acknowledge my husband, Michael, and son, Marc, for their ongoing love and support!

Editor

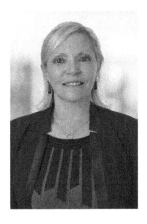

Renée J.G. Arnold completed her undergraduate training at the University of Maryland and earned her Doctor of Clinical Pharmacy degree from the University of Southern California in Los Angeles. She also completed a post-doctoral residency at University Hospital in San Diego, which is affiliated with the University of California at San Francisco School of Pharmacy. She is currently President and CEO of Arnold Consultancy & Technology LLC, as well as Adjunct Professor, Department of Environmental Medicine and Public Health, Master of Public Health program, Icahn School of Medicine at Mount Sinai in New York City, where she developed and teaches the pharmacoeconomics coursework. Her special interest in evidence-based health derives from her research that deals with the use of technology to collect and/or model real-world data for use in rational decision-making by healthcare practitioners and policy makers.

Dr. Arnold was previously Vice President, Health Economics and Outcomes Research at Quorum Consulting, Inc./Navigant Consulting; Principal, IMS Health (IQVIA); and President and Cofounder of Pharmacon International, Inc. Center for Health Outcomes Excellence. She is a founding member and former Chair of the Education Committee of the International Society for Pharmacoeconomics and Outcomes Research (ISPOR). Currently, she chairs both the ISPOR Distance Learning Program and the newly developed Open Source Models Special Interest Group. At no time have healthcare models been more relevant than the present, where many coronavirus forecasting models, sometimes with wildly diverging predictions, have been referenced for morbidity, mortality, and the like. The problem she and others see is that the code and inputs are unavailable to understand how these results were derived. The use of open source models (OSMs), those for which all data and programming associated with the model are made openly available to enhance transparency and, perhaps, facilitate replication and ongoing modifications of the model, have the potential to allow for faster access to critical knowledge. Use of OSMs, perhaps in an easily accessible database, could allow for a "crowdsourced" model review and more accurate/timely models, at least as far as the existing data allow. Dr. Arnold is an author/coauthor of numerous articles, book chapters, and books in the areas of pharmacology, pharmacoeconomics, and cost containment strategies. She is also a reviewer for National Institutes of Health Small Business Innovation Research (SBIR) applications, for Patient-Centered Outcomes Research Institute (PCORI) applications, for numerous journals, including *Pharmacoeconomics, Journal of Managed Care Pharmacy, Value in Health, American Journal of Pharmacy Benefits, Nature Biotechnology,* and *Annals of Internal Medicine,* and is on the editorial board of *Pharmacoeconomics Open.* She is also a volunteer for the Medical Reserve Corps in New York City. In addition, Dr. Arnold is a licensed pharmacist.

Contributors

Mark S. Roberts, MD, MPP
Professor and Chair, Department of
  Health Policy and Management
Graduate School of Public Health
Professor of Medicine, Industrial
  Engineering, Business
  Administration and Clinical and
  Translational Science
University of Pittsburgh
Pittsburgh, PA, USA

Ken Smith, MD, MS
Professor of Medicine
Section of Decision Sciences and
  Clinical Systems Modeling
Division of General Internal
  Medicine, Department of Medicine
University of Pittsburgh
Pittsburgh, PA, USA

William F. McGhan, PharmD, PhD
President and Senior Researcher
Health Decision Strategies, LLC
Tampa, FL, USA

Professor Emeritus, Philadelphia
  College of Pharmacy and Health
  Policy
University of the Sciences
Philadelphia, PA, USA

Renée J.G. Arnold, PharmD, RPh
Adjunct Professor
Master of Public Health Program
  Department of Environmental
  Medicine and Public Health, Icahn
  School of Medicine at Mount Sinai
New York, NY, USA

President
Arnold Consultancy & Technology,
  LLC
New York, NY, USA

J. Robert Beck, M.D.
Deputy Director
Fox Chase Cancer Center
Philadelphia, PA, USA

Elizabeth A. Handorf, Ph.D.
Associate Research Professor
Fox Chase Cancer Center
Philadelphia, PA, USA

Sanjeev Balu, PhD
Senior Director, HEOR
US Oncology, Breast and Lung
  Cancer Franchises
Novartis Pharmaceuticals Corporation
East Hanover, NJ, USA

Alan Haycox, MD
Honorary Reader
University of Liverpool Management
  School

Director
Liverpool Health Economics
Liverpool, UK

Josephine Mauskopf, MA, MHA, PhD
Vice President, Health Economics
RTI International
Research Triangle Park, NC, USA

Lieven Annemans, MSc, MMan, PhD
Professor of Health Economics
Ghent University, Brussels
  University
Brussels, Belgium

Sumitra Sri Bhashyam, PhD
Operational Team Lead, Modelling
  and Optimisation
Decision Lab UK
London, UK

Kevin Marsh, PhD
Executive Director, Patient-Centered
    Research
Evidera
London, UK

**J. Jaime Caro, MDCD, FRCPC,
    FACP**
McGill University
Montreal, Canada
Evidera, Boston, USA
LSE, London, UK

Jörgen Möller, MSc
Vice President, Modeling
    Technologies, Evidence Synthesis,
    Modeling & Communication
Evidera
London, UK

Stuart Birks, PhD
Director, Centre for Public Policy
    Evaluation, Massey University
Palmerston North, NZ

Dianne Bryant, MSc, PhD
Clinical Epidemiologist
Professor
Assistant Dean of Graduate
    Programs, Faculty of Health
    Sciences
Faculty of Health Sciences, School of
    Physical Therapy
Schulich School of Medicine &
    Dentistry, Department of Surgery
Western University
London, Ontario, Canada

Andrew Firth, MSc
Fowler Kennedy Sports Medicine
    Clinic
Western University
London, Ontario, Canada

Gordon Guyatt, MD, MSc
Department of Clinical Epidemiology
    & Biostatistics
Hamilton Health Sciences Centre

McMaster University
Hamilton, Ontario, Canada

Prof Maarten J Postma
Unit of PharmacoEpidemiology &
    PharmacoEconomics (PE^2)
Department of Pharmacy
University of Groningen
Groningen, Netherlands

Chris Sampson, MSc, PhD
Principal Economist
Office of Health Economics
London, UK

Margherita Neri, MSc
Senior Economist
Office of Health Economics
London, UK

Kyann Zhang, MSc
Economist
Office of Health Economics
London, UK

Neil X. Hawkins, PhD, MBA, MSc
Professor
University of Glasgow
Scotland, UK

Ryung Suh, MD
Chair and Associate Professor,
    Department of Health Systems
    Administration
Georgetown University
Washington, DC, USA

David Atkins, MD, MPH
Director, Quality Enhancement
    Research Initiative (QUERI)
Department of Veterans Affairs
Washington, DC, USA

Sean Ekins, PhD
Founder, Board member, Chief
    Executive Officer
Collaborations Pharmaceuticals, Inc.
Raleigh, NC, USA

1 Introduction to Pharmacoeconomics

William F. McGhan, PharmD, PhD
Health Decision Strategies, LLC
Tampa, FL, USA

University of the Sciences
Philadelphia, PA, USA

Renée J.G. Arnold, PharmD, RPh
Icahn School of Medicine at Mount Sinai
Arnold Consultancy & Technology, LLC
New York, NY, USA

TABLE OF CONTENTS

1.1   INTRODUCTION

Practitioners, patients, and health agencies face a multitude of conundrums as the development of new therapies seems boundless; however, the funding for these cures is limited. How does one decide which are the best medicines to use within restricted budgets? The continuing impact of cost-containment is causing administrators and policy makers in all health fields to closely examine the costs and benefits of both proposed and existing interventions. It is increasingly obvious that purchasers and public agencies are demanding that health treatments be evaluated in terms of clinical and humanistic outcomes against the costs incurred.

Pharmacoeconomics is the field of study that evaluates the behavior or welfare of individuals, firms, and markets relevant to the use of pharmaceutical products, services, and programs [1]. The focus is frequently on the cost (inputs) and consequences (outcomes) of that use. Of necessity, it addresses the clinical, economic, and humanistic aspects of healthcare interventions in the prevention, diagnosis, treatment, and management of disease. Pharmacoeconomics is a collection of descriptive and analytic techniques for evaluating pharmaceutical interventions, encompassing the spectrum of individual patients to the healthcare system as a whole. Pharmacoeconomic techniques include cost-minimisation, cost-effectiveness, cost–utility, cost–benefit, cost of illness, cost-consequence, and any other economic analytic technique that provides valuable information to healthcare decision makers for the allocation of scarce resources. Pharmacoeconomics is often referred to as "health economics" or "health outcomes research," especially when it includes (a) comparison(s) with non-pharmaceutical therapy or preventive strategies such as surgical interventions, medical devices, or screening techniques.

Pharmacoeconomic tools are vitally important in analyzing the potential value for individual patients and the public. These methods supplement the traditional marketplace value as measured by the prices that the patient or patron is willing to pay. With government agencies and third parties' continuing concern about the higher expenditures for prescriptions, pharmaceutical manufacturers and pharmacy managers are highly cognizant that pharmaceutical interventions and services require comparative cost-justification and continual surveillance to assure cost-effective outcomes [2–5].

From pharmaceutical research, we have seen significant therapeutic advances and breakthroughs. From healthcare delivery entrepreneurs, we have seen numerous expanding roles for pharmacists, nurses, and physician assistants, with services such as home intravenous therapy, drug-level monitoring, parenteral nutrition management, hospice care, self-care counseling, and genetic screening for customizing therapy, among other innovations. The use of valid economic evaluation methods to measure the value and impact of new interventions can increase acceptance and appropriate use of such programs by third-party payers, government agencies, and consumers [2–5].

There is increasing scrutiny over all aspects of health care as we attempt to balance limited finances and resources against optimal outcomes. Cost-effectiveness evaluations of pharmaceutical options are becoming mandatory for attaining adequate reimbursement and payment for services [2–6]. Pharmacoeconomic methods document the costs and benefits of therapies and pharmaceutical services and establish priorities for those options to help in appropriately allocating resources in ever-changing healthcare landscapes and reimbursement environments/schema.

1.2 ANALYTICAL PERSPECTIVES

Point of view is a vital consideration in pharmacoeconomics. If a medicine is providing a positive benefit in relation to cost in terms of value to society as a whole, the service may not be valued in the same way by separate segments of society. For example, a drug therapy that reduces the number of admissions or patient days in an acute care institution is positive from society's point of view but not necessarily from that of the institution's administrator, who depends on a high number of patient admissions to meet expenses. Thus, one must determine whose interests are being served when identifying outcome criteria for evaluation. When considering pharmacoeconomic perspectives, one must always consider who pays the costs and who receives the benefits. A favorable economic analysis that showed savings in clinic utilization from the employer perspective would probably not be viewed positively from the clinic's budget perspective. More broadly, what is viewed as saving money for society may be viewed differently by private third-party payers, administrators, health providers, governmental agencies, or even the individual patient. Historically, it has been suggested among health economists that the societal perspective be discussed in an evaluative report, even though the focus of the report might deal with other segments such as hospitals or insurance agencies. Recent articles, books, and healthcare frameworks, however, discuss the importance of the individual payer perspective as well [5, 7]. Indeed, although the societal perspective is appropriate in single-payer countries, in the United States, with many different healthcare delivery and payer approaches, this can be complicated, and analyses are often done from multiple perspectives to assist adjudication by myriad stakeholders.

1.3 CODE OF ETHICS

The International Society for Pharmacoeconomics and Outcomes Research (ISPOR) has published a code of ethics that is vital to the honesty and transparency of the discipline [8]. The code encourages pharmacoeconomists to maintain the highest ethical standards because the organization recognizes that activities of its members affect many constituencies. These include but are not limited to: (1) patients, caregivers, and patients' associations, who are ultimately going to experience the greatest impact of the research; (2) healthcare professionals who will be treating or not treating patients with therapies, medications, and procedures made available or not made available because of the research; (3) healthcare organizations; (4) decision makers and payers, including governments, employers, and administrators, who must decide what is covered so as to optimize the health of the patient and resource utilization; (5) professional outcomes researchers; (6) industries/manufacturers, whose products are often the subject of this research; (7) academic institutions where research is conducted and students are trained; (8) colleagues, whose relationships in conducting research and related activities are particularly critical; (9) research employees concerned about how they are regarded, compensated, and treated by the researchers for whom they work;

(10) students, whose respect and appropriate behavior are important; and (11) clients for whom the research is conducted, and researcher relationships are developed and maintained.

The ISPOR code of ethics lists many standards for researchers, but a (paraphrased) sample section of the code related to "research design considerations," divided into primary and secondary concerns, is as follows:

1. Primary:
   A. In terms of participant recruitment, researchers should provide potential subjects information about study intentions, funding, and Institutional Review Board (IRB)/Ethics Committee (EC) rulings;
   B. In terms of population and research setting, researchers should describe and justify the chosen population;
   C. Sample size and site selection should be adequate to meet the study objectives and be statistically justified;
   D. Safety and adverse event reporting should be followed, as appropriate; and,
   E. Any incentive/honorarium should be appropriate, vetted with the IRB/EC, and not so large as to induce study participation.
2. Secondary:
   A. When using secondary data sources, such as large administrative datasets, ensure that intellectual property rights are respected and referenced, with all permissions being secured;
   B. Ensure reasonableness and transparency to minimize bias;
   C. Appropriate statistical and other methods should be employed and disclosed to ensure data completeness and validity, as well as study result reproducibility 9;
   D. In terms of transparency, consider study registration in clinicaltrials.gov or other appropriate source; and,
   E. In terms of modeling studies that often make use of secondary data, typically through incorporation into a decision-analytic model, ensure that inputs are derived via a comprehensive review of the literature, be transparent about assumptions, and employ sensitivity analyses to examine the impact of assumptions and data inputs on model outcomes.

1.4 OVERVIEW OF ECONOMIC EVALUATION METHODS

This section will give the reader a brief overview of the methodologies based on the two core pharmacoeconomic approaches, namely cost-effectiveness analysis (CEA) and cost–utility analysis (CUA). Table 1.1 provides a basic comparison of the following methods: cost-of-illness, cost-minimisation, and cost–benefit analysis (CBA). One can differentiate between the various approaches according to the units used to measure the inputs and outputs, as shown in the table. In general, the outputs in CEA are related to various natural units of measure, such as

TABLE 1.1

Comparison of Pharmacoeconomic Methods and Calculations

Method	Abbr	Basic Formula	Discounting Math	Input	Output	Results Expressed	Goal Determine:	Advantage/ Disadvantage	Example
Cost of Illness	COI	DC+IC	$\sum_{t=1}^{n}[C_t/(1+r)^t]$	$	$	Total cost of illness	Total cost of illness	Does not look at TXs separately	Cost of migraine in U.S.
Cost-Minimisation Analysis	CMA	$C_1 - C_2$ or [Preferred Formula] $(DC_1+IC_1) - (DC_2+IC_2)$	$\sum_{t=1}^{n}[C_t/(1+r)^t]$	$	Assumed equal	Net cost savings	Lowest cost TX	Assume both TXs have same effectiveness	Assume two antibiotics have the same effects for killing infection but differ on nursing and intravenous cost
Cost-Effectiveness Analysis	CEA	$(C_1-C_2)/(E_1-E_2)$ or [Preferred Formula] $(DC_1+IC_1) - (DC_2+IC_2)/(E_1 - E_2)$	$\sum_{t=1}^{n}[C_t/(1+r)^t]/\sum_{t=1}^{n}[E_t/(1+r)^t]$	$	Health effect	Incremental cost against change in unit of outcome	TX attaining effect for lower cost	Compare TXs that have same type of effect units	Compare two HTN prescriptions for life years gained

(Continued)

TABLE 1.1 (Cont.)

Method	Abbr	Basic Formula	Discounting Math	Input	Output	Results Expressed	Goal Determine:	Advantage/ Disadvantage	Example
Cost–Benefit Analysis or Net Benefit	CBA	$(B_1 - B_2)/(DC_1+IC_1) - (DC_2-IC_2)$ or [Preferred Formula] Net Benefit = $(B_1-B_2) - (DC_1+IC_1) - (DC_2+IC_2)$	$\sum_{t=1}^{n}[B_t/(1+r)^t]/\sum_{t=1}^{n}[C_t/(1+r)^t]$ or $\sum_{t=1}^{n}[(B_t-C_t)/(1+r)^t]$	$	Dollars	Net benefit or ratio of incremental benefits to incremental costs	TX giving best net benefit or higher B/C ratio (or return on investment)	TXs can have different effects, but must be put into dollars	Compare two cholesterol prescriptions and convert life years to wages
Cost– Utility Analysis	CUA	$(C_1-C_2)/(U_1-U_2)$ or [Preferred Formula] $(DC_1+IC_1) - (DC_2+IC_2)/(U_1 - U_2)$	$\sum_{t=1}^{n}[C_t/(1+r)^t]/\sum_{t=1}^{n}[U_t/(1+r)^t]$	$	Health effect, including Patient Preference	Incremental cost against change in unit of outcome adjusted by patient preference	TX attaining effect (adjusted for patient preference) for lower cost	Preferences are difficult to measure	Compare two cancer prescriptions and use QoL adjusted life years gained (QALYs)

Note: DC = Direct Cost; IC = Indirect Cost; R = Discount Rate; T = Time; HTN = Hypertension; QoL = Quality of Life; TX = Treatment or Intervention.

lives saved, life years added, disability days prevented, blood pressure (change in mmHg), lipid level, and so on. CBA uses monetary values (e.g., euros, dollars, pounds, yen) to measure both inputs and outputs of the respective interventions. Further discussion and examples of these techniques have been presented elsewhere [9]. It is hoped that the evaluation mechanisms delineated further in this book will be helpful in managing pharmaceutical interventions toward improving societal value and generate greater acceptance by health authorities, administrators, and the public. The first edition of this book used the human papillomavirus vaccine as an example for case studies. This has been supplemented with additional examples outside of that narrow focus. Other chapters in this book will further illustrate the various analytical methodologies related to CEA, CUA, CBA, etc. See Chapters 2, 4, 7, and 9 for more information on these techniques.

1.5 QUALITY OF LIFE AND PATIENT PREFERENCES

Significant components in pharmacoeconomics are patient outcomes and quality of life (QoL), with an expanding list of related factors to consider (Table 1.2) [10–14]. Although it is recognized that there are physical, mental, and social impairments associated with disease, there is not always consensus on how to accurately measure many of these factors. Consequently, the concept of satisfaction with care is often overlooked in cost-effectiveness studies and even during the approval process of the U.S. Food and Drug Administration. Generally, pharmacoeconomic and outcomes researchers consider QoL a vital factor in creating a full model of survival and service improvement. QoL is related to clinical outcomes as much as drugs, practitioners, settings, and types of disease. The question becomes how to select and utilize the most appropriate instruments for measuring QoL and satisfaction with care in a meaningful way.

The quality-adjusted life year (QALY) has become a major concept in pharmacoeconomics. It is a measure of health improvement used in CUA, which combines mortality and QoL gains and considers the outcome of a treatment measured as the number of years of life saved, adjusted for quality.

One approach to conceptualizing QoL and outcomes data collected in clinical trials is to consider the source of the data. There are several potential sources of data to evaluate the safety and efficacy of a new drug. Potential sources and examples are listed below:

Patient-reported outcomes (PROs) – e.g., global impression, functional status, health-related QoL, symptoms (see Chapter 12 on PRO measures)[15]

Caregiver-reported outcomes – e.g., dependency, functional status

Clinician-reported outcomes – e.g., global impressions, observations, tests of function

Physiological outcomes – e.g., pulmonary function, blood glucose, tumor size

TABLE 1.2

Outcomes and Quality of Life Measurement.

Approaches

  I. Basic Outcomes List — Six D's

    A. Death

    B. Disease

    C. Disability

    D. Discomfort

    E. Dissatisfaction

    F. Dollars (Euros, Pounds, Yen)

 II. Major Quality of Life Domains

    A. Physical status and functional abilities

    B. Psychological status and well-being

    C. Social interactions

    D. Economic status and factors

III. Expanded Outcomes List

    A. Clinical End Points

      1. Symptoms and Signs

      2. Laboratory Values

      3. Death

    B. General Well-being

      1. Pain/Discomfort

      2. Energy/Fatigue

      3. Health Perceptions

      4. Opportunity (future)

      5. Life Satisfaction

    C. Satisfaction with Care/Providers

      1. Access

      2. Convenience

      3. Financial Coverage

      4. Quality

      5. General

1.6   DECISION ANALYSIS AND MODELING

Decision analysis is defined as "... a systematic approach to decision making under conditions of uncertainty." Decision analysis, which is explored further in Chapter 2, is an approach that is explicit, quantitative, and prescriptive [1, 16, 17].

It is explicit in that it forces the decision maker to separate the logical structure into its component parts so that they can be analyzed individually, then recombined systematically to suggest a decision. It is quantitative in that the decision maker is compelled to be precise about values placed on outcomes. Finally, it is prescriptive in that it aids in deciding what a person should do under a given set of circumstances. The basic steps in decision analysis include identifying and bounding the decision problem; structuring the decision problem over time; characterizing the information needed to fill in the structure; and then choosing the preferred course of action.

Pharmacoeconomic models can involve decision trees, spreadsheets, Markov analyses, discrete event simulation, basic forecasting, multi-criteria decision analysis, and many other approaches [9, 18]. See Chapters 4 and 9 for more information.

In a simplified form, a decision tree can double as an educational tool for presenting available therapeutic options and probable consequences to patients and decision makers [9, 18]. Wennberg and colleagues have explored ways to involve patients in a shared decision-making process [19, 20]. One of his projects involved a computer interactive program on prostate surgery education. The program explains to patients the probability of success, the degree of pain that might be encountered at each step, and what the procedure actually entails. After viewing this program with visual graphic depictions of the surgery, most patients changed their decisions about wanting surgery rather than watchful waiting. This reduction in a major procedure resulted from a greater focus on QoL and patient satisfaction. With further evaluation and perhaps modification of the computer program, it should also produce more cost-effective care. More recently, Wennberg and colleagues undertook a year-long randomized investigation to compare the effects on patients who received a usual level of support in making a medical treatment decision with the effects on patients who received enhanced support, which included more contact with trained health coaches through telephone, mail, e-mail, and the Internet. They found that patients who received enhanced support had 5.3% lower overall medical costs, 12.5% fewer hospital admissions and 9.9% fewer preference-sensitive surgeries than patients who received the usual level of support. These findings indicate that support for shared decision-making can generate savings. Wennberg's work is an application of outcomes research that helped to weigh costs, utilities, and QoL for the patient and shows that shared decision-making can generate savings as well as enhanced patient satisfaction.

1.7 RANKING PRIORITIES: DEVELOPING A FORMULARY LIST

Table 1.3 illustrates how cost–utility ratios can be used to rank alternative therapies as one might do for a drug formulary (see Chapter 8 for more information on Budget Impact Analysis). The numbers in the second column of the table list the total QALYs for all of a decision maker's patient population that is expected to benefit from the treatment options in each row. The numbers in the third column detail the total cost of treatment for all of one's targeted patient population for each treatment option in each row. For the next step in the selection process, rank the therapy options by their cost–utility ratios. Options have already been ranked appropriately in this table. For the final selection step, add each therapy option into one's formulary, moving down each row

TABLE 1.3

Health Economic Selections* with Fixed Budget.

Therapy or Program	QALYS[1]	Cost[2]($thousand)	Cost–Utility Ratio ($thousand)
A	50	100	2
B	50	200	4
C	20	120	6
D	25	200	8
E	10	120	12
F	5	80	16
G	10	180	18
H	10	220	22
I	15	450	30

1 Total Quality-Adjusted Life Years (QALYs) for all of patient population benefiting.

2 Total cost of treatment for all of targeted patient population.

* Selection procedure: first, rank therapies by cost–utility ratios, then add therapeutic options until budget is exhausted.

until your allocated budget (using the cost column) is exhausted. In other words, if you have only $420,000, you would be able to fund therapies A, B, and C. These options have the best cost–utility for one's population given one's available budget. Cost-effectiveness and cost–utility ratios are sometimes presented in similar fashion and are called League Tables. Tengs et al. [21] have published an extensive list of interventions, and Neumann and colleagues [22] maintain a website with a substantial list of cost–utility ratios based on health economic studies, with a sample in Table 1.4. These listings must be used with caution because there are multiple criticisms of rankings with league tables, including:

- Different reports use different methods
- What the comparators were (e.g., which drugs, which surgeries)
- Difficult to be flexible about future comparators
- Orphan and rare disease versus more prevalent diseases
- Randomized prospective trials versus retrospective studies
- Regional and international differences in clinical resource use
- Regional and international differences in direct and indirect costs of treatment
- Statistical confidence intervals of cost and outcomes results
- Difficult to test statistical significance between the pharmacoeconomic ratios of treatments listed

TABLE 1.4

Selected Cost–Utility Ratios from the CEA Registry.[1]

Intervention vs. Comparator in Target Population	C/U (cost/QALY) Ratio in 2017 US$
Naloxone distribution plus pre-exposure prophylaxis (PrEP) and linkage to addiction treatment vs. Naloxone distribution plus linkage to addiction treatment in 19 to 40 years, 41 to 64 years, ≥65 years Injection drug use, HIV-negative patients in the US not on pre-exposure prophylaxis (PrEP)[36].	$99,000
Daclatasvir+Sofosbuvir vs. Standard/Usual Care- Sofosbuvir+Ribavirin in Interferon-ineligible/intolerant adults with Hepatitis C Virus (genotype 3) in the United Kingdom [37]	Cost saving
Haemophilus influenzae Type b (HiB) vaccination vs. None in Healthy children in Thailand [38]	$35
American College of Cardiology/American Heart Association strategy vs. Standard/Usual Care – Base case (status quo): current use of statin treatment among adults 35 to 94 years old per NHANES 2007–2010 in healthy 41 to 64 years, ≥65 years in the US [39]	Cost saving
Polypill vs. Optimal guideline care for men aged 50–59/women aged 60–69 who were prescribed a statin and/or blood pressure lowering therapy with no history of cardiovascular disease in the UK [40]	$11,000/18,000
Current investment (all currently implemented smoking cessation interventions) vs. Zero investment (standard/usual care): only the top-level policies (i.e. indoor smoking ban in public places and tobacco taxes; both at their current levels) in adult smokers in Germany [41]	$370
Fulverstrant vs Standard/Usual Care- Generic aromatase inhibitor anastrozole 1mg in postmenopausal women with estrogen receptor-positive locally advanced or metastatic breast cancer whose disease progressed or relapsed while on/after previous endocrine therapies in Sweden [42]	$39,000
Postpartum depression (PPD) screening and treatment vs. standard/usual care in patients <65 years old with PPD and psychosis who have experienced one birth in the past year.in the US [43]	$14,000
Combined exercise and bisphosphonates vs. bisphosphonates in fracture prevention in women aged ≥65 years in the US [44]	$18,000–160,000
Transcatheter aortic valve replacement (TAVR) vs. standard/usual care in surgical aortic valve replacement (SAVR) adults with severe stage aortic stenosis in the US [45]	$62,091
Herpes zoster virus vaccine booster at 10 years vs. None in healthy patients vaccinated with a single dose of herpes zoster virus vaccine (HZV) at age 60/70/80 in the US [46]	$34,000–66,000

(Continued)

TABLE 1.4 (Cont.)

Intervention vs. Comparator in Target Population	C/U (cost/QALY) Ratio in 2017 US$
Biologic therapy (etanercept) combined with methotrexate first vs. standard/ usual care (first-line treatment with triple therapy of a combination of conventional disease-modifying anti-rheumatic drugs (DMARDs)) adult patients with active rheumatoid arthritis unresponsive to methotrexate monotherapy in Canada [47]	$540,000

Source: With permission from Center for the Evaluation of Value and Risk in Health, The Cost-Effectiveness Analysis Registry [Internet]. (Boston), Institute for Clinical Research and Health Policy Studies, Tufts Medical Center. Available from: www.cearegistry.org. Accessed on January 20, 2019 [48].
[1] With quality scores of 5 or above on a scale of 1 to 7.

Indeed, Kvizhinadze determined that age, discount rate employed, and choice of cost-effectiveness threshold were factors for the maximum intervention cost a society could invest in a life-saving intervention at different ages while remaining cost-effective, with results varying from US$880,000 for an intervention to save the life of a child, US$540,000 for a 50-year-old, and US$158,000 for an 80-year-old [23].

1.8 INCREMENTAL ANALYSIS AND QUADRANTS

Whether one is dealing with cost analyses or decision analysis, it is important to properly compare one treatment with another, and one should understand the concepts in incremental analysis. Incremental analysis does not mean that one is adding a second therapy to the patient's regimen, but it is a technique for comparing one therapy with another. The basic incremental formulas are as follows:

$$CEA : (Cost_1 - Cost_2)/(Effectiveness_1 - Effectiveness_2)$$

or

$$CUA : (Cost_1 - Cost_2)/(QALYs_1 - QALYs_2)$$

An interesting way of displaying this information is illustrated in Figure 1.1. By displaying this information in quadrants, one can more easily visualize the relationship between therapies. Drugs that are cheaper and more effective would fall in the "accept" or "dominant" sector, while drugs that are more expensive and less effective would be "dominated." The slopes of the lines represent the incremental cost–effectiveness ratios and, in general, therapies between $20,000 and $100,000 per life year saved (or per QALY) are often considered acceptable in public policy reports (see more about value frameworks in Chapter 15).

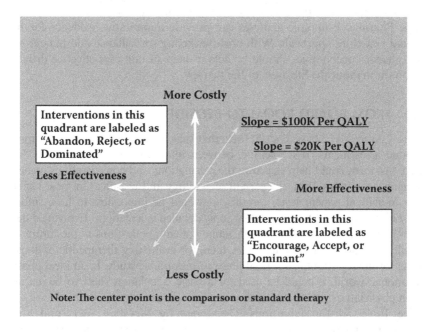

FIGURE 1.1 Incremental ratios and quadrants. QALY=quality-adjusted life year.

A classic paper involving incremental analysis deals with the comparison of tissue plasminogen activator (TPA) to streptokinase [24]. In this study, the important question did not involve looking at the CEA ratio of each drug individually; instead, it analyzed the incremental differences of the new drug, TPA, over the standard therapy at the time. The analysis demonstrated that TPA, when compared with streptokinase, had an incremental cost per life year saved of about $40,000, which was considered a socially acceptable value.

1.9 FOURTH HURDLE AND DRUG APPROVALS

The classic basic elements required for approval of new drugs are (1) therapeutic efficacy, (2) drug safety, and (3) product quality. But more recently, with the realization of limited national and global financial resources, another drug approval step has been added that considers factors related to pricing and reimbursement. Therefore, in at least two dozen countries, there is an additional jump before the marketing of pharmaceuticals that is often called "the fourth hurdle" [25]. This criterion, usually involving cost-effectiveness and pharmacoeconomic analyses, is required even when efficacy, safety, and quality have been demonstrated. Such a fourth hurdle was initially introduced in Australia for the reimbursement of new drugs and has been extended to multiple countries in Europe, Asia, and Latin America. Despite the extra development costs to conduct these studies, and concern from the pharmaceutical industry, the fourth step can also be viewed as a positive opportunity to better support more innovative medicines over me-too drugs. Pharmacoeconomic analyses can provide quantitative evidence for more rational new drug approvals. With post-marketing surveillance and patient registries, pharmacoeconomics should be able to help sustain cost-effective drug utilization throughout the life cycle of the therapy.

1.10 FROM BOARD ROOM TO BEDSIDE

Figure 1.2 provides a basic consult form that suggests a framework for pharmacoeconomic assessments. If a decision between alternative treatments needs to be made, this form could help structure the calculations and considerations related to pharmacoeconomics. With the current technology and resources in most facilities, at an individual patient level, certainly, it would be impossible to have sufficient time with each patient to individually apply detailed calculations. Evolving e-health technologies and the Internet may facilitate patient applications in the future. This consult worksheet is a basic template, then, for evaluating therapeutic options for a drug formulary, framing a formal pharmacoeconomic study. In an ideal pharmacoeconomic world, it could be used for a basic calculation sheet to be discussed with a physician or patient and maintained in a patient's medical record.

See Table 1.1 for definitions. Developed by McGhan, W.F. and Smith, M.D. Reprinted with permission. Interactive version available through www. healthstrategy.com

PHARMACOECONOMICS CONSULT: BASIC CALCULATION SHEET						
I. ID NUMBER:						
II. TREATMENT OBJECTIVES:						
III. PERSPECTIVE:	☐Society	☐Patient	☐Payer	☐Provider	☐Hospital	☐Other
IV. TYPE OF ANALYSIS:[1]	☐COI	☐CMA	☐CBA	☐CEA	☐CUA	☐Other
V. TREATMENT OPTIONS:	Treatment A			Treatment B		
Names of Treatment:						
Disease/Symptom:						
Major Outcome Measure:						
VI. COST FACTORS	Treatment A		Treatment B		Incremental	
A. DIRECT COSTS: (HEALTH CARE RESOURCES)						
Practitioner						
Clinic/Hospital						
Acquisition						
Administration						
Monitoring						
Managing ADRs						
B. DIRECT COSTS: (NON-HEALTH CARE RESOURCES)						
Transport						
Telephone						

FIGURE 1.2   Pharmacoeconomic consult template.

	Treatment A	Treatment B	Incremental
C. INDIRECT COSTS			
Morbidity Costs (time lost from work in dollars)			
Mortality Costs (time lost from work in dollars)			
D. INTANGIBLE COSTS (difficult to put into dollars)			
Discomfort/Pain			
Emotional			
QoL Quality of Life Index (as percentage of full health)			
TOTAL COST			

VII. MEASUREMENT CONSIDERATIONS
   of effectiveness, benefit, or utility.

   Unit of measurement
   COI   (direct and indirect costs of illness)
   CMA   (input costs only, outcomes assumed equivalent)
   CBA & NB   (input = $, outcomes all in dollars)
   CEA   (input = $, outcomes in natural units, mmHg, etc.)
   CUA   (input = $, outcomes in utilities, QALYs)
   Other

VIII. CALCULATED RESULTS:		Treatment A	Treatment B		Incremental
(Ratios are results of Outcomes divided by Inputs.)					
COI	(direct & indirect costs of illness)				
CMA:	(total direct & indirect costs)				
CBA:	(benefit over cost ratio)				
NB:	(benefit minus cost)]				
CEA:	(cost over effectiveness ratio)				
CUA:	(cost over utility ratio)				
Other:					

1 See calculation formula Table 1 for definitions

Developed by McGhan WF and Smith MD. Reprinted with permission.
Interactive version available through www.healthstrategy.com

FIGURE 1.2   (Continued)

Although a pharmacoeconomic analysis of a new treatment may indicate that the intervention is cost-effective compared to existing therapy, the continued clinical success of the new treatment is paramount [26]. The least cost-effective drug, from an individual patient perspective, is the drug that does not work. Substantially more research needs to be performed not only on future drugs in the pipeline but also on existing interventions in the marketplace so that we can maximize patient outcomes and enhance cost-effectiveness. Computer technology and the Internet are tremendous resources for disseminating and applying pharmacoeconomic techniques, and then continually documenting outcomes for practitioners and patients [2]. It is expected that reimbursement plans will include more incentives (paying for performance or value-based outcomes – see Chapter

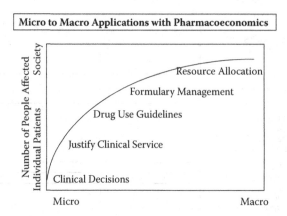

FIGURE 1.3   Micro to macro applications with Pharmacoeconomics.

15) for improvements in these economic, clinical, and humanistic outcomes [3, 27–33], although these schema may be difficult to implement. Nonetheless, pharmacoeconomics reaches from the societal (macro) and board room level out to the clinical and patient (micro) level, as envisioned in Figure 1.3.

Even health practitioners will be increasingly expected to allocate scarce resources based on pharmacoeconomic principles. Using pharmacoeconomics and disease management concepts, health providers can produce more cost-effective outcomes in a number of ways [34]. For example:

- Decrease drug–drug and drug–lab interactions.
- Increase the percentage of patients in therapeutic control.
- Reduce the overall costs of the treatment by utilizing more efficient modes of therapy.
- Reduce the unnecessary use of emergency rooms and medical facilities.
- Reduce the rate of hospitalization attributable to or affected by the improper use of drugs.
- Contribute to better use of health manpower by utilizing automation, telemedicine, and technicians.
- Decrease the incidence and intensity of iatrogenic disease, such as adverse drug reactions.

By improved monitoring and assessment of drug therapy outcomes, practitioners can provide early detection of therapy failure and provide cost-effective prescribing.

1.11   CONCLUSIONS

In this chapter, we provided a general introduction to pharmacoeconomics. There are many reports in the literature that demonstrate that the benefit of medicines is worth the cost to the payer(s) for numerous disease states. Still, it must be realized that even though most research is positive, there is a need to continue to develop interventions and services that maximize the benefit-to-cost ratio to society. Even though new drugs can demonstrate positive ratios of benefit to cost, society or agencies will ultimately invest their resources in programs that have the higher benefit-to-cost or the best cost-to-utility ratio. Similarly, the health system must be convinced that any new therapy is worth utilizing, with a resultant modification or even deletion of other, less effective, therapeutic options, if necessary. All sectors of society, and certainly the pharmaceutical arena, must fully understand pharmacoeconomics if everyone around the globe is to have optimal health care and a better future [2, 26, 35].

REFERENCES

[1] D. Hu, S. Goldie, The economic burden of noncervical human papillomavirus disease in the United States. *Am J Obstet Gynecol* 198(5) (2008) 500 e1–7.

[2] R.J.G. Arnold, S. Ekins, Ahead of our time: Collaboration in modeling then and now. *PharmacoEconomics* 35 (2017) 975–976.

[3] L.P. Garrison, Jr., P.J. Neumann, R.J. Willke, A. Basu, P.M. Danzon, J.A. Doshi, M.F. Drummond, D.N. Lakdawalla, M.V. Pauly, C.E. Phelps, et al, A health economics approach to us value assessment frameworks-summary and recommendations of the ISPOR special task force report [7]. *Value Health* 21(2) (2018) 161–65.

[4] P.J. Neumann, J.T. Cohen, Measuring the value of prescription drugs. *N Engl J Med* 373(27) (2015) 2595–97.

[5] P.J. Neumann, G.D. Sanders, Cost-effectiveness analysis 2.0. *N Engl J Med* 376(3) (2017) 203–05.

[6] A. Angelis, A. Lange, P. Kanavos, Using health technology assessment to assess the value of new medicines: Results of a systematic review and expert consultation across eight European countries. *The European Journal of Health Economics: HEPAC: Health Economics in Prevention and Care* 19(1) (2018) 123–52.

[7] P. Neumann, G. Sanders, L. Russell, J. Siegel, T. Ganiats, *Cost-effectiveness in health and medicine*, 2nd ed., Oxford University Press, New York, 2017.

[8] J. Santos, F. Palumbo, E. Molsen-David, R.J. Willke, L. Binder, M. Drummond, A. Ho, W.D. Marder, L. Parmenter, G. Sandhu, et al, ISPOR code of ethics 2017 (4th Edition). *Value Health* 20(10) (2017) 1227–42.

[9] M.F. Drummond, M.J. Sculpher, K. Claxton, G.L. Stoddart, G.W. Torrance, *Methods for the economic evaluation of health care programmes*, 4th ed., Oxford University Press, Oxford, UK, 2015.

[10] CDC, Health-related quality of life (HRQoL), 2018. www.cdc.gov/hrqol/index.htm. (Accessed December 27 2018).

[11] P.M. Ellwood, Shattuck lecture–outcomes management. A technology of patient experience. *N Engl J Med* 318(23) (1988) 1549–56.

[12] L.D. MacKeigan, D.S. Pathak, Overview of health-related quality-of-life measures. *Am J Hosp Pharm* 49(9) (1992) 2236–45.

[13] D.A. Revicki, L. Kleinman, D. Cella, A history of health-related quality of life outcomes in psychiatry. *Dialogues in Clinical Neuroscience* 16(2) (2014) 127–35.

[14] M. Zach, Health-related quality of life — United States, 2006 and 2010. *MMWR* 62(03) (2013) 105–11.

[15] D.C. Lavallee, K.E. Chenok, R.M. Love, C. Petersen, E. Holve, C.D. Segal, P.D. Franklin, Incorporating patient-reported outcomes into health care to engage patients and enhance care. *Health Aff (Millwood)* 35(4) (2016) 575–82.

[16] J. Beck, Markov modeling in decision analysis, in: R. Arnold (Ed.), *Pharmacoeconomics: From theory to practice*, CRC Press (Taylor & Francis Group LLC), Boca Raton, 2010, pp. 47–58.

[17] M. Roberts, K. Smith, Decision modeling techniques, in: R. Arnold (Ed.), *Pharmacoeconomics: From theory to practice*, CRC Press (Taylor & Francis Group LLC), Boca Raton, 2010, pp. 17–36.

[18] A. Briggs, K. Claxton, M. Sculpher, *Decision modeling for health economic evaluation*, 1st ed., Oxford University Press, New York, 2006.

[19] D. Veroff, A. Marr, D.E. Wennberg, Enhanced support for shared decision making reduced costs of care for patients with preference-sensitive conditions. *Health Aff (Millwood)* 32(2) (2013) 285–93.

[20] J.E. Wennberg, The paradox of appropriate care. *JAMA* 258(18) (1987) 2568–69.

[21] T.O. Tengs, M.E. Adams, J.S. Pliskin, D.G. Safran, J.E. Siegel, M.C. Weinstein, J.D. Graham, Five-hundred life-saving interventions and their cost-effectiveness. *Risk Anal* 15(3) (1995) 369–90.

[22] S.M. Hunt, J. McEwen, The development of a subjective health indicator. *Sociology of Health and Illness* 2(3) (1980) 231–46.

[23] G. Kvizhinadze, N. Wilson, N. Nair, M. McLeod, T. Blakely, How much might a society spend on life-saving interventions at different ages while remaining cost-effective? A case study in a country with detailed data. *Population Health Metrics* 13(1) (2015) 15.

[24] D.B. Mark, M.A. Hlatky, R.M. Califf, C.D. Naylor, K.L. Lee, P.W. Armstrong, G. Barbash, H. White, M.L. Simoons, C.L. Nelson, Cost effectiveness of thrombolytic therapy with tissue plasminogen activator as compared with streptokinase for acute myocardial infarction. *N Engl J Med* 332(21) (1995) 1418–24.

[25] M.D. Rawlins, Crossing the fourth hurdle. *British Journal of Clinical Pharmacology* 73(6) (2012) 855–60.

[26] R.J. Arnold, Cost-effectiveness analysis: Should it be required for drug registration and beyond? *Drug Discov Today* 12(21-22) (2007) 960–65.

[27] P.M. Danzon, Affordability challenges to value-based pricing: Mass diseases. *Orphan Diseases, and Cures, Value Health* 21(3) (2018) 252–57.

[28] S.K. Schaffer, D. Messner, J. Mestre-Ferrandiz, E. Tambor, A. Towse, Paying for Cures: Perspectives on solutions to the "Affordability Issue". *Value Health* 21(3) (2018) 276–79.

[29] P.M. Danzon, M.F. Drummond, A. Towse, M.V. Pauly, Objectives, budgets, thresholds, and opportunity costs-A health economics approach: An ISPOR special task force report [4]. *Value Health* 21(2) (2018) 140–45.

[30] D.N. Lakdawalla, J.A. Doshi, L.P. Garrison, Jr., C.E. Phelps, A. Basu, P.M. Danzon, Defining elements of value in health care-a health economics approach: An ISPOR special task force report [3]. *Value Health* 21(2) (2018) 131–39.

[31] S.D. Pearson, The ICER value framework: Integrating cost effectiveness and affordability in the assessment of health care value. *Value Health* 21(3) (2018) 258–65.

[32] A. Towse, J.A. Mauskopf, Affordability of new technologies: The next frontier. *Value Health* 21(3) (2018) 249–51.

[33] J.B. Watkins, Affordability of health care: A global crisis. *Value Health* 21(3) (2018) 280–82.

[34] R.M. Kaplan, J.P. Anderson, T.G. Ganiats, The Quality of Well-being Scale: Rationale for a single quality of life index, in: S.M. Walter, R.M. Rosser (Eds.), *Quality of life assessment: key issues in the 1990s*, Springer Netherlands, Dordrecht, Netherlands, 1993, 65–94.

[35] G.W. Torrance, D.H. Feeny, W.J. Furlong, R.D. Barr, Y. Zhang, Q. Wang, Multiattribute utility function for a comprehensive health status classification system. Health utilities index mark 2. *Medical Care* 34(7) (1996) 702–22.

[36] J. Uyei, D.A. Fiellin, M. Buchelli, R. Rodriguez-Santana, R.S. Braithwaite, Effects of naloxone distribution alone or in combination with addiction treatment with or without pre-exposure prophylaxis for HIV prevention in people who inject drugs: A cost-effectiveness modelling study. *Lancet Public Health* 2(3) (2017) e133–e140. doi:10.1016/S2468-2667(17)30006-3.

[37] P. McEwan, S. Webster, T. Ward, M. Brenner, A. Kalsekar, Y. Yuan, Estimating the cost-effectiveness of daclatasvir + sofosbuvir versus sofosbuvir + ribavirin for patients with genotype 3 hepatitis C virus. *Cost Eff Resour Alloc* 15(15) (2017) doi:10.1186/s12962-017-0077-4.

[38] S. Kotirum, C. Muangchana, S. Techathawat, P. Dilokthornsakul, D.B. Wu, N. Chaiyakunapruk, Economic evaluation and budget impact analysis of vaccination against haemophilus influenzae type b infection in Thailand. *Front Public Health* 5 (2017) 289. doi:10.3389/fpubh.2017.00289.

[39] D.J. Heller, P.G. Coxson, J. Penko, M.J. Pletcher, L. Goldman, M.C. Odden, D.S. Kazi, K. Bibbins-Domingo, Evaluating the impact and cost-effectiveness of statin use guidelines for primary prevention of coronary heart disease and stroke. *Circulation* 136(12) (2017) 1087–98. doi:10.1161/CIRCULATIONAHA.117.027067.

[40] S. Jowett, P. Barton, A. Roalfe, K. Fletcher, F.D.R. Hobbs, R.J. McManus, J. Mant, Cost-effectiveness analysis of use of a polypill versus usual care or best practice for primary prevention in people at high risk of cardiovascular disease. *PLoS One* 12(9) (2017) e0182625. doi:10.1371/journal.pone.0182625.

[41] M.B. Huber, M. Prager, K. Coyle, D. Coyle, A. Lester-George, M. Trapero-Bertran, B. Nemeth, K.L. Cheung, R. Stark, M. Vogl, et al, Cost-effectiveness of increasing the reach of smoking cessation interventions in Germany: Results from the EQUIPTMOD. *Addiction* 113(Suppl 1) (2018) 52–64. doi:10.1111/add.14062.

[42] U. Sabale, M. Ekman, D. Thunstrom, C. Telford, C. Livings, Economic evaluation of fulvestrant 500 mg compared to generic aromatase inhibitors in patients with advanced breast cancer in Sweden. *Pharmacoecon Open* 1(4) (2017) 279–90. doi:10.1007/s41669-017-0031-6.

[43] A. Wilkinson, S. Anderson, S.B. Wheeler, Screening for and treating postpartum depression and psychosis: A Cost-Effectiveness Analysis. *Matern Child Health J* 21 (4) (2017) 903–14. doi:10.1007/s10995-016-2192-9.

[44] T. Mori, C.J. Crandall, D.A. Ganz, Cost-effectiveness of combined oral bisphosphonate therapy and falls prevention exercise for fracture prevention in the USA. *Osteoporos Int* 28(2) (2017) 585–95. doi:10.1007/s00198-016-3772-7.

[45] M.R. Reynolds, Y. Lei, K. Wang, K. Chinnakondepalli, K.A. Vilain, E.A. Magnuson, B.Z. Galper, C.U. Meduri, S.V. Arnold, S.J. Baron, et al, U.S.H.R.P.T.I. CoreValve, Cost-Effectiveness of transcatheter aortic valve replacement with a self-expanding prosthesis versus surgical aortic valve replacement. *J Am Coll Cardiol* 67(1) (2016) 29–38. doi:10.1016/j.jacc.2015.10.046.

[46] P. Le, M.B. Rothberg, Cost effectiveness of a shingles vaccine booster for currently vaccinated adults in the U.S. *Am J Prev Med* 53(6) (2017) 829–36. doi:10.1016/j. amepre.2017.08.029.

[47] N. Bansback, C.S. Phibbs, H. Sun, J.R. O'Dell, M. Brophy, E.C. Keystone, S. Leatherman, T.R. Mikuls, A.H. Anis, C.R. Investigators, Triple therapy versus biologic therapy for active rheumatoid arthritis: A cost-effectiveness analysis. *Ann Intern Med* 167(1) (2017) 8–16. doi:10.7326/M16-0713.

[48] Center for the Evaluation of Value and Risk in Health, The cost-effectiveness analysis registry [Internet]. (Boston), Institute for Clinical Research and Health Policy Studies, Tufts Medical Center. www.cearegistry.org. (Accessed January 20 2019).

2 Decision Modeling Techniques

Mark S. Roberts, MD, MPP
University of Pittsburgh
Pittsburgh, PA, USA

Ken Smith, MD, MS
University of Pittsburgh
Pittsburgh, PA, USA

TABLE OF CONTENTS

2.1 INTRODUCTION

The fundamental purpose of a pharmacoeconomic model is to evaluate the expected costs and outcomes of a decision (or a series of decisions) about the use of a pharmacotherapy compared to one or many alternatives. Decision modeling provides an excellent framework for developing estimates of these outcomes in a flexible analytic framework that allows the investigator to test many alternative assumptions and scenarios. In addition to providing an "answer" to a specific pharmacoeconomic decision, one of the major advantages of having a model of a particular decision is that the model can provide significant information regarding how the answer changes with different basic assumptions or under different conditions. It is this power to evaluate multiple "what if" scenarios that provides a substantial amount of the power of pharmacoeconomic modeling.

This chapter provides a brief introduction to the many methods of constructing decision models for the purpose of pharmacoeconomic analyses. After describing the basic methods of decision analysis, basic branch and node decision trees are described in the context of an actual pharmacoeconomic problem. Many of the techniques used to make these models more clinically detailed and realistic are detailed in other chapters in this book, and these chapters are referenced where appropriate. In addition, a list of more detailed articles, books and tutorials is provided at the end of the chapter for the reader who wishes to have more detailed explanations of these techniques.

2.1.1 DECISION MODELING PARADIGM

The most important aspect of the decision modeling process is that it must represent the choice that is being made. When constructing a model of a clinical or pharmacological decision, there is a series of characteristics of the actual problem that must be represented in the model structure and method. First, the model should represent the set of reasonable choices from which the decision maker can choose. Leaving out reasonable potential or common strategies subjects the model to criticisms of bias and selecting comparators that make the superiority of a particular strategy more likely. Even if "doing nothing" is not a viable clinical alternative, it is often useful to include such a strategy as a baseline check of the model's ability to predict the outcomes of the natural history of untreated disease.

Once the strategies are outlined, the modeler must enumerate the possible outcomes implied by each strategy. These outcomes are not always symmetric: a surgical therapy may have an operative mortality, whereas a medical therapy may not. However, all potential outcomes that can occur and are considered relevant to clinicians taking care of the problem should be included. Pharmacoeconomic models are characterized by their simultaneous assessment of the clinical and cost consequences of various strategies, so even clinically insignificant outcomes that incur significant costs may need to be modeled. In order to make an appropriate decision regarding what consequences and outcomes to include, the modeler must make decisions regarding four characteristics: the *perspective* of the analysis, the *setting* or context of the analysis, the appropriate level of detail or *granularity*, and the appropriate *time horizon* [1].

Perspective: The perspective of the analysis (Table 2.1) determines from whose point of view the decision is being made. Defining the perspective of the analysis is especially important in pharmacoeconomic analyses because the costs that are incurred depend heavily on the perspective. The most typical perspectives used in pharmacoeconomic analyses are that of the *payer* (insurance companies, HMOs, and Medicare), in which only those costs that are incurred by the payer are

TABLE 2.1

Characteristics of Potential Perspectives

Perspective	Characteristics
Societal	Broadest perspective includes all costs and benefits, regardless of who bears them. Considered the appropriate perspective for a reference case from the US Panel (US Panel) on Cost Effectiveness in Health Care
Payer	Typical perspective for payment/coverage decisions. Now also included as a secondary perspective by the US Panel.
Health Plan/HMO	
Individual	Appropriate perspective for understanding optimal decisions or strategies for individual patients or groups of patients

included; a *provider* (hospital, health system, and provider group), in which the costs and reimbursements for providing a particular service are included; and society, in which all costs and effects are included, irrespective of who has borne them. A more detailed description of perspective is provided in standard texts [2] and in multiple areas in this book. For example, an analysis conducted from the payers' perspective on a particular treatment for a neurological condition might not take into account the differential effects of the various therapies being studied on the patients' ability to return to work, as these are not costs or benefits that are borne by the payer. However, these costs and benefits should be included if the analysis is being conducted from the perspective of society.

Setting: The setting defines the characteristics for which a particular decision is being made. Just as any study design needs to define the population the study will evaluate by inclusion and exclusion criteria in randomized controlled trials or by case and control definition in many observational designs, a decision model must explicitly state the type of patient(s) to which the decision will be applied. For example, in developing a pharmacoeconomic model of the use of statins in hyper-cholesterolemia, the modeler must decide the distribution of age, gender, lipid levels, comorbid disease, and other variables that are important and must be represented in the model. A model that demonstrated a particular result in one group of patients is not likely to have the same result in populations with different characteristics.

Granularity: The correct amount of detail to include in a model of a given clinical situation is one of the most difficult decisions a modeler must make in the development of a representation of a particular decision and its consequences. Albert Einstein once said: "things should be made as simple as possible ... but not simpler." Although this concept is directly translatable to building decision models, it provides little actual guidance: the clinical and pharmacoeconomic characteristics of the problem dictate the level of detail required to represent the problem. For example, in many analyses of medications, the modeler must represent side effects of the medication. Should a model contain all of the individual potential side effects and their likelihoods of occurring, or can they be grouped into side effects of various severities such as mild (which might only be assumed to change the quality of life of the patient and perhaps decrease medication adherence) and major (which might be assumed to require some form of medical intervention)? One of the best methods to decide the appropriate level of detail is to engage in discussions and collaborations with clinicians who treat the particular condition in question such that the areas of importance to them can be sufficiently detailed. The model itself can sometimes be used to test whether more detail is necessary. Conducting sensitivity analyses (see Chapter 13) on a particular aspect of the model can indicate whether more detail is required. If multiple sensitivity analyses on the parameters of a more aggregated or simplistic section of a model do not have a significant impact on the results, it is not likely that expanding the detail of that section of the model will provide new or important insights.

Time horizon: The time horizon indicates the period of time over which the specific strategies are chosen, and the relevant outcomes occur. This time frame is generally determined by the biology of the particular problem. If an analysis is being done comparing different treatments for acute dysuria in young women, the time frame of the analysis may be as short as a week, as long-term sequelae are extremely uncommon in this condition. In contrast, in an analysis of the effects of various interventions to alter cardiovascular risk, the time frame might very likely be the entire lifetime of the patient. It is important to remember that the time frame does not include only those events directly related to the various strategies, but all of the future events implied by choosing each strategy. If a particular intervention increases the risk of a life-changing complication (stroke, heart attack, pulmonary embolism), the long-term effects of the complications must be considered as well.

2.1.1.1 Types of Decision Modeling Techniques

There are many methodologies and modeling types that can be used to create and evaluate decision models and the modeler should use the method most appropriate to the particular problem being addressed. The choice is dependent upon the complexity of the problem, the need to model outcomes over extended periods of time, and whether or not resource constraints and interactions of various elements in the model are required. We will describe in detail the development of simple branch and node decision trees, which set the context for many of the other techniques. A brief review of several methodologies is then provided; more detailed descriptions of many of these techniques can be found in other chapters in this book.

2.1.1.2 Decision Trees

The classic decision analysis structure is the branch and node decision tree, which is illustrated in Figure 2.1. The decision tree has several components that are always present and need to be carefully developed. A decision model comprises the modeling structure itself (the decision tree), which represents the decision that is being made and the outcomes that can occur as the result of each decision, the probabilities that the various outcomes will occur, and the values of

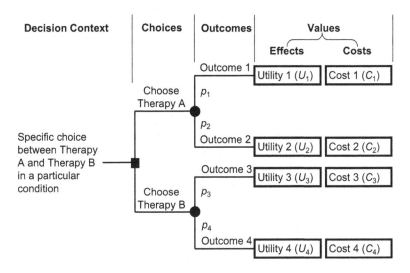

FIGURE 2.1 Basic structure of a branch and node decision tree, illustrating two choices in a particular clinical situation. After each choice is made, outcomes occur with specific probabilities, these outcomes are associated with values, which may be measured in clinical or cost metrics.

the outcomes if they do occur. Similar to any other research problem, the decision tree should start with a specific problem formulation, which in the figure is a choice between therapy A and therapy B in a particular condition. In pharmacoeconomic models, these should represent the actual choice being made, and should include the necessary descriptors of the population in which the decision is being made to allow the reader to understand the context of the choice. The context is followed by a decision node (represented in the figure as a square), and should include as comparators the relevant, real choices the decision maker has at his/her disposal. In the figure, this particular decision has only two choices represented by the branches off the decision node labeled Choose Therapy A and Choose Therapy B. Each choice is followed by a series of chance nodes (represented in the figure by circles), which describe the possible outcomes that are implied by making each of the respective choices. Each outcome occurs with a specific probability (p_1 through p_4 in the figure). Each outcome is also associated with one or more values (represented in the figure by the rectangles), which describe the clinical effects and costs of arriving at that particular outcome. We will use this figure in the following description of the basic steps that should be conducted each time a decision analysis or pharmacoeconomic model is developed.

2.1.1.2.1 Steps in Conducting a Decision Analysis

In the following sections, we describe the basic steps through which the modeler should proceed in the construction of a model of a pharmacoeconomic decision. The basic question should be framed and the perspective chosen, the structure of the problem should be developed, the probabilities and values for the outcomes should be estimated, the tree should be analyzed to obtain the expected value of the outcomes, and sensitivity analysis should be conducted to evaluate the effect of assumptions on the results. These are not necessarily linear: often evaluation of the tree or sensitivity analysis will indicate that a particular part of the structure of the model needs either more or less detail. Often several of these steps are cycled through many times during the development of a model. We illustrate a specific example of these steps for the development of a published pharmacoeconomic model for the use of low molecular weight heparin (LMWH) as prophylaxis for thromboembolism in patients with cancer (details given in Section 2.1.1.4).

2.1.1.2.2 Step 1: Frame the Question
As in any study design, the modeler must decide several basic details regarding for whom the decision is being made and from whose perspective the decision is being made. Deciding for whom the decision is being made is similar to the development of inclusion and exclusion criteria for a typical randomized controlled trial: the decision problem must specify exactly who would be affected by the decision. The description should be as detailed as necessary to describe the problem at hand, and should specify, if important, the age and gender of the population being studied, the specific disease and comorbid conditions that the patients may have, and the specific treatments or strategies that are being evaluated.

Choosing the perspective of the decision maker is also very important, as it determines the appropriate metric in which to measure the outcomes and costs of the analysis. As described in Section 2.2, typical perspectives from which to conduct analyses are society, the payer, or the patient.

2.1.1.2.3 Step 2: Structure the Clinical Problem
The structuring of the problem entails diagramming the branches and nodes that represent the particular problem being modeled. There are several aspects of the process that are important to remember. The first is that the choices one makes from the decision node must be mutually exclusive: one and only one of the choices (branches of the decision node) can be made. If there are several aspects to the choice, then these aspects should be described as a series of mutually exclusive options, rather than described as sequential or embedded decisions. This is illustrated in Figure 2.2, which describes a decision to treat a particular cancer with surgery, medical therapy, or both, and also investigates the order in which the two therapies are applied. The structure on the top of the panel describes all of the possibilities, but at a decision node, all of the decisions should be listed as branches of the initial decision node itself, as in the bottom panel of the figure. This allows for a comparison between all of the specific choices individually, and allows for direct comparisons across each of the choices. However, the appropriate construction for chance nodes is different. For example, Figure 2.3 describes a portion of a model of a surgical therapy that has several possible outcomes; for

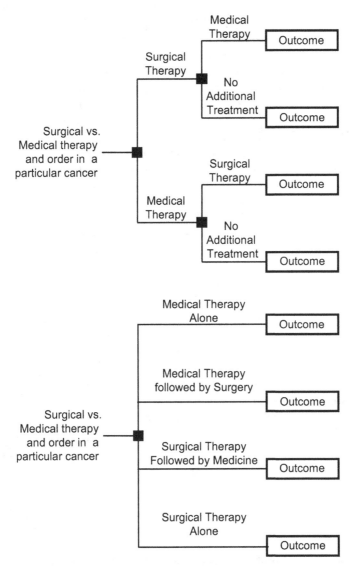

FIGURE 2.2 Embedded decisions. It is very difficult to analyze trees with embedded or sequential decisions, as drawn in the top panel. Each *strategy* should be its own choice, as shown in the lower panel.

example, the patient may die or have a major surgical complication, a minor surgical publication, or no surgical complication. In the top panel of Figure 2.3 all possible outcomes are drawn as branches of the root node. As shown, the probabilities of each complication are indicated separately and the probabilities of all four branches must sum to one. If this structure is used, it becomes somewhat

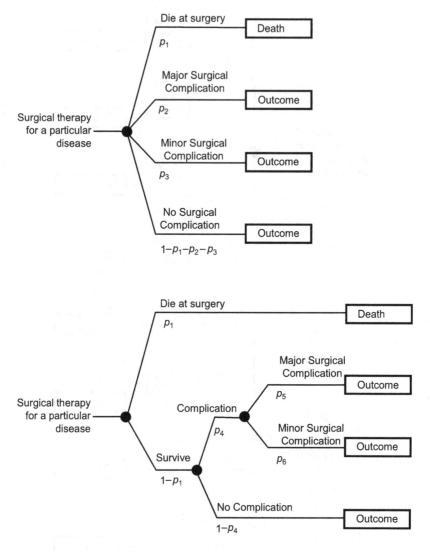

FIGURE 2.3 Superiority of binary chance nodes. It is generally preferable to make complex chance nodes a sequence of individual binary nodes (bottom panel) rather than a complex multi-branch node (top panel).

complicated to conduct sensitivity analysis on the probability of surgical death or major or minor surgical complications. However, if this same tree is drawn as a series of binary chance nodes, as shown in the lower panel of Figure 2.3, sensitivity analysis and the ability to vary prospective probabilities become easier. The first chance node indicates whether the patient dies or survives. If the patient survives, they have a complication or not. If the patient has a complication, that complication is either a major or a minor complication. In this setting, it is much easier to directly model the relationships between complication rates, survival rates, and normal outcomes.

It is important to remember that the structure drawn into a decision tree represents the disease process, treatments, and outcomes that the modeler has decided are important in this particular representation of the disease. Any particular model represents a specific version of the reality that the modeler is trying to evaluate. The art of modeling is the ability to have the model, as created in software, depict the version of reality that the modeler is hoping to represent.

2.1.1.2.4 Step 3: Estimate the Probabilities

Once the structure of the decision tree has been developed, the probabilities must be estimated for the various chance nodes in the tree. There are several sources that modelers can use to find and estimate probabilities for various parameters in a decision model. It is important to understand that the typical hierarchy of evidence-based grading does not necessarily apply to all of the various parameters that are necessary to calibrate a decision analysis or a pharmacoeconomic model. For example, the typical hierarchy for evidence-based medicine ranks randomized, controlled trials as the best type of evidence for efficacy. However, as mentioned in Chapter 5, retrospective database analysis, randomized, controlled trials are very poor at estimating many other types of the parameters that are important in a decision model. For example, neither the incidence of a particular disease can be estimated by a randomized, controlled trial, nor can the complication rate of a particular therapy when it is applied in general practice. Therefore, the quality of the evidence that a modeler uses to calibrate a decision model is entirely dependent upon the type of data necessary for a particular parameter in the model. Indeed, parameters on effectiveness of therapy may well be best derived from the reports of randomized, controlled trials or meta-analyses of randomized, controlled trials, whereas incidence and prevalence data may best come from observational studies and large cohort or administrative database analyses, and medication use data may best come from claims databases maintained by large health insurance plans. The important concept is that a model requires the best, unbiased estimates of the specific parameters in the model: these parameters do not need to come from the same source, nor do they all need to be of the same type of study or accuracy of data. These sorts of differences can be investigated in sensitivity analyses.

2.1.1.2.5 Step 4: Estimate the Values of the Outcomes

Similar to estimating the probabilities of various events, the modeler needs to assess the values for the outcomes that occur as a consequence of each one of the choices. The appropriate outcome measure will have previously been determined in the framing of the question when the perspective of the analysis is decided. This will direct the modeler to choose the appropriate outcome measure for the analysis. For example, in an analysis conducted from a societal point of view, the appropriate outcome measure is usually QALYs (see Chapter 1: Introduction). The choice of outcome is also determined by the particular disease that the treatment is designed to ameliorate. For example, in a pharmacoeconomic model of a treatment for depression, it may be that the appropriate outcome measure is depression-free days or a similar disease-related outcome metric. In a model of a particular intervention for oral hygiene, the appropriate outcome might simply be the number of cavities avoided. The outcomes used must be those that are clinically relevant to the particular decision makers involved in the decision. One of the advantages of developing a model of a pharmacoeconomic problem is that clinical and cost outcomes may be evaluated and modeled simultaneously. Therefore, in most economic models, the model will simultaneously account for the clinical and cost consequences of each potential decision.

2.1.1.2.6 Step 5: Analyze the Tree (Average Out/Fold Back)

The evaluation of the decision tree is conceptually quite simple. The overall goal is to calculate the expected value of the outcomes implied by choosing each branch of the root decision node. For example, in Figure 2.1 there are two choices: Therapy A and Therapy B. If Therapy A is chosen, a portion of the population (indicated by p_1) will experience Outcome 1, which has a utility U_1 and another portion of the population (indicated by p_2) will experience Outcome 2, which has a utility U_2. Assume the utilities represent life expectancies, then the expected value of choosing Therapy A represents the life expectancy of a cohort of people who would be given that therapy, p_1 of them living U_1 years, p_2 of them living U_2 years. Mathematically, the expected value of choosing Therapy A is:

$$E(\text{TherapyA}) = (p_1 \times U_1) + (p_2 \times U_2).$$

Similarly, the expected value of choosing Therapy B is:

$$E(\text{TherapyB}) = (p_3 \times U_3) + (p_4 \times U_4).$$

The choice that has the highest expected value is then chosen as superior.

Essentially, no matter how complicated the tree becomes, the process of finding the expected value is the same. Starting with the terminal nodes, each chance node is replaced by the expectation of that chance node (the expected value of the outcome at that chance node), and that process is continued until one is left with the expected value of each branch of the initial decision node. Pragmatically, a modeler never is required to do this calculation by hand; there are several decision analysis software packages that do the analysis and calculations automatically.

2.1.1.2.7 Step 6: Test Assumptions (Sensitivity Analysis)

After the model has been developed, calibrated and the initial analyses completed, one of the most useful steps in modeling is conducting sensitivity analyses. In its simplest form, the definition of sensitivity analysis is the evaluation of the outcomes of the model for various different levels of one or more input variables. Sensitivity analyses have several purposes. They can be used to "debug" a model to make sure that the model behaves as it is designed to behave. It is often the case that the modeler and the content experts with whom the modeler has developed a model will be able to predict the optimal choice under certain specified conditions. Similar to basic theoretical principles or knowledge of the given disease process, the modeler may be able to make predictions about the direction the value of a particular strategy should move under different assumptions. For example, in a decision between surgical and medical therapy, it seems obvious that the relative value of the medical therapy choice should increase compared to the surgical therapy choice, as the mortality from surgery increases. If a sensitivity analysis on surgical mortality is conducted and the expected finding does not occur, this may indicate programming or structural errors in the development of the model.

Another important use of sensitivity analysis is in the determination of which variables in the model have the most impact on the outcomes. This is the traditional use of sensitivity analysis and is the basis for many initial valuations of the stability of a particular decision modeling result over a wider range of underlying assumptions and probabilities. There are many types of sensitivity analyses, the simplest of which is a one-way sensitivity analysis in which the changes in the outcomes are evaluated as the value of a single variable is changed. Slightly more complicated is a two-way sensitivity analysis, which plots the optimal choice implied with various combinations of two different input variables, and a multi-way sensitivity analysis is conducted by changing and evaluating the results across many input variables simultaneously. Finally, probabilistic sensitivity analyses are used to test the stability of the results over ranges of variability in the input parameters. We describe a simple sensitivity analysis from published work in Section 2.3.6. A more complete description of sensitivity analysis in pharmacoeconomic analyses is provided in Chapter 13.

2.1.1.2.8 Step 7: Interpret the Results
Once the analysis has been completed, the stability of the model has been tested with sensitivity analysis, and a modeler is convinced that the model represents the clinical and pharmacoeconomic characteristics of the problem adequately, the results must be interpreted and summarized. It is often the case that a specific answer that the model gives under one particular set of conditions is not the most important attribute of the model itself. Often times it is the manner in which the answer varies with changes in underlying parameter estimates and underlying probabilities and values for outcomes that are the most interesting aspect of the interpretation of an analysis.

However, most pharmacoeconomic analyses will result in an estimate of a cost-effectiveness ratio or similar metric of each choice as its major finding.

2.1.1.3 Markov Models
In a traditional branch and node decision tree, as illustrated in Figure 2.1, the terminal nodes are all single outcomes. For example, the value of the outcome might be measured as a life expectancy and quality-adjusted life expectancy or a cost. However, for any model the outcomes that are expected to occur after each choice are actually quite complex combinations of events that happen in

the people's lives proceeding down that path. Many times the intervention being modeled at a decision node affects the risks of future events, such as heart attacks and strokes in the case of cholesterol-modifying therapy, or might affect the rate of recurrence of a particular event, such as asthma episodes in an analysis of the use of corticosteroids in patients with reactive airway disease. When a model must consider events that occur over time or events that may recur in time, the traditional branch and node structure is an inefficient method for representing these events. Standard decision analytic methods typically use a Markov process to represent events that occur over time. As illustrated in the upper panel of Figure 2.4, a simple decision tree would terminate in single values such as a life expectancy. However, that life expectancy is actually determined by the average life histories of many people who would proceed down that choice. This can be represented as seen in the lower half of Figure 2.4 by replacing the single life expectancy value with a Markov process that represents the events the modeler wants to detect that occur after the decision is made and certain outcomes occur. A Markov process is simply a mathematical representation of the health states in which a patient might find himself or herself and the likelihood of transitioning between those states. The Markov process itself, when it is evaluated, calculates the average life expectancy of a cohort proceeding through the Markov process. Markov processes are described in much more detail in Chapter 4. Discretely integrated condition event (DICE) simulation, a novel modeling approach described in Chapter 10, transparently unifies the common modeling techniques, thus making it possible to create Survival Partition, Cohort and Individual Markov as well as unconstrained Discrete Event Simulation models in a single framework.

2.1.1.4 Simulation Models

Over the past 10–15 years, the decision analytic and pharmacoeconomic investigators have started to rely more on simulation methodologies to create progressively more complicated and clinically realistic models of disease processes and treatments. Although a detailed exposition of these methods is beyond the scope of this chapter, we will briefly describe the three most common simulation methodologies used in current pharmacoeconomic analysis. They differ by their ability to model progressively more complicated clinical situations and their ability to model interactions between individual patients in the model.

2.1.1.4.1 Microsimulation

The term microsimulation has come to represent those models in which individual patients are modeled, one at a time, as they proceed through the model. The advantage of microsimulation is that it eliminates a problem with standard Markov process models in that it releases the assumption of path-independent transition probabilities. Although this is discussed in more detail in Chapter 4, the basic problem is that in standard Markov decision models, transition probabilities are dependent only upon the state the patient is in: information regarding

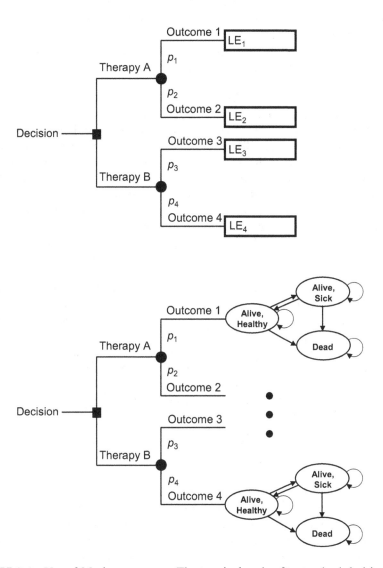

FIGURE 2.4 Use of Markov processes. The terminal node of a standard decision tree typically represents life expectancy, which is a complex summary of many possible paths and events. These can often be represented by a Markov process, in which the actual events that occur over time are specifically modeled. The dots in the lower model represent the same health states and transitions as outcome 1 for outcomes 2 and 3. See text and Chapter 4 for details on Markov processes.

where the patient was in the prior time period is lost. Because only one patient is in the model at any given time in a microsimulation, the patient's specific history can be recorded and transition probabilities can be made to depend on those variables, allowing for remarkable clinical complexity in the development of a model. There are several examples of the use of microsimulation in the literature: Freedberg has used microsimulation to evaluate the cost-effectiveness of various treatment and prevention strategies in HIV disease [3]. Details of simulation methodology can be found in several texts [4, 5].

2.1.1.4.2 Discrete Event Simulation

One of the problems with many of the modeling systems previously discussed is that they cannot easily model the competition for resources. Therefore, although a decision analysis or a cost-effectiveness analysis might be able to determine that a particular diagnostic or therapeutic strategy should be adopted, these analyses cannot tell whether the resources, delivery systems, geographic constraints, or other problems allow for the optimal strategy to actually be implemented. Discrete event simulation, which was originally developed over 50 years ago by industrial engineering to model production processes in factories, provides the modeler with a set of tools that can represent queues, resource limitations, geographic distribution, and many other physical structures or limitations that constrain the implementation of a particular strategy or therapy.

In health care, discrete event simulation has been used for many years to allow for understanding flows and bottlenecks in operating room scheduling, emergency vehicle distribution and response time, throughput in emergency rooms, and many other resource constraint problems. More recently, as the ability to blend highly detailed clinical data with discrete event simulation models has improved, discrete event simulation has been used to address and evaluate more clinically interesting problems. For example, we have used discrete event simulation to model the US organ allocation process and evaluate the effects of various organ allocation policy changes prior to their implementation [1, 6]. The advantage of discrete event simulation, in this case, is that it has specific structures to allow for the formation of queues, waiting lists, and arrival of both patients and donated organs.

2.1.1.4.3 Agent-Based Simulation

One of the purposes of making models more complex is to represent more realistic physiological or biological systems. Many components of biological systems act entirely independently and simply respond to their environments based on internal sets of processes that govern their behavior. Cells respond to cytokines, hormones and other biological signals, organs (the pancreas) respond to levels of hormones (insulin) and a myriad of other factors and signals. Agent-based models, in which each "agent" or component of the model independently contains all of the information it needs to interact with and respond to the actions of the other agents in the model, have been increasingly used to understand and model complex biological systems, from individual cells and organs to populations. One fundamental concept of agent-based models is that the aggregated behavior of multiple individual autonomous agents can replicate and predict very complex social and group behaviors. In the realm of medicine and public health, agent-based models have been used in the modeling of epidemics and population reactions to epidemics [7–9].

2.1.1.5 Deterministic (Mechanistic) Models

Deterministic models seek to capture and characterize specific biological relationships and causes and effects directly through series' of equations. Some of the first medical problems to be evaluated using deterministic models were what are termed "compartment models" that represented the spread of infectious diseases in a community. Also called "susceptible, infected, recovered" (SIR) models, they have been widely used over the past 50 years to model the effects of interventions, such as quarantines and vaccines, on epidemic and pandemic infections. Basically, the relevant population is divided into compartments, and the flows between those compartments are represented as series' of differential equations that are related to both the level and rates of flow of each of the compartments.

More recently, these sorts of models have been used to model physiological processes. At their highest level of abstraction, these models represent physiology and disease as one might see in a physiology textbook, with diagrams that indicate how one hormone or cytokine, or level of some electrolyte or other substance, affects the production and level of another. These typically form feedback loops; examples might be that thyroid stimulating hormone (TSH) is produced in response to low thyroid hormone levels and TSH acts on the thyroid to produce more thyroid hormone. Examples of the application of deterministic modeling to health care include the development of complex system models of sepsis and injury [10–13]. More physiologically complex, and more directly applicable to problems in pharmacoeconomics, the Archimedes model of disease uses a very complex system of mathematical and differential equations in the concept of an agent-based model to represent multiple metabolic processes and diseases that include diabetes, heart disease, and some cancers [14, 15]. It has been used to compare and evaluate the cost-effectiveness of different strategies for the prevention of diabetes [16].

2.1.1.6 Summary of Modeling Types

There are a wide variety of mathematical modeling types available to the modeler to represent disease, treatments, and costs, and a tradeoff exists between complexity of the process being modeled and the type of model that should be used to represent the problem. In general, the simplest modeling technique that accurately represents the components of the problem according to a clinical expert is sufficient. It is our experience that most problems can be addressed with either simple branch or node decision trees or standard Markov process-based state transition models. In the next section, we will illustrate the development and analysis of a simple branch and node decision tree model to evaluate a clinical treatment problem.

2.1.2 EXAMPLE

To illustrate the 7 steps used to conduct a decision analysis, we will use an analysis performed by Aujesky et al. [17] examining the use of low molecular weight heparin (LMWH) as secondary prophylaxis for venous thromboembolism in patients with cancer.

2.1.2.1   Step 1: Framing the Question

Venous thromboembolism frequently occurs in patients with cancer and carries a poor prognosis. In addition, cancer patients who have had an episode of venous thromboembolism are prone to recurrent episodes. Because of this recurrence risk, prolonged use of anticoagulants as secondary prophylaxis has been advocated, typically for 6 months or longer. Data suggest that LMWH is more effective than warfarin for this patient group, leading to recommendations for LMWH as first-line therapy in this clinical scenario. However, the costs of LMWH and the potential need for home nursing to administer daily subcutaneous injections raise questions about whether effectiveness gained through LMWH use is worth its significantly increased cost.

Thus, the question this analysis seeks to answer is what the costs and benefits of using LMWH are as compared to warfarin for secondary prophylaxis of venous thromboembolic disease in cancer patients. In the base case analysis, patient cohorts were 65 years old, based on the mean patient age in studies of cancer-related venous thromboembolism. Since venous thromboembolism can recur throughout the remaining life span of cancer patients, a lifetime time horizon was chosen for the analysis. However, the life expectancy of cancer patients with venous thromboembolism averages only 1–2 years due to venous thromboembolism itself, the high prevalence of advanced cancer in patients with thromboembolism, and the age of the patient group.

This analysis sought to inform physicians and policy makers about the incremental value, defined broadly, of LMWH use compared to warfarin use. For decisions framed in this fashion, cost and effectiveness metrics should be as comprehensive and generalizable as possible. With this in mind, the analysis took the societal perspective, where costs included both direct medical costs and the costs of seeking and receiving care, and used life expectancy and quality-adjusted life expectancy as the effectiveness measures.

2.1.2.2   Step 2: Structuring the Clinical Problem

A decision tree model was chosen to depict this problem, based on the relatively short time horizon of the model and the concentration on outcomes related to venous thromboembolism and its treatment. If a longer time horizon or more outcomes had been required to adequately model the problem, another model structure, such as a Markov process, could have been used. The decision tree model is shown in Figure 2.5. This model assumes that all events that are not related to venous thromboembolism or its treatment are unaffected by the choice between LMWH and warfarin.

In the decision tree, the square node on the left depicts the decision to use either LMWH or warfarin. Circular nodes depict chance nodes, where events occur based on their probabilities. All patients are at risk for early complications, whose probabilities differ based on treatment choice. Patients who survive the first 6 months after a venous thromboembolism episode are at risk for late complications. The triangular nodes on the right represent the cost and effectiveness values associated with that particular path through the model. In addition, the

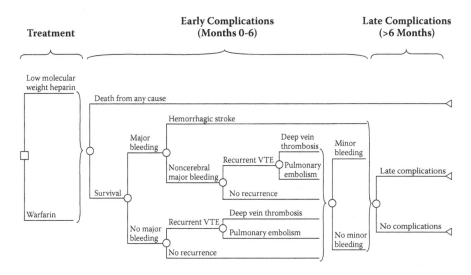

FIGURE 2.5 Basic decision tree for LMWH as secondary prevention for cancer-induced thromboembolism. Reproduced with permission.

model assumes that patients suffering a hemorrhagic stroke had anticoagulation permanently discontinued, with only transient interruption of anticoagulation with noncerebral bleeding, and that a second venous thromboembolic episode resulted in permanent inferior vena cava filter placement.

2.1.2.3   Step 3: Estimate the Probabilities

Probabilities for the model were obtained from a variety of sources. A large clinical trial of cancer patients with venous thromboembolism provided data on mortality, recurrent thromboembolism, and major bleeding associated with LMWH or warfarin use [18]. Anticoagulation-related intracranial bleeding rates, which could not be reliably estimated from single trials, were obtained from a meta-analysis of venous thromboembolism therapy in a wide variety of patient groups [19]; its base case value (9%) was varied over a broad range (5–30%) in sensitivity analyses to account for the possibility of greater risk in cancer patients. Intracranial bleeding risk was assumed to be the same with either anticoagulation regimen. In the model, an estimated 20% of patients receiving LMWH required daily home nursing and 50% of patients with deep venous thrombosis received outpatient treatment.

2.1.2.4   Step 4: Estimate the Values of the Outcomes

Model outcomes were cost and effectiveness. US Medicare reimbursement data were used to estimate costs for hospitalization, emergency department, physician and home nursing visits, laboratory tests, and medical procedures. Anticoagulant drug costs were average wholesale prices; base case daily pharmacy costs for LMWH and warfarin averaged $48 and $1, respectively. Costs related to intracranial bleeding and late complications were obtained from medical literature sources. Since the analysis took the societal perspective, patient costs for seeking and receiving care were incorporated into the analysis, including patient transportation expenses for care visits and anticoagulation monitoring and patient time costs related to continuing care needs.

Effectiveness was measured as life expectancy and quality-adjusted life expectancy. Life expectancy was estimated using 6- and 12-month mortality data from randomized trials of secondary venous thromboembolism prophylaxis in cancer patients [18, 20] and longer-term survival data from a cohort study of cancer patients with venous thromboembolism [21]. Quality-adjusted life expectancy was calculated by multiplying quality of life utility values (see Chapter 12: Patient-Reported Outcomes) for chronic health states by the length of time spent in those states. These utilities were obtained from the medical literature. In addition, decreases in utility from acute complications were accounted for by subtracting days of illness, based on US average hospital length of stay data, from quality-adjusted life expectancy totals.

2.1.2.5   Step 5: Analyze the Tree

Averaging out and folding back the tree resulted in Table 2.2. The LMWH strategy was more effective than warfarin, whether in terms of life expectancy or quality-adjusted life expectancy, while also being nearly twice the cost of the warfarin strategy. Effectiveness differences between strategies translated to about 24 days in the unadjusted life expectancy analysis or about 19 quality-adjusted days in quality-adjusted life expectancy. Two incremental cost-effectiveness ratios resulted, since two effectiveness metrics were used, both of which were more than $100,000 per effectiveness unit gained.

2.1.2.6   Step 6: Test Assumptions (Sensitivity Analysis)

In a series of one-way sensitivity analyses, varying parameter values over clinically plausible ranges, individual variation of 11 parameters was found to change base case results by 10% or more. These parameters and the incremental cost-effectiveness ratios resulting from their variation are shown in Figure 2.6 as a tornado diagram, where the range of incremental cost-effectiveness results that occurred with variation of that parameter are shown as horizontal bars arranged from the greatest range to the least. Results were most sensitive to variation of parameters at the top of the figure: low values for early mortality

---

TABLE 2.2

Example Analysis Results

	Low Molecular Weight Heparin	Warfarin	Difference
Life expectancy, years	1.442	1.377	0.066
Quality-adjusted life expectancy, years	1.097	1.046	0.051
Total costs	$15,239	$7,720	$7,609
Incremental cost-effectiveness ratio, $/life-year	—	—	$115,847
Incremental cost-effectiveness ratio, $/QALY	—	—	$149,865

with warfarin or high values for early mortality with LMWH caused the LMWH strategy to be dominated, that is, to cost more and be less effective than the warfarin strategy. Variation of an individual parameter did not cause cost per QALY gained for the LMWH strategy to fall below $50,000. However, when simultaneously varying early mortality both due to LMWH and to warfarin in a two-way sensitivity analysis, cost per QALY gained was <$50,000 if mortality differences between the two agents were >8%. The LMWH strategy cost <$100,000/QALY gained if the utility for warfarin was <0.93, daily pharmacy cost for LMWH was <$41, or if the early mortality difference between agents was >3%.

A probabilistic sensitivity analysis was also performed, where all sensitive parameters were varied simultaneously over distributions 1000 times. In this analysis, warfarin was favored in 97% of model iterations if the societal willingness-to-pay threshold was $50,000/QALY, or in 72% when the threshold was $100,000/QALY gained.

2.1.2.7 Step 7: Interpret the Results

The results of this analysis suggested that treatment with LMWH in cancer patients with a history of venous thromboembolism was relatively expensive when compared to warfarin therapy, with gains in effectiveness and decreased costs resulting from fewer early complications with LMWH offset by its much higher pharmacy costs. These results were relatively robust in sensitivity analyses when parameters were varied individually and collectively over clinically

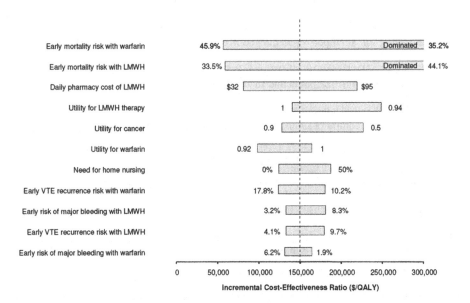

FIGURE 2.6 Tornado diagram of multiple one-way sensitivity analyses of the important variables in the LMWH example. Reproduced with permission.

reasonable ranges. A key exception was when the cost of LMWH was varied; this agent became more economically reasonable when its daily cost was in the range of $40 or less. Interestingly, in many countries other than the United States, LMWH costs are well below this range.

Thus, we can conclude that LMWH for secondary prophylaxis of venous thromboembolism in US cancer patients is relatively expensive, calling into question whether the documented improvement in outcomes is worth the added cost. However, the added expense of the newer intervention is largely driven by the cost of the agent itself, making LMWH a much more economically reasonable strategy when (and where) it costs less.

REFERENCES

[1] Roberts MS, Sonnenberg FA. Decision modeling techniques. In: Chapman GB, Sonnenberg FA, eds. *Decision Making in Health Care. Theory, Psychology, and Applications.* Cambridge, UK: Cambridge University Press; 2000:20–64.

[2] Drummond MF, Sculpher MJ, Torrance GW, O'Brien BJ, Stoddart GL. *Methods for the Economic Evaluation of Health Care Programmes.* Oxford, UK: Oxford Medical Publications, Oxford University Press; 2005.

[3] Freedberg KA, Losina E, Weinstein MC, et al. The cost effectiveness of combination antiretroviral therapy for HIV disease. *N Engl J Med.* 2001;344(11):824–31.

[4] Bratley P, Fox BL, Schrange LE. *A Guide to Simulation, Second Edition.* New York, NY: Springer; 1987.

[5] Law AM. *Simulation Modeling and Analysis, Fourth Edition.* New York, NY: McGraw-Hill; 2007.

[6] Shechter SM, Bryce CL, Alagoz O, et al. A clinically based discrete-event simulation of end-stage liver disease and the organ allocation process. *Med Decis Making.* 2005;25(2):199–209.

[7] Burke DS, Epstein JM, Cummings DA, et al. Individual-based computational modeling of smallpox epidemic control strategies. *Acad Emerg Med.* 2006;13 (11):1142–9.

[8] Halloran ME, Ferguson NM, Eubank S, et al. Modeling targeted layered containment of an influenza pandemic in the United States. *Proc Natl Acad Sci U S A.* 2008;105(12):4639–44.

[9] Longini IM, Jr., Halloran ME, Nizam A, et al. Containing a large bioterrorist smallpox attack: a computer simulation approach. *Int J Infect Dis.* 2007;11(2):98–108.

[10] Clermont G, Neugebauer EA. Systems biology and translational research. *J Crit Care.* 2005;20(4):381–2.

[11] Vodovotz Y, Chow CC, Bartels J, et al. In silico models of acute inflammation in animals. *Shock.* 2006;26(3):235–44.

[12] Vodovotz Y, Clermont G, Hunt CA, et al. Evidence-based modeling of critical illness: an initial consensus from the society for complexity in acute illness. *J Crit Care.* 2007;22(1):77–84.

[13] Kumar R, Chow CC, Bartels JD, Clermont G, Vodovotz Y. A mathematical simulation of the inflammatory response to anthrax infection. *Shock.* 2008;29 (1):104–11.

[14] Eddy DM, Schlessinger L. Validation of the Archimedes diabetes model. *Diabetes Care.* 2003;26(11):3102–10.

[15] Eddy DM, Schlessinger L. Archimedes: a trial-validated model of diabetes. *Diabetes Care.* 2003;26(11):3093–101.

[16] Eddy DM, Schlessinger L, Kahn R. Clinical outcomes and cost-effectiveness of strategies for managing people at high risk for diabetes. *Ann Intern Med*. 2005;143 (4):251–64.

[17] Aujesky D, Smith KJ, Cornuz J, Roberts MS. Cost-effectiveness of low-molecular-weight heparin for secondary prophylaxis of cancer-related venous thromboembolism. *Thromb Haemost*. 2005;93(3):592–9.

[18] Lee AY, Levine MN, Baker RI, **et al**. Low-molecular-weight heparin versus a coumarin for the prevention of recurrent venous thromboembolism in patients with cancer. *N Engl J Med*. 2003;349(2):146–53.

[19] Linkins LA, Choi PT, Douketis JD. Clinical impact of bleeding in patients taking oral anticoagulant therapy for venous thromboembolism: a meta-analysis. *Ann Intern Med*. 2003;139(11):893–900.

[20] Lee AY, Rickles FR, Julian JA, **et al**. Randomized comparison of low molecular weight heparin and coumarin derivatives on the survival of patients with cancer and venous thromboembolism. *J Clin Oncol*. 2005;23(10):2123–9.

[21] Cook N, Thomas DM. Retrospective survey of unselected hospital patients with and without cancer comparing outcomes following venous thromboembolism. *Intern Med J*. 2002;32(9–10):437–44.

3 Cost of Illness

Renée J.G. Arnold, PharmD, RPh
Icahn School of Medicine at Mount Sinai
Arnold Consultancy & Technology, LLC
New York, NY, USA

TABLE OF CONTENTS

3.1 INTRODUCTION

Cost-of-illness (COI) analysis [1–14] measures the economic burden of disease and illness on society. It is often also called burden-of-illness (BOI) or burden-of-disease (BOD) analysis. COI analyses may encompass multiple aspects of a disease's impact on direct or indirect medical costs, influence on quality of life, and as the basis for opportunity cost, that is, is the disease costly enough that monies should be spent to ameliorate the condition or should the monies be better spent elsewhere? [15–17] COI studies are, therefore, used to aid in policy making, for example, resource allocation—that is, prioritizing resource use for disease treatment and prevention—and as baseline research to determine the potential benefit of new therapies. For example, governments may use COI research to estimate the financial impact of a disease on public budgets and to determine if the cause is worthwhile for the greater good, while pharmaceutical companies may determine if the societal burden is large enough to justify directing their research efforts toward a disease's treatment [15–17]. They are often used in conjunction with other types of economic analyses, namely cost-effectiveness (Chapter 7) or budgetary impact analyses (Chapter 8), that are covered in later chapters in this book.

Costs can be divided into direct, indirect and intangible costs. Direct *medical* costs are those related to providing medical services, such as a hospital stay, emergency department (ED) visits, physician fees for outpatient visits, rehabilitation costs, home healthcare costs and drug costs (including the cost of the medication itself and any downstream adverse events that may arise as a result of drug administration). Direct *nonmedical* costs are those related to expenses, such as transportation costs, household expenditures, relocating, property losses and informal care [16], that are a direct result of the illness and are required for direct interaction with the healthcare system, but are not specifically healthcare related. Direct costs are most frequently included in a COI study, whereas indirect costs, those associated with changes of individual productivity, are often not included in a COI study, because they are difficult to obtain. Examples of indirect costs are lost time from work (absenteeism) and unpaid assistance from a family member. While absenteeism means that the person is not physically able to work at their job, presenteeism means that although the person is physically present, they may not be functioning to their fullest capacity due to the disease or treatment. An example of the latter may be nausea due to chemotherapy or drowsiness due to antihistamine treatment of allergies. In addition, intangible costs, such as pain and suffering, may be included in the analysis. Analyses can be done from one or several perspectives, which will help in determining the distribution of disease costs across multiple stakeholders [16–18]. The societal perspective typically includes indirect, as well as direct, medical costs because these are costs to society, that is, as previously mentioned, lost time from work. The payer's perspective typically includes only direct costs (see Chapters 1 and 2 for more on perspective).

3.1.1 APPROACHES

There are two approaches to conducting COI analyses, the prevalence-based approach and the incidence-based approach. The prevalence-based approach considers the cost of disease within a specified time period. This approach is most appropriate for diseases or illnesses that are measured within the time period of analysis, usually 1–2 years, and that do not change much over time (e.g., migraine, arrhythmia [2], heart failure [11]) or acute diseases (e.g., asthma [3], eczema [1, 5]).

This is in contrast to the incidence-based approach, which calculates the lifetime costs of disease from onset until cure or death. This approach is most appropriate for chronic diseases, such as hypertension, or diseases that take a long time to progress, such as diabetes, because it considers disease progression and survival probability. Such an approach may be particularly useful to determine how costs vary over time and when therapies are targeted for specific stages of a disease [17]. The disease is first defined using existing disease definitions or classification systems, such as International Classification of Diseases–Ninth (ICD-9-CM) or Tenth (ICD-10-CM) Revision codes. To accurately capture the disease COI over the appropriate time frame, depending on the aforementioned approaches, one must take into consideration the epidemiology of the disease under study and the demographic profiles of the typical patient population.

There are three methods typically employed to calculate indirect costs—human capital, friction cost and willingness to pay (WTP). The human capital method values the individual's productivity in society and estimates the hours of work lost by the person due to the disease and multiplies them by an hourly wage; this method, therefore, takes the patient perspective. The human capital method may be problematic for several reasons as follows:

- It is uncertain what figure to use for the hourly wage, although in the United States often a figure from the Bureau of Labor Statistics is used for average hourly wage.
- It may underestimate costs in the extremes of age (children/elderly) [17].
- It may overestimate costs in cases of long-term absence, disability or premature death; in fact, it is the assumption that a worker cannot be replaced even if the unemployment rate is significantly high that results in this overestimation [16, 17].

Nonetheless, this is the method commonly employed. It may be operationalized using the Work Productivity and Activity Impairment (WPAI) questionnaire. The WPAI was created as a patient-reported quantitative assessment of the amount of absenteeism, presenteeism and daily activity impairment attributable to general health (WPAI:GH) or a specific health problem (WPAI:SHP). It is readily modifiable to address any health condition.

The friction cost method "estimates the value of human capital when another person from the unemployment pool replaces the present value of a worker's future earnings until the sick or impaired worker returns or is eventually replaced [16]." Thus, it is a function of the availability of labor. The friction cost is characterized by the initial disruption costs plus training costs. It is viewed from the employer's perspective and may underestimate productivity costs.

The WTP method suggests that the avoidance of a disease can be estimated from the amount people would be willing to pay to reduce the probability of morbidity or mortality due to a disease [16, 17]. There are various ways to determine and estimate an individual's WTP such as conducting surveys, examining the extra wages for highly risky jobs, and estimating the demand for products that lead to a greater level of health or safety [16]. An example of a WTP analysis might use the following scenario: suppose that in a population of 100,000, a new heart failure medication is expected to result in 1 fewer death per year from heart failure. You've elicited the fact that each person in that population of 100,000 is willing to pay US$20 a year for the reduction in mortality risks (maximum premium WTP). What is the implied value of life? The equation for this is dV/dR, where dV = maximum premium WTP and dR = risk reduction. We have reduced the annual risk of dying by 0.00001 (1/100,000). Thus, the implied value of life = US$20/.00001 = US$2,000,000 and the total WTP is US$2 million for an annual risk reduction that can be expected in the statistical sense to save one life.

3.1.2 Methods

A micro-costing method has been used in many studies to examine COI. The direct costs included in this method typically comprise out-of-pocket expenses for noninsured items (over-the-counter medications, visits to out-of-plan health practitioners, laundry/clothing and specialty items) and co-payments for prescription medications and clinic visits determined from insurance claims databases as well as the usual direct cost items previously outlined.

Several examples of COI studies, atopic dermatitis (AD), human papillomavirus (HPV), asthma and arrhythmia, will now be examined.

3.2   ATOPIC DERMATITIS

AD is a chronic disease that affects the skin of children and adults. It results in itchy, flaky skin and demonstrates a considerable impact on patient quality of life, as well as a substantial monetary burden [1, 9, 19–28]. Direct and indirect costs for AD have been measured in various countries and are substantial from both patient and societal perspectives. The direct costs have been reported to range from US$71 to US$2,559 per patient per year [29]. This variation in cost is due to the differences in study methodology as well as differences in healthcare systems of the various countries. Most of the costs of AD consist of indirect costs associated with time lost from work, lifestyle changes, and nontraditional or over-the-counter treatments for AD [29]. According to Drucker et al. [30], "a conservative estimate of the annual costs of atopic dermatitis in the United States is US$5.297 billion (in 2015 US$)". The financial burden on the health care system and on society is expected to grow because the prevalence of the disease is increasing.

Indeed, using a prevalence-based approach to calculate COI, studies have demonstrated direct costs ranging from US$150 [21] (using the approximate US$ equivalent in 2005) to US$580 [22] per patient per year, and even up to US$19,462 [31], with differences varying due to different cost-accounting methods and categories of costs included. Filanovsky et al. [32] recently calculated a mean *monthly* personal cost of AD in the month before an office visit as US$274 (median US$114; IQR US$29, US$276), with US$75 from direct costs (median US$45; IQR US$20, US$110) and US$199 from indirect costs (median US$0; IQR US$0, US$208). Table 3.1 lists numerous references in which US$ (or equivalent) per patient COI were calculated.

Typically, outpatient visits and medications compose the majority of direct costs [9, 28], ranging from approximately 62% to >90% [9]. The distribution of AD-associated direct costs from Fivenson et al. [9] is shown in Figure 3.1. In those studies that examined indirect costs (e.g., the patient out-of-pocket costs for co-pays, medications, household items, loss of productivity), they made up substantial percentages of the total, for example, 36% [23], 38% [30] or 73%, respectively [9]. Several studies showed increasing costs with worsening disease severity in adults. Using a micro cost-accounting approach, whereby costs of hospitalizations, consultations, drug therapy, treatment procedures, diagnostic tests, laboratory tests, clinic visits and urgent care visits were summed, Fivenson, Arnold, and colleagues (Table 3.2) reported an average annual per patient direct cost ranging from US$435 in mild patients to US$3,229 in severe patients. This association of higher costs

TABLE 3.1

Selected References of Cost of Illness of Atopic Dermatitis

Reference	Year	Direct	Indirect	Perspective (Payer)	Total[1]
Ehlken [1]	2005	US$150[2]	US$1589	Societal	US$1739
Ellis [2]	2002	US$580	Not measured	Private insurer	
Ellis [2]	2002	US$1250	Not measured	Medicaid	
Fivenson [3]	2002	US$167	US$147	Health plan	US$609
Emerson [4]	2001	US$73[2]	US$42	Societal	US$115
Jenner [5]	2004		US$281[2]	Patient	
Ricci [6]	2006		US$1540	Patient	
Verboom [7]	2002	US$71		Country	

1 If both direct and indirect available
2 US$ equivalent for 2005 calculated using www.gocurrency.com historic EU to US$ converter

[1] B. Ehlken, M. Mohrenschlager, B. Kugland, K. Berger, K. Quednau, J. Ring, [Cost-of-illness study in patients suffering from atopic eczema in Germany], *Hautarzt* 56(12) (2005) 1144–51.

[2] C.N. Ellis, L.A. Drake, M.M. Prendergast, W. Abramovits, M. Boguniewicz, C.R. Daniel, M. Lebwohl, S.R. Stevens, D.L. Whitaker-Worth, J.W. Cheng, K.B. Tong, Cost of atopic dermatitis and eczema in the United States, *J Am Acad Dermatol* 46(3) (2002) 361–70.

[3] D. Fivenson, R.J. Arnold, D.J. Kaniecki, J.L. Cohen, F. Frech, A.Y. Finlay, The effect of atopic dermatitis on total burden of illness and quality of life on adults and children in a large managed care organization, *J Manag Care Pharm* 8(5) (2002) 333–42.

[4] R.M. Emerson, H.C. Williams, B.R. Allen, What is the cost of atopic dermatitis in preschool children?, *Br J Dermatol* 144(3) (2001) 514–22.

[5] N. Jenner, J. Campbell, R. Marks, Morbidity and cost of atopic eczema in Australia, *Australas J Dermatol* 45(1) (2004) 16–22.

[6] G. Ricci, B. Bendandi, L. Pagliara, A. Patrizi, M. Masi, Atopic dermatitis in Italian children: Evaluation of its economic impact, *J Pediatr Health Care* 20(5) (2006) 311–15.

[7] P. Verboom, L. Hakkaart-Van, M. Sturkenboom, R. De Zeeuw, H. Menke, F. Rutten, The cost of atopic dermatitis in the Netherlands: An international comparison, *Br J Dermatol* 147(4) (2002) 716–24.

among patients with greater disease severity was found in an analysis of patients with commercial, Medicaid and Medicare insurance [31].

Indirect costs also increased by worsening disease severity—by more than twofold [19, 27] to threefold [26] to as much as almost tenfold [9]. Similarly, Ehlken et al. [21] showed a greater than twofold increase in total (both direct and indirect) costs for patients with mild vs. severe disease.

3.2.1 THERAPY-SPECIFIC COST

Several studies have compared the cost of different uses of topical corticosteroids (TCS) vs. topical immunomodulators (i.e., pimecrolimus and tacrolimus) and of the topical immunomodulators against each other. Some of these are detailed in the following sections.

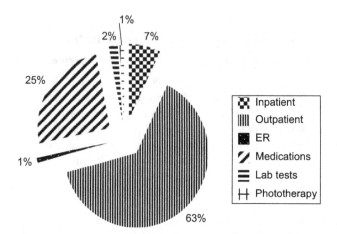

FIGURE 3.1   Distribution of atopic-dermatitis-associated direct costs in a US health plan.

3.2.1.1   Topical Corticosteroids

Green and colleagues undertook a systematic review of 10 RCTs in patients with AD [24, 25]. Their literature search at the time revealed no published studies of this nature. The authors noted a wide variation in price and product availability, with the lowest price being generic hydrocortisone (£0.60 [approximately US$1.09]) to the highest at that time being mometasone furoate (Elocon) of £4.88 (approximate US$8.80 equivalent).

Six of the RCT studies favored the once-daily option as the lowest-cost treatment and four favored a twice-daily option, with successful outcome being defined by overall response to treatment, relapse or flare-up rate, adverse effects, compliance, tolerability, patient preference measures, and impact on quality of life. One of the twice-daily-favored studies achieved a greater benefit (number of successful treatment responders) at a greater cost. However, it was felt that this greater cost would still likely be very cost-effective, given the relatively low prices of TCS. The limitations noted in the review were those of potentially low generalizability due to 80% of the RCTs referring to potent TCS in patients with moderate-to-severe disease, whereas the majority of patients with AD have mild disease and lack of information on quantity of product usage.

3.2.1.2   Topical Immunomodulators

Clinical data show that topical immunomodulators are effective in AD, yet do not cause the significant adverse effects associated with TCS [19]. Delea et al. [20] retrospectively compared 157 pimecrolimus patients with 157 tacrolimus patients previously receiving TCS in a large claims database of managed care patients in terms of resource utilization (concomitant medications) and AD-related follow-up costs. They used propensity matching to control for differences between the groups in baseline demographic and

TABLE 3.2

Total Annual Costs for Adults by Provider-assessed Severity

	Mild (N=55)		Moderate (N=31)		Severe (N=3)		Unknown (N=18)	
	Total US$	Mean per patient US$ ± SE	Total US$	Mean per patient US$ ± SE	Total US$	Mean per patient US$ ± SE	Total US$	Mean per patient US$ ± SE
Direct Costs								
Inpatient	1,082	19.68 ± 19.68	0	0	0	0	0	0
Outpatient	4,947	89.95 ± 7.54	3,605	116.29 ± 15.7	884	294.67 ± 49.67	1,406	78.11 ± 11.56
Emergency room	0	0	0	0	0	0	0	0
Medications	1,873	.06 ± 9.86	1,765	56.95 ± 14.14	1,189	396.40 ± 349.59	764	42.44 ± 11.57
Labs	24	0.44 ± 0.44	0	0	0	0	0	0
Phototherapy	0	0	63	2.03 ± 1.44	0	0	0	0
Subtotal	**7,926**	**144.13 ± 23.97**	**5,433**	**175.27 ± 25.84**	**2,073**	**691.07 ± 389.36**	**2,170**	**120.55 ± 17.08**
Indirect Costs								
Practitioner visits	575	10.45 ± 6.75	100	3.23 ± 2.29	0	0	1,510	83.89 ± 58.39
Visit copays	380	6.91 ± 0.59	280	9.03 ± 1.28	70	23.33 ± 4.41	110	6.11 ± 0.86
Medications	3,740	68.00 ± 25.83	1,306	42.13 ± 13.52	357	119.00 ± 55.32	1,808	100.44 ± 48.73
Medication copays	316	5.74 ± 0.99	254	8.21 ± 1.73	88	29.33 ± 19.06	83	4.61 ± 1.25
Household Items	1,024	18.62 ± 10.37	1,863	60.10 ± 29.52	620	206.67 ± 206.67	1,000	55.56 ± 25.66
Child Care	0	0	0	0	0	0	0	0
Subtotal	**6,035**	**109.72 ± 35.34**	**3,803**	**122.70 ± 34.49**	**1,135**	**378.33 ± 244.31**	**4,511**	**250.61 ± 84.65**
Productivity								
Days lost from work	9,983	181.51 ± 120.62	8,705	280.82 ± 113.89	6,476	2,159.65 ± 1,033.12	4,138	229.90 ± 93.63
Subtotal	9,983	181.51 ± 120.62	8,705	280.82 ± 113.89	6,476	2,159.65 ± 1,033.12	4,138	229.90 ± 93.63
TOTAL	**23,944**	**435.35 ± 156.40**	**17,941**	**578.79 ± 131.27**	**9,684**	**3,229.05 ± 1,306.96**	**10,819**	**601.06 ± 137.26**

clinical characteristics and utilization of AD-related services prior to assessment of disease severity. Patients in the pimecrolimus group had fewer pharmacy claims for TCS (mean 1.37 vs. 2.04, $P = 0.021$); this occurred primarily in the high-potency topical corticosteroid category. Fewer patients in the pimecrolimus group also received antistaphylococcal antibiotics during the follow-up period (16% vs. 27%, $P = 0.014$) and total AD-related costs during this time were lower in this group than in the tacrolimus group (mean US\$263 vs. US\$361, $P = 0.012$).

3.3 HUMAN PAPILLOMAVIRUS

Persistent infection with cancer-associated HPV (termed oncogenic or high-risk HPV) causes the majority of squamous cell cervical cancer, the most common type of cervical cancer, and its histologic precursor lesions, the low-grade cervical dysplasia Cervical Intraepithelial Neoplasia-1 (CIN 1) and the moderate-to-high-grade dysplasia CIN 2/3. Multiple HPV strains cause varying degrees of invasive cervical cancer (ICC) and its CIN precursors. HPV strains 16 and 18 cause approximately 70% of all cervical cancers [33, 34] CIN3, specifically, and 50% of CIN 2 cases. In addition, HPV 16 and 18 cause approximately 35–50% of all CIN 1. Low-oncogenic HPV risk types 6 and 11 account for 90% of genital wart cases [35]. Unfortunately, cytological and histological examinations cannot reliably distinguish between those patients who will progress from cervical dysplasia to ICC from those whose dysplasias will regress spontaneously, the latter being the vast majority of cases [36]. This inability to definitely ascertain the natural history of HPV infection is one of the primary reasons for the dilemma with HPV vaccination.

Although cervical cancer screening programs, such as the use of routine screening via the Papanicolaou (Pap) cervical smear, have substantially reduced the incidence and mortality of ICC in developed countries over the past 50 years [35, 37], there has been a slowing of these declines in recent years due to poor sensitivity of cervical cytology, anxiety and morbidity of screening investigations, poor access to and attendance of screening programs, falling screening coverage and poor predictive value for adenocarcinoma, an increasingly common cause of ICC [37]. HPV is the most common sexually transmitted disease in the United States and virtually 100% of cervical cancer is due to HPV. HPV is also linked to head and neck cancer in men. There are more than 100 HPV strains (thereby potentially reducing vaccine efficacy for oncogenic strains not covered by the vaccine); HPV infection is often self-limited. A mitigating factor for the argument against using the vaccine is the fact that the cost-effectiveness of screening with Pap smears is reduced (improves) from US\$1 million/QALY if patients continue to be screened annually, as is the common current recommendation, to US\$150,000/QALY if patients are screened every 3 years, the latter a likely scenario if the vaccine is used [33, 38–40].

Worldwide, the incidence of cervical cancer is 570,000 new cases in 2018 [41] and 266,000 deaths per year [42]; it is the fourth-leading cause of cancer deaths, with 90% of these cases observed in developing countries [41]. Women in developing countries are especially vulnerable as they lack access to both cervical cancer screening and treatment. The demographics of cervical cancer in the United States show that 13,240 new cases of ICC were expected to be diagnosed in 2018 and about 4,170 deaths in women were expected from ICC [43]. The National Cancer Institute estimates an annual incidence of new genital HPV infections of 14 million [44]. There are three vaccines currently available—Gardasil®, Gardasil 9® and Cervarix®—in the United States and Europe that cover the two major oncogenic HPV strains (16 and 18) for cervical cancer. In addition, Gardasil covers HPV strains 6 and 11, the primary causes of genital warts and Gardasil 9 covers five additional strains (31, 33, 45, 52 and 58). As of May 2017, Gardasil 9 is the only HPV vaccine available in the United States; the others are still available outside of the United States [44]. To significantly reduce the rate of cervical cancer in the population as a whole, 70% of girls need to be vaccinated to achieve what is called "herd immunity"—when the vaccine's impact goes beyond just people who are inoculated. The concept of herd immunity has been a "hot topic" regarding the novel coronavirus pandemic, as well, since the more people have contracted the disease and recovered, the fewer will be available to infect others. So far, it is unknown if HPV strains will mutate as the vaccine is introduced, although this is not very likely, seeing that HPV is a DNA-based virus [36].

Insinga et al. [45] used administrative and laboratory data from a large US health plan to examine costs, resource utilization and annual health plan expenditures for cervical HPV-related disease. An episode of care was defined as beginning with a routine cervical smear, that is, one that required no evidence of follow-up for a previous Pap smear abnormality or ICD-9 diagnosis of a cervical abnormality during the previous 9 months. If CIN or cancer was not detected during an episode of care, biopsy results were termed false-positive. Because the data source was a prepaid health plan without direct billing for procedures or services, service-specific costs were assigned from the Medstat Marketscan database (now IBM Marketscan) as a proxy for the health plan costs. Because of the small number of cervical cancer cases in the data set, costs were assigned on an age- and stage-specific basis using the Surveillance Epidemiology and End Results Program (SEER; National Cancer Institute; US Department of Health and Human Services, Bethesda, MD) database and an Agency for Healthcare Research and Quality evidence report. All cost estimates were converted to 2002 US$ using the Medical Care component of the Consumer Price Index.

The authors found that episodes of care after an abnormal routine cervical smear were US$732 on average, compared with US$57 for visits with negative results, with a statistically significant trend toward higher costs with increasing grade of initial cytologic abnormality. False-positive cervical smears cost US$376 annually, while incomplete follow-up was US$79. Regardless of age group, cervical HPV-related disease annual healthcare costs were US$26,415 per 1,000 enrollees, with the greatest costs of US$51,863 being observed in the 20- to 29-year-old age group. The largest cost contribution was that of routine screening at 63.4% of total costs (range by age group of 54.1% to 70.8%), followed by cost of CIN 2/3, then cancer, false-positive smear, CIN 1 and incomplete follow-up (see Figure 3.2) [45, 46].

Insinga and co-authors extrapolated their results to the general US population to derive a total healthcare cost of US$3.4 billion for HPV-related disease in 1998, with expenditures for routine screening accounting for US$2.1 billion, false-positive Pap test US$300 million, CIN 1 US$150 million, CIN 2/3 US$450 million and ICC US$350 million in 2002 US$. A follow-up study by the same authors estimated the annual direct costs of abnormal cervical findings and treating cancer at US$3.5 billion in 2005 US$ [48]. Annual direct cost estimates in 2005 US$ have been as high as $4.6 billion [47] and adding in costs of anogenital warts and other cancers associated with oncogenic HPV strains raises the total estimated economic burden to as high as US$5 billion in 2006 US$ [45,46].

Chesson et al. [48] estimated an overall annual direct medical cost burden of preventing and treating HPV-associated disease to be US$8.0 billion (2010 US$). Of this total cost, about US$6.6 billion (82.3%) was for routine cervical cancer screening and follow-up, US$1.0 billion (12.0%) was for cancer (including US$0.4 billion for cervical cancer and US$0.3 billion for oropharyngeal cancer), US$0.3 billion (3.6%) was for genital warts and US$0.2 billion (2.1%) was for recurrent respiratory papillomatosis.

Insinga and colleagues also estimated indirect costs, assuming that there were 130,377 women who would have been alive during 2000 had they not died from cervical cancer during that or a previous year, >75% of these women died before age 60, with >25% dying prior to age 40, and that 37,594 (29%) of these women would have had labor force earnings during 2000. Using these data, the total productivity loss in 2000 owing to cervical cancer mortality was estimated at US$1.3 billion, several times higher than estimates of the annual US direct medical costs of US$300 to US$400 million associated with cervical cancer [49]. As in the AD studies, therefore, indirect costs are thought to account for a much greater burden than direct costs of HPV [9].

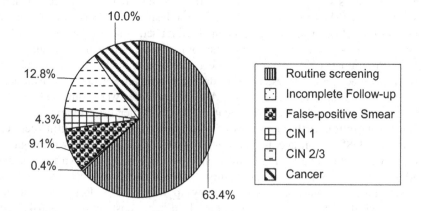

FIGURE 3.2 Distribution of cervical HPV-related disease direct costs in a commercial US health plan.

3.4 ASTHMA

Asthma is a chronic disease with acute exacerbations (flare-ups), similar to the epidemiology of AD. Although a minority of patients today with asthma experience disease-related ED visits and hospitalizations, these events continue to result in significantly disproportionate use of healthcare resources and expenses [50]. Asthma guidelines recommend periodic assessment of impairment and risk factors to prevent exacerbations, which can lead to hospitalization, increased healthcare utilization and cost. Fractional exhaled nitric oxide (FeNO) testing assists in the management of asthma by providing clinicians with an objective assessment of underlying type 2 helper cells (Th2)/type 2 driven airway inflammation and corresponding corticosteroid sensitivity. In addition, FeNO is one of the several risk factors that has been shown to predict the likelihood of a future asthma exacerbation [51, 52]. According to Cochrane meta-analysis data, FeNO monitoring is associated with a 40–50% reduction in the risk of exacerbations [53, 54]. Cost modeling indicated the potential for significant cost savings with FeNO use [55] and, as such, Arnold et al [3] attempted to verify this potential for cost savings within a real-world database of Medicare beneficiaries [3]. This retrospective observational study investigated asthma-related claims from the Centers for Medicare and Medicaid Services (CMS)' 5% Standard Analytic Files (SAFs) from January 1, 2012 through December 31, 2015. The CMS 5% SAFs contain every fully adjudicated Medicare claim filed for 5% of the Medicare fee-for-service population. Medicare beneficiaries are randomly selected by their beneficiary ID, which usually is a form of the social security number. While the beneficiary ID is encrypted, it is consistent between all claims in a year and across years, allowing for longitudinal analysis. A denominator file provides demographic and coverage data about the beneficiaries in the data set. These data include approximately 5 million claims annually, of which a large majority is Carrier Part B claims for physician services. Arnold et al. chose those patients who had a history of exacerbation so as to best study the potential impact of the FeNO intervention since frequency of future exacerbation is best determined by past history of exacerbation [51]. The moderate-to-severe exacerbator cohort was identified using guidelines from the American Thoracic Society (ATS) addressing asthma clinical research and included beneficiaries who had at least one inpatient (IP) hospitalization or ED visit with a primary diagnosis of asthma (ICD-9-CM Dx 493.xx) in 2013 [56, 57]. The date of the first identified asthma IP or ED visit was the index date.

Beneficiaries were included who had 2 years of records following an asthma-related IP hospitalization or ED claim. All-cause and asthma-related healthcare resource utilization and costs were assessed at baseline and during follow-up periods. All-cause healthcare resource utilization and costs included all medical encounters; asthma-related healthcare resource utilization and costs were limited to medical encounters with a primary diagnosis of asthma. Costs were calculated as the sum of the amount paid by the health plan, the beneficiary and any third-party payer. Costs were also reported as per patient per day. Index events claims and costs were excluded from all pre-FeNO analyses. All costs were adjusted to 2016 US$ using the annual figure for the Medical Care Component of the Consumer Price Index. A case-crossover analysis was completed of asthma-related IP/ED events before and after FeNO use during the two-year study period. Study design was of utmost importance when determining how best to assess any influence of an intervention such as FeNO on asthma exacerbations. Indeed, the researchers stated that they considered using a case–cohort analysis, but were concerned that there may be associated confounding/unmeasurable factors that would result in biases that would undermine the integrity of the study. Because of the matched nature of a case-crossover study design, all time-invariant confounders are automatically corrected for without having to measure the confounders [58]. Case–control analyses are especially relevant in cases such as this study where there was an acute "exposure" (FeNO) and an outcome defined by an acute event (asthma exacerbation). Employing a similar methodology, Sadatsafavi and colleagues found an increased 30-day risk of asthma-related hospital readmission after an episode of asthma-related hospitalization. Interestingly, similar to Arnold and colleagues [3], where nonasthma-related events ("All claims") were less likely to be as highly statistically significant than asthma-related events, there was no correlation of readmission after an episode of hospitalization not related to asthma [59].

In the Arnold et al. study, 100 of the 5,911 asthma beneficiaries who met the inclusion criteria within the database had a FeNO test during the two-year study period. During the period before FeNO use, 98/101 (97%) beneficiaries had an asthma-related IP/ED event compared to 46/101 (46%) during the FeNO period. Asthma-related IP/ED claims and charges per beneficiary per day during the period before FeNO were 0.004 and US$16.21 compared to 0.002 and US$6.46 during the FeNO period ($p = 0.0433$ and $p = 0.0133$, respectively). While the analysis consistently demonstrated that, while asthma-related claims and asthma-related ED/IP claims and charges per patient per day were statistically significantly lower after FeNO use, this was not the case with all-cause claims, where the opposite occurred, that is, that these figures were higher post-FeNO than pre-FeNO. This make sense if one considers that it is the more difficult asthma cases (in terms of place of treatment), regardless of comorbidities or other reasons why beneficiaries would be hospitalized, that account for FeNO use resulting in positive outcomes, hence the authors' concentration on beneficiaries with frequent moderate-to-severe exacerbations in the study.

Thus, the authors found that FeNO monitoring in beneficiaries with a history of exacerbations was associated with a substantial reduction in asthma-related IP/ED claims and charges.

3.5   ARRHYTHMIA

Arrhythmias, such as atrial fibrillation (AF), are often asymptomatic, yet are associated with critical adverse outcomes, such as stroke. Moreover, survivors of a stroke with AF have a high risk of recurrent stroke [60]. Their management is expensive, with one source citing a cost of approximately US$26 billion associated with AF [61]. Additionally, 25% of strokes are of unknown cause and subclinical AF is often suspected to be the cause under these circumstances [61–63]. AF has been reported to be the most common type of arrhythmia and the incidence and prevalence of AF are exhibiting a continuing upward trend [64]. If an arrhythmia is suspected, Holter monitoring may be ordered. The Holter monitor was first introduced into clinical practice in the 1960s and is a type of ambulatory electrocardiogram (AECG) [61, 65–67]. It is used to monitor ECG tracing continuously for a period of 24–48 hours after a patient experiences an arrhythmia that is not observed during an in-office ECG [62, 64]. These types of events are often categorized as subclinical or asymptomatic.

Despite the popularity of this test, the diagnostic yield (i.e., the detection of arrhythmias) may be low, varying from 1% to 22% in various case series [67–70]. Indeed, the common belief (although not well documented) is that repeat cardiac monitoring is frequent. Overall, the diagnostic sequence and its associated costs for arrhythmia detection utilizing Holter ambulatory ECG monitoring have not been studied to any extent. It was the authors' goal, then, to characterize the diagnosis, additional monitoring, clinical events and sequelae of this detection system for arrhythmias. These were translated into costs that occurred after an initial Holter monitor with a particular focus on Medicare patients using the same type of Medicare SAFs indicated in the asthma study. Arnold and colleagues executed a retrospective, longitudinal claims analysis limited to 24- or 48-hour Holter patients with no prior arrhythmia and who underwent a "new" Holter monitor [2]. Patients were followed over time to identify related diagnoses, additional monitoring events and related clinical events. The study period was defined for each patient as the two-year window from the first Holter event reported in 2009. Two years is a relevant time frame to identify related follow-up events; a shorter time frame may undercount such events, while a longer study period may identify fewer relevant events. Additionally, all monitoring codes were used to capture follow-up monitoring events, including global and technical components, hook-up and interpretation. Repeat monitor events (by AMA Current Procedural Terminology [CPT] code and date of service) must have been billed more than seven days apart from another monitoring event of the same type to limit the risk of double counting a single event. The research studied years 2008 through 2011 in Medicare Fee-For-Service (FFS) Carrier (Part B), Inpatient, Outpatient and Denominator files.

Patients were included in the evaluation if the beneficiary had an index Holter in 2009 and enrolled in Medicare FFS Parts A and B in the 1 year prior to the date of the first Holter to date of death or 2 years after the date of the index Holter event in 2009. Exclusion criteria for a given beneficiary included the use of a Holter or other cardiac monitoring device 1 year prior to the purported date of the first Holter use event in 2009, diagnosis of AF 1 year prior to the date of the first Holter event in 2009, a cardiac ablation procedure in the 1 year prior to the date of the first Holter event in 2009 (unless specified for supraventricular tachycardia, Wolff–Parkinson–White or accessory bypass tract). To illustrate how these criteria worked, consider the following example. A patient whose first Holter event occurred on February 1,

2009 would be retrospectively evaluated over the period February 1, 2008 through January 31, 2009 for exclusion criteria. The follow-up period for analyses would cover February 1, 2009 through February 1, 2011.

There were 46,840 beneficiaries with an initial Holter performed in 2009. After application of the exclusion criteria, the study cohort was reduced to 17,887 patients. Diagnosis was identified by appropriate ICD-9 codes and additional ambulatory ECG monitoring by CPT codes and date of service. Clinical events were identified through site of service and ICD-9 codes for ED, IP and Observation (OBS) unit stays and ICD-9 codes for stroke, transient ischemic attack (TIA) and cardiac arrests. The principal diagnosis was used to determine clinical events. Costs were derived from the claims data in the Medicare SAFs. The diagnostic sequence of events (which was characterized as the "Diagnostic Odyssey") was used to group patients into one of the eight possible outcome categories based on the occurrence of a clinical event, the ability of the Holter monitoring to provide a diagnosis, the use of repeat monitoring and the ultimate success in diagnosis and preventing clinical events. The 17,887 patients in the study sample were classified into eight categories based on their diagnostic odyssey (Figure 3.3) and the numbers and percentages tabulated. These were further subclassified into survival through the study period (as described earlier). Finally, the cost of care for the eight cohorts was determined from the Medicare SAF through the allowable charges in that database. From the combination of the percentage of patients in each

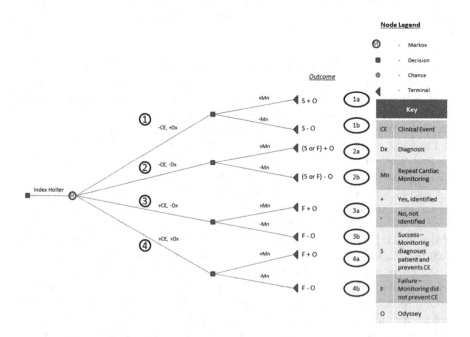

FIGURE 3.3   Outcomes Categories: Decision Tree – "Diagnostic Odyssey"

TABLE 3.3

"Diagnostic Odyssey" Patient Counts and Allowed Charges

Branch	N patients	Total	Average Per Patient	Allowed Charges		
				Total inpatient	Total Outpatient	Total Part B
2b −CE, −Dx, −Mn	8,074	$115,244,713	$14,274	$29,210,291	$28,792,599	$57,241,823
3b +CE, −Dx, −Mn	2,385	$63,144,546	$26,476	$22,073,938	$14,748,296	$26,322,311
2a −CE, −Dx, +Mn	1,976	$45,987,782	$23,273	$14,150,566	$10,424,886	$21,412,330
1b −CE, +Dx, −Mn	1,924	$48,291,936	$25,100	$19,400,990	$10,684,998	$18,205,949
4b +CE, +Dx, −Mn	1,459	$65,653,071	$44,999	$34,017,088	$11,397,619	$20,238,364
1a −CE, +Dx, +Mn	1,156	$30,187,408	$26,114	$11,344,771	$6,323,153	$12,519,484
4a +CE, +Dx, +Mn	465	$19,170,535	$41,227	$7,810,190	$4,055,323	$7,305,021
2b +CE, −Dx, +Mn	448	$14,620,310	$32,635	$5,418,757	$3,696,332	$5,505,220
Total	17,887	$402,300,299	$22,491	$143,426,591	$90,123,207	$168,750,501

Mn = repeat cardiac monitoring; CE = clinical event; blue highlighted group (group 2a) is the "No odyssey" category.

category and their corresponding charges, it was possible to extrapolate to the general population of Holter monitor use. The study's focus was on the group of patients who, despite undergoing repeat cardiac monitoring, demonstrated no diagnoses or clinical events (group 2a in Table 3.3).

Table 3.3 provides a summary of the patient counts and allowed charges for the entire study period for the eight categories ("Diagnostic Odyssey").

The 1,976 patients (11.1% of the total) in group 2a reflected the failure of repeat Holter monitoring to either detect clinical events or diagnose disease. In spite of this failure, there was a total allowed charge of more than US$45 million or slightly more than US$23,000 per involved patient. When extrapolated over the entire Medicare FFS population with the given study criteria, this category was estimated to cost more than US$900 million over the two-year study period.

Further examination of this group showed that Holter monitoring was the most commonly repeated test during the 2 years of follow-up. When a repeat test was performed, the majority of the time it occurred in the first 3 months after the initial Holter test. Moreover, only one repeat test was typically performed. This suggests that a large degree of effort, time and expense is spent on a relatively large group of individuals for which no obvious discernible clinical benefit is engendered. In agreement with Kuhne [70], the diagnostic yield of Holter monitoring may not be as substantial as the prevailing clinical sentiment suggests. As a consequence, Healey et al. [63] have pointed out that subclinical outcomes such as tachyarrythmias have a significant association with the increased risk of AF along with stroke and systemic embolism. In the current study, it was noted that repeat monitoring, often of the same type as done initially, frequently did not yield a diagnosis and patients continued to experience clinical events. Arnold and colleagues concluded that additional diagnostic paradigms must be explored to improve these patient and system outcomes.

3.6 SUMMARY

In summary, COI or BOI lays the foundation on which the different types of analyses that are used to make decisions in allocation of healthcare resources are framed. As indirect costs, that is, productivity, often account for a substantial portion of the burden, these should be assessed as part of the COI computation whenever possible. The major limitation of COI studies is that they neither consider the effectiveness of treatment, nor the ease with which that treatment may reduce the burden of disease on society or the individual. Thus, these studies should be performed in conjunction with cost-effectiveness analyses, whenever possible.

REFERENCES

[1] R. Arnold, R. Kuan, Quality-of-life and costs in atopic dermatitis, *Handbook of Disease Burdens and Quality of Life Measures*, Springer, Heidelberg, 2008.

[2] R. Arnold, A. Layton, Cost analysis and clinical outcomes of ambulatory care monitoring in Medicare patients: describing the diagnostic odyssey, *JHEOR* 2(2) (2015) 161–9.

[3] R. Arnold, A. Layton, M. Massanari, Cost impact of monitoring exhaled nitric oxide in asthma management, *Allergy Asthma Proc* 39 (2018) 337–43.

[4] R. Arnold, K. Pettit, J. DiCesare, J. Fastenau, D. Kaniecki, Prospective economic evaluation in a Phase IIIb renal transplant clinical trial, *Value Health* 1 (1998) 36.

[5] R. Arnold, Y. Zhou, K. Wong, J. Sung, Burden of illness and impact of atopic dermatitis on parents' quality of life among children with atopic dermatitis (P704), 63rd Annual Meeting of the American Academy of Dermatology, 2005.

[6] R.J.G. Arnold, Y. Han, R. Balakrishnan, A. Layton, C.E. Lok, M. Glickman, D.K. Rajan, Comparison between surgical and endovascular hemodialysis arteriovenous fistula interventions and associated costs, *J Vasc Interv Radiol* 29(11) (2018) 1558–66 e2.

[7] R.J.G. Arnold, J. Tang, J. Schrecker, C. Hild, Impact of definitive drug-drug interaction testing on medication management and patient care, *Drugs Real World Outcomes* 5(4) (2018) 217–24.

[8] S. Bansilal, J.M. Castellano, E. Garrido, H.G. Wei, A. Freeman, C. Spettell, F. Garcia-Alonso, I. Lizano, R.J. Arnold, J. Rajda, et al., Assessing the impact of medication adherence on long-term cardiovascular outcomes, *J Am Coll Cardiol* 68 (8) (2016) 789–801.

[9] D. Fivenson, R.J. Arnold, D.J. Kaniecki, J.L. Cohen, F. Frech, A.Y. Finlay, The effect of atopic dermatitis on total burden of illness and quality of life on adults and children in a large managed care organization, *J Manag Care Pharm* 8(5) (2002) 333–42.

[10] H. Lachmann, R. Arnold, M. Gattorno, I. Kone-Paut, A. Ferreira, J. Kummerle-Deschner, A retrospective patient chart review and survey in patients with cryopyrin-associated periodic syndromes treated with anakinra, *JHEOR* 1(2) (2013) 123–33.

[11] M.M. Najib, R.J. Goldberg Arnold, D.J. Kaniecki, K.G. Pettit, D. Roth, L. Antell, J. Xuan, Medical resource use and costs of congestive heart failure after carvedilol use, *Heart Dis* 4(2) (2002) 70–7.

[12] S. Pokras, V. Divino, C. Ferrufino, R. Arnold, H. Huang, The economic burden of dasatinib and nilotinib treatment failure in chronic myeloid leukemia (CML) patients: a real-world analysis, *Value Health* 16 (2013) A137.

[13] S. Yang, C. Lok, R. Arnold, D. Rajan, M. Glickman, Comparison of post-creation procedures and costs between surgical and an endovascular approach to arteriovenous fistula creation, *J Vasc Access* 18(Suppl. 2) (2017) 8–14.

[14] A. Zaman, R.J. Goldberg, K.G. Pettit, D.J. Kaniecki, K. Benner, C. Zacker, J. DiCesare, M. Helfand, Cost of treating an episode of variceal bleeding in a VA setting, *Am J Gastroenterol* 95(5) (2000) 1323–30.

[15] A. Angelis, D. Tordrup, P. Kanavos, Socio-economic burden of rare diseases: a systematic review of cost of illness evidence, *Health Policy* 119(7) (2015) 964–79.

[16] C. Jo, Cost-of-illness studies: concepts, scopes, and methods, *Clinical and Molecular Hepatology* 20(4) (2014) 327–37.

[17] R. Linertova, L. Garcia-Perez, I. Gorostiza, Cost-of-illness in rare diseases, *Adv Exp Med Biol* 1031 (2017) 283–97.

[18] A.A. Honeycutt, J.E. Segel, T.J. Hoerger, E.A. Finkelstein, Comparing cost-of-illness estimates from alternative approaches: an application to diabetes, *Health Serv Res* 44(1) (2009) 303–20.

[19] W. Abramovits, M. Boguniewicz, A.S. Paller, D.L. Whitaker-Worth, M.M. Prender-gast, M. Tokar, K.B. Tong, The economics of topical immunomodulators for the treatment of atopic dermatitis, *Pharmacoeconomics* 23(6) (2005) 543–66.

[20] T.E. Delea, M. Gokhale, C. Makin, M.A. Hussein, J. Vanderpoel, T. Sandman, J. Chang, J. Sung, P. Pinkston, D. Gause, et al., Administrative claims analysis of utilization and costs of care in health plan members with atopic dermatitis who had prior use of a topical corticosteroid and who initiate therapy with pimecrolimus or tacrolimus, *J Manag Care Pharm* 13(4) (2007) 349–59.

[21] B. Ehlken, M. Mohrenschlager, B. Kugland, K. Berger, K. Quednau, J. Ring, [Cost-of-illness study in patients suffering from atopic eczema in Germany], *Hautarzt* 56 (12) (2005) 1144–51.

[22] C.N. Ellis, L.A. Drake, M.M. Prendergast, W. Abramovits, M. Boguniewicz, C.R. Daniel, M. Lebwohl, S.R. Stevens, D.L. Whitaker-Worth, J.W. Cheng, et al., Cost of atopic dermatitis and eczema in the United States, *J Am Acad Dermatol* 46(3) (2002) 361–70.

[23] R.M. Emerson, H.C. Williams, B.R. Allen, What is the cost of atopic dermatitis in preschool children? *Br J Dermatol* 144(3) (2001) 514–22.

[24] C. Green, J.L. Colquitt, J. Kirby, P. Davidson, Topical corticosteroids for atopic eczema: clinical and cost effectiveness of once-daily vs. more frequent use, *Br J Dermatol* 152(1) (2005) 130–41.

[25] C. Green, J.L. Colquitt, J. Kirby, P. Davidson, E. Payne, Clinical and cost-effectiveness of once-daily versus more frequent use of same potency topical corticosteroids for atopic eczema: a systematic review and economic evaluation, *Health Technol Assess* 8(47) (2004) iii,iv, 1–120.

[26] N. Jenner, J. Campbell, R. Marks, Morbidity and cost of atopic eczema in Australia, *Australas J Dermatol* 45(1) (2004) 16–22.

[27] A.S. Kemp, Cost of illness of atopic dermatitis in children: a societal perspective, *Pharmacoeconomics* 21(2) (2003) 105–13.

[28] P. Verboom, L. Hakkaart-Van, M. Sturkenboom, R. De Zeeuw, H. Menke, F. Rutten, The cost of atopic dermatitis in the Netherlands: an international comparison, *Br J Dermatol* 147(4) (2002) 716–24.

[29] C.L. Carroll, R. Balkrishnan, S.R. Feldman, A.B. Fleischer, Jr., J.C. Manuel, The burden of atopic dermatitis: impact on the patient, family, and society, *Pediatr Dermatol* 22(3) (2005) 192–9.

[30] A.M. Drucker, A.R. Wang, W.-Q. Li, E. Sevetson, J.K. Block, A.A. Qureshi, The burden of atopic dermatitis: summary of a report for the National Eczema Association, *J Investig Dermatol* 137(1) (2017) 26–30.

[31] S. Shrestha, R. Miao, L. Wang, J. Chao, H. Yuce, W. Wei, Burden of atopic dermatitis in the United States: analysis of healthcare claims data in the commercial, *Medicare Medi Cal Databases Adv Ther* 34(8) (2017) 1989–2006.

[32] M.G. Filanovsky, S. Pootongkam, J.E. Tamburro, M.C. Smith, S.J. Ganocy, S.T. Nedorost, The financial and emotional impact of atopic dermatitis on children and their families, *J Pediatr* 169 (2016) 284–90.e5.

[33] S.L. Kulasingam, E.R. Myers, Potential health and economic impact of adding a human papillomavirus vaccine to screening programs, *Jama* 290(6) (2003) 781–9.

[34] N. Van de Velde, M. Brisson, M.C. Boily, Modeling human papillomavirus vaccine effectiveness: quantifying the impact of parameter uncertainty, *Am J Epidemiol* 165 (7) (2007) 762–75.

[35] M. Brisson, N. Van de Velde, P. De Wals, M.C. Boily, The potential cost-effectiveness of prophylactic human papillomavirus vaccines in Canada, *Vaccine* 25(29) (2007) 5399–408.

[36] C.B. Woodman, S.I. Collins, L.S. Young, The natural history of cervical HPV infection: unresolved issues, *Nat Rev Cancer* 7(1) (2007) 11–22.

[37] M. Adams, B. Jasani, A. Fiander, Human papilloma virus (HPV) prophylactic vaccination: challenges for public health and implications for screening, *Vaccine* 25(16) (2007) 3007–13.

[38] S.J. Goldie, M. Kohli, D. Grima, M.C. Weinstein, T.C. Wright, F.X. Bosch, E. Franco, Projected clinical benefits and cost-effectiveness of a human papillomavirus 16/18 vaccine, *J Natl Cancer Inst* 96(8) (2004) 604–15.

[39] G.D. Sanders, A.V. Taira, Cost-effectiveness of a potential vaccine for human papillomavirus, *Emerg Infect Dis* 9(1) (2003) 37–48.

[40] A.V. Taira, C.P. Neukermans, G.D. Sanders, Evaluating human papillomavirus vaccination programs, *Emerg Infect Dis* 10(11) (2004) 1915–23.

[41] World Health Organization, *Cervical Cancer*, 2018. www.who.int/cancer/preven tion/diagnosis-screening/cervical-cancer/en/. (Accessed December 31 2018).

[42] Guttmacher-Lancer Commission, *Guttmacher-Lancer Commission on Sexual and Reproductive Health and Rights*, 2018. www.guttmacher.org/infographic/2018/ number-deaths-worldwide-cervical-cancer-each-year. (Accessed December 31 2018).

[43] American Cancer Society, *Key Statistics about Cervical Cancer*, 2018. www.cancer. org/cancer/cervical-cancer/about/key-statistics.html. (Accessed December 31 2018).

[44] US National Institutes of Health/National Cancer Institute, *HPV and Cancer*, 2018. www.cancer.gov/about-cancer/causes-prevention/risk/infectious-agents/hpv-fact-sheet. (Accessed December 31 2018).

[45] R.P. Insinga, A.G. Glass, B.B. Rush, The health care costs of cervical human papillomavirus–related disease, *Am J Obstet Gynecol* 191(1) (2004) 114–20.

[46] R.J. Lipsy, Assessing the short-term and long-term burden of illness in cervical cancer, *Am J Manag Care* 14(6 Suppl 1) (2008) S177–84.

[47] Insinga RP, Dasbach EJ, Elbasha EH. 2005. Assessing the annual economic burden of preventing and treating anogenital human papillomavirus-related disease in the US: analytic framework and review of the literature. *Pharmacoeconomics*; 23(11):1107–22.

[48] H.W. Chesson, D.U. Ekwueme, M. Saraiya, M. Watson, D.R. Lowy, L.E. Markowitz, Estimates of the annual direct medical costs of the prevention and treatment of disease associated with human papillomavirus in the United States, *Vaccine* 30 (42) (2012) 6016–19.

[49] R.P. Insinga, Annual productivity costs due to cervical cancer mortality in the United States, *Womens Health Issues* 16(5) (2006) 236–42.

[50] G.J. Rodrigo, C. Rodrigo, J.B. Hall, Acute asthma in adults: a review, *Chest* 125(3) (2004) 1081–102.

[51] J.F. Donohue, N. Jain, Exhaled nitric oxide to predict corticosteroid responsiveness and reduce asthma exacerbation rates, *Respir Med* 107(7) (2013) 943–52.

[52] M. Essat, S. Harnan, T. Gomersall, P. Tappenden, R. Wong, I. Pavord, R. Lawson, M.L. Everard, Fractional exhaled nitric oxide for the management of asthma in adults: a systematic review, *Eur Respir J* 47(3) (2016) 751–68.

[53] H.L. Petsky, K.M. Kew, A.B. Chang, Exhaled nitric oxide levels to guide treatment for children with asthma, *Cochrane Database Syst Rev* 11 (2016) CD011439.

[54] H.L. Petsky, K.M. Kew, C. Turner, A.B. Chang, Exhaled nitric oxide levels to guide treatment for adults with asthma, *Cochrane Database Syst Rev* 9 (2016) CD011440.

[55] E.A. Brooks, M. Massanari, Cost-effectiveness analysis of monitoring fractional exhaled nitric oxide (FeNO) in the management of asthma, *Manag Care* 27(7) (2018) 42–8.

[56] International Classification of Diseases, Ninth Revision, Clinical Modification (ICD-9-CM).

[57] H.K. Reddel, D.R. Taylor, E.D. Bateman, L.P. Boulet, H.A. Boushey, W.W. Busse, T.B. Casale, P. Chanez, P.L. Enright, P.G. Gibson, et al, C. American Thoracic Society/European Respiratory Society Task Force on Asthma, Exacerbations, An official American Thoracic Society/European Respiratory Society statement: asthma control and exacerbations: standardizing endpoints for clinical asthma trials and clinical practice, *Am J Respir Crit Care Med* 180(1) (2009) 59–99.

[58] J.A. Delaney, S. Suissa, The case-crossover study design in pharmacoepidemiology, *Stat Methods Med Res* 18(1) (2009) 53–65.

[59] M. Sadatsafavi, L.D. Lynd, J.M. Fitzgerald, Post-hospital syndrome in adults with asthma: a case-crossover study, *Allergy Asthma Clin Immunol* 9(1) (2013) 49.

[60] R.G. Hart, L.A. Pearce, M.I. Aguilar, Adjusted-dose warfarin versus aspirin for preventing stroke in patients with atrial fibrillation, *Ann Intern Med* 147(8) (2007) 590–2.

[61] P.M. Barrett, R. Komatireddy, S. Haaser, S. Topol, J. Sheard, J. Encinas, A.J. Fought, E.J. Topol, Comparison of 24-hour Holter monitoring with 14-day novel adhesive patch electrocardiographic monitoring, *Am J Med* 127(1) (2014) 95. e11–17.

[62] M. Grond, M. Jauss, G. Hamann, E. Stark, R. Veltkamp, D. Nabavi, M. Horn, C. Weimar, M. Kohrmann, R. Wachter, et al., Improved detection of silent atrial fibrillation using 72-hour Holter ECG in patients with ischemic stroke: a prospective multicenter cohort study, *Stroke* 44(12) (2013) 3357–64.

[63] J.S. Healey, S.J. Connolly, M.R. Gold, C.W. Israel, I.C. Van Gelder, A. Capucci, C. P. Lau, E. Fain, S. Yang, C. Bailleul, et al., Subclinical atrial fibrillation and the risk of stroke, *N Engl J Med* 366(2) (2012) 120–9.

[64] S.Z. Rosero, V. Kutyifa, B. Olshansky, W. Zareba, Ambulatory ECG monitoring in atrial fibrillation management, *Prog Cardiovasc Dis* 56(2) (2013) 143–52.

[65] S.L. Higgins, A novel patch for heart rhythm monitoring: is the Holter monitor obsolete? *Future Cardiology* 9(3) (2013) 325–33.

[66] H.L. Kennedy, The evolution of ambulatory ECG monitoring, *Prog Cardiovasc Dis* 56(2) (2013) 127–32.

[67] P. Zimetbaum, A. Goldman, Ambulatory arrhythmia monitoring: choosing the right device, *Circulation* 122(16) (2010) 1629–36.

[68] E.B. Bass, E.I. Curtiss, V.C. Arena, B.H. Hanusa, A. Cecchetti, M. Karpf, W. N. Kapoor, The duration of Holter monitoring in patients with syncope. Is 24 hours enough? *Arch Intern Med* 150(5) (1990) 1073–8.

[69] S. Kinlay, J.W. Leitch, A. Neil, B.L. Chapman, D.B. Hardy, P.J. Fletcher, Cardiac event recorders yield more diagnoses and are more cost-effective than 48-hour Holter monitoring in patients with palpitations. A controlled clinical trial, *Ann Intern Med* 124(1 Pt 1) (1996) 16–20.

[70] M. Kuhne, B. Schaer, N. Moulay, C. Sticherling, S. Osswald, Holter monitoring for syncope: diagnostic yield in different patient groups and impact on device implantation, *QJM* 100(12) (2007) 771–7.

4 Markov Modeling in Decision Analysis

J. Robert Beck, M.D.
Fox Chase Cancer Center
Philadelphia, PA, USA

Elizabeth A. Handorf, Ph.D.
Fox Chase Cancer Center
Philadelphia, PA, USA

TABLE OF CONTENTS

4.1 INTRODUCTION

A pharmacoeconomic problem is tackled using a formal process that begins with constructing a mathematical model. In this book a number of pharmacoeconomic constructs are presented, ranging from spreadsheets to sophisticated numerical approximations to continuous compartment models. For nearly 50 years, the decision tree has been the most common and simplest formalism, comprising choices, chances, and outcomes. As discussed in Chapter 2, the modeler crafts a tree that represents near-term events within a population or cohort as structure and attempts to balance realism and attendant complexity with simplicity. In problems that lead to long-term differences in outcome, the decision model must have a definite time horizon, up to which the events are characterized explicitly. At the horizon, the future health of a cohort must be summed and averaged to "subsequent prognosis." For problems involving quantity and quality of life, where the future natural history is well characterized, techniques such as the declining exponential approximation of life expectancy [1, 2] or differential equations may be used to generate outcome measures. Life tables may be used directly or the results from clinical trials may be adopted to generate relevant values. Costs in decision trees are generally aggregated, collapsing substantial intrinsic variation into single monetary estimates.

Most pharmacoeconomic problems are less amenable to these summarizing techniques. In particular, clinical scenarios that involve a risk that is ongoing over time, competing risks that occur at different rates, or costs that need to be assessed incrementally lead to either rapidly branching decision trees or unrealistic pruning of possible outcomes for the sake of simplicity. In these cases, a more sophisticated mathematical model is employed to characterize the natural history of the problem and its treatment. This chapter explores the pharmacoeconomic modeling of cohorts using a relatively simple probabilistic characterization of natural history that can substitute for the outcome node of a decision tree. Beck and Pauker introduced the Markov process as a solution for the natural history modeling problem in 1983, building on their and others' work with stochastic models over the previous six years [3]. During the ensuing 36 years, over 2,000 articles have directly cited either this paper or a tutorial published a decade later [4], and over 6,000 records in PubMed can be retrieved using (Markov decision model) OR (Markov cost-effectiveness) as a search criterion. This chapter will define the Markov process model by its properties and illustrate its use in pharmacoeconomics by exploring a simplified example from the field of advanced prostate cancer [5].

4.2 THE MARKOV PROCESS AND TRANSITION PROBABILITIES

4.2.1 Stochastic Processes

A Markov process is a special type of stochastic model. A stochastic process is a mathematical system that evolves over time with some element of uncertainty. This contrasts with a deterministic system, in which the model and its parameters specify the outcomes completely. The simplest example of a stochastic process is coin flipping. If a fair coin is flipped a number of times and a record of the result kept (H="heads," T="tails"), a sequence such as THHTTHHHHTTHHHTHTHHTTHTTTTHTHTHH might arise. At each flip (or trial), either T or H would result with equal probability of one-half. Dice rolling is another example of this type of stochastic system, known as an independent trial experiment. Each flip or roll is independent of all that have come before, because dice and coins have no memory of prior results. Independent trials have been studied and described for nearly three centuries [6].

4.2.2 Markov Processes

The Markov process relaxes this assumption a bit. In a Markov model, the probability of a trial outcome varies depending on the current result (generally known as a "state"). Andrei Andreevich Markov, a Russian mathematician, originally characterized such processes in the first decade of the 20th century [7]. It is easy to see how this model works via a simple example. Consider a clerk who assigns case report forms to three reviewers: Larry, Maureen, and Nell. The clerk assigns charts to these readers using a peculiar method. If the last chart was given to Larry, the clerk assigns the current one to Larry with probability one-quarter, and to Maureen or Nell with equal probability of three-eighths. Maureen never gets two charts in a row; after Maureen, the clerk assigns the next chart to Larry with probability one-quarter and Nell three-quarters. After Nell gets a chart, the next chart goes to Larry with probability one-half, and Nell and Maureen each one-quarter. Thus, the last assignment (Larry, Maureen, or Nell) must be known to determine the probability of the current assignment.

4.2.2.1 Transition Probabilities

Table 4.1 shows this behavior as a matrix of *transition probabilities*. Each cell of Table 4.1 shows the probability of a chart being assigned to the reviewer named as column head if the last chart was assigned to the reviewer named as row head. An $n \times n$ matrix is a *probability matrix* if each row element is nonnegative and each row sums to 1. Since the row headings and column headings refer to states of the process, Table 4.1 is a special form of probability matrix: a transition probability matrix.

This stochastic model differs from independent trials because of the *Markov Property*: the distribution of the probability of future states of a stochastic process depends on the current state (and only on the current state, not the prior natural history). That is, one does not need to know what has happened with scheduling in the past, but only needs to know who was most recently assigned a chart. For example, if Larry got the last review, the next one will be assigned to any of the three readers with equal probability.

4.2.2.2 Working with a Transition Probability Matrix

The Markov property leads to some interesting results. What is the likelihood that, if Maureen is assigned a patient chart, that Maureen will get the patient chart after next? This can be calculated as follows:

TABLE 4.1

Chart Assignment Probability Table

Current	Next		
	Larry	**Maureen**	**Nell**
Larry	0.250	0.375	0.375
Maureen	0.250	0.000	0.750
Nell	0.500	0.250	0.250

After Maureen, the probability of Larry is one-quarter and Nell three-quarters. After Larry, the probability of Maureen is three-eighths, and after Nell it is one-quarter. So, the probability of Maureen–(anyone)–Maureen is (one-quarter × three-eighths) + (three-quarters × one-quarter), or 0.281. A complete table of probabilities at two assignments after a known one is shown in Table 4.2. This table is obtained using matrix multiplication, treating Table 4.1 as a 3 × 3 matrix and multiplying it by itself.[1] Note that the probability of Maureen going to Maureen in two steps is found in the corresponding cell of Table 4.2.

This process can be continued because Table 4.2 is also a probability matrix, in that the rows all sum to 1. In fact, after two more multiplications by Table 4.1, the matrix is represented by Table 4.3.

The probabilities in each row are converging, and by the seventh cycle, after a known assignment, the probability matrix is shown in Table 4.4. This is also a probability matrix, with all of the rows identical, and it has a straightforward interpretation. Seven or more charts after a known assignment, the probability that the next chart review would go to Larry is 0.353, to Maureen 0.235, and to Nell 0.412. Or, if someone observes the clerk at any random time, the likelihood of the next chart going to Larry is 0.353, and so on. This is the limiting Markov matrix, or the steady state of the process. Over time Larry would be issued 35.3% of the charts, Maureen fewer, and Nell somewhat more.

TABLE 4.2

Two-Step Markov Probabilities

Current	Chart After Next		
	Larry	Maureen	Nell
Larry	0.344	0.188	0.469
Maureen	0.438	0.281	0.251
Nell	0.313	0.250	0.438

TABLE 4.3

Assignment Model After Four Cycles

Current	After Four Cycles		
	Larry	Maureen	Nell
Larry	0.355	0.235	0.411
Maureen	0.352	0.237	0.411
Nell	0.352	0.235	0.413

1 Matrix multiplication can be reviewed in any elementary textbook of probability or finite mathematics, or at http://en.wikipedia.org/wiki/Matrix_multiplication.

TABLE 4.4

Steady-State or Limiting Markov Matrix

	Larry	Maureen	Nell
Larry	0.353	0.235	0.412
Maureen	0.353	0.235	0.412
Nell	0.353	0.235	0.412

4.2.3 ABSORBING MARKOV MODELS

The chart review example is known as a *regular* Markov chain. The transition probabilities are constant, and depend only on the state of the process. Any state can be reached from any other state, although not necessarily in one step (e.g., Maureen cannot be followed immediately by Maureen, but can in two or more cycles). Regular chains converge to a limiting set of probabilities. The other principal category of Markov models is *absorbing*. In these systems the process has a state that is possible to enter, in a finite set of moves, from any other state, but from which no movement is possible. Once the process enters the absorbing state, it terminates (i.e., stays in that state forever). The analogy with clinical decision models is obvious—an absorbing Markov model has a state equivalent to death in the clinical problem.

4.2.3.1 Behavior of the Absorbing Model

This is shown in Figure 4.1, a simplified three-state absorbing clinical Markov model. In a clinical model, the notion of time appears naturally. Assume that a clinical process is modeled where definitive disease progression is possible and that death often ensues from progressive disease. At any given month the patient may be in a Well state, shown in the upper left of Figure 4.1, the Sick state in the upper right, or Dead in the lower center. If in the Well state, the most likely result for the patient is that he/she would remain well for the ensuing month and next be still found in the Well state. Alternatively, the patient could become sick and enter the Progressive state or die and move to the Dead state. If in Progressive, the patient would most likely stay in that state, but could also die from the Progressive state, presumably at a higher probability than from the Well state. There is also a very small probability of returning to the Well state.

A possible transition probability matrix for this model is shown in Table 4.5. In the upper row, a Well patient remains so with probability 80%, has a 15% chance of having progressive disease over one cycle, and a 5% chance of dying in the cycle. A sick patient with progressive disease is shown with a 2% chance of returning to the Well state, a 28% chance of dying in one month, and the remainder (i.e., 70% chance) staying in the Progressive state. Of course, the Dead state is *absorbing*, reflected by a 100% chance of staying Dead.

Table 4.5 is a probability matrix, so it can be multiplied as in the prior example. After two cycles, the matrix is shown in Table 4.6. Thus, after two

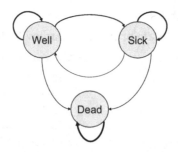

FIGURE 4.1   Simple Three-State Absorbing Markov Model.

TABLE 4.5

Transition Probability Matrix for Clinical Example

Current	Next		
	Well	**Progressive**	**Dead**
Well	0.80	0.15	0.05
Progressive	0.02	0.70	0.28
Dead	0.00	0.00	1.00

TABLE 4.6

Two-Cycle State Matrix for Clinical Example

	Well	**Progressive**	**Dead**
Well	0.643	0.225	0.132
Progressive	0.030	0.493	0.477
Dead	0.000	0.000	1.000

---

cycles of the Markov process, someone who started in the Well state has slightly less than a two-thirds chance of staying well, and a 22.5% chance of having Progressive disease. By the 10th cycle, the top row of the transition matrix is

Well	**Progressive**	**Dead**
0.124	0.126	0.750

So, someone starting well has a 75% chance of being dead within 10 cycles and, of the remaining 25%, roughly an even chance of being well or having Progressive disease. This matrix converges slowly because of the moderate

probability of death in any one cycle, but eventually this matrix would end up
as a set of rows:

$$0 \qquad\qquad 0 \qquad\qquad 1$$

Everyone in this process eventually dies.

Clinical Markov models offer interesting insights into the natural history of
a process. If the top row of the transition matrix is taken at each cycle and
graphed, Figure 4.2 results. This graph can be interpreted as the fate of a cohort
of patients beginning together at Well. The membership of the Well state
decreases rapidly, as the forward transitions to Progressive and Dead overwhelm
the back transition from Progressive to Well. The Progressive state grows at first,
as it collects patients transitioning from Well, but soon the transitions to Dead,
which, of course, are permanent, cause the state to lose members. The Progressive
state peaks at Cycle 4, with 25.6% of the cohort. The Dead state actually is
a sigmoid (S-shaped) curve, rising moderately for a few cycles because most
people are Well, but as soon as the 28% mortality from the Progressive state
takes effect, the curve gets steeper. Finally, it flattens, as few people remain alive.
This graph is typical of absorbing Markov process models.

4.2.3.2   Use of Absorbing Markov Models in Clinical Decision Analysis

The Markov formalism can substitute for an outcome in a typical decision tree.
The simplest outcome structure is life expectancy. This has a natural expression
in a Markov cohort model: life expectancy is a summed experience of the
cohort over time. If we assign credit for being in a state at the end of a cycle, the
value of each state function in Figure 4.2 represents the probability of being

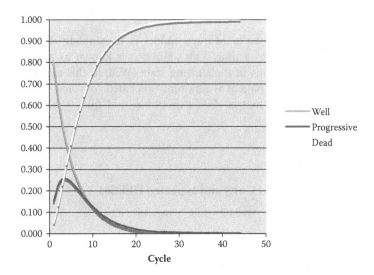

FIGURE 4.2   Absorbing Markov chain natural history.

alive in that state in that cycle. At the start of the process, all members of the cohort are in the Well state. At Cycle One (Table 4.5), 80% are still Well and 15% have progressive disease, so the cohort would have experienced 0.8 average cycles Well, and 0.15 cycles in Progressive disease. At Cycle Two (Table 4.6), 64.3% are Well and 22.5% have Progressive disease. Thus, after two cycles, the cohort experience is 0.8 + 0.643, or 1.443 cycles Well and 0.15 + 0.225, or 0.375 cycles in Progressive disease. Summing the process over 45 cycles, until all are in the Dead state, the results are 4.262 cycles Well and 2.630 cycles in Progressive. So, the life expectancy of this cohort, transitioning according to the probability matrix in Table 4.5, is 6.892 cycles, roughly 2:1 in Well versus Progressive disease. Refinements to this approach, involving correction for initial state membership, can be found in Sonnenberg and Beck [4].

Whereas a traditional outcome node is assigned a value, or in Chapters 2, 7, 8, 10, and 12, a *utility*, the Markov model is used to calculate the value by summing adjusted cohort membership. For this to work, each Markov state is assigned an incremental utility for being in that state for one model cycle. In the example above, the Well state might be given a value of 1, the Progressive state a value of 0.7. That is, the utility for being in the Progressive state is 70% of the value of the Well state for each cycle in it. In most models Dead is worth 0. Incremental costs can also be applied for Markov cost-effectiveness or cost-utility analysis. For this tutorial example, assume the costs of being in the Well state are $5,000 per cycle, and in the Progressive state $8,000 per cycle. Summing the cohort over 45 cycles leads to the results in Table 4.7. In the second column, the overall cost in the Well state is calculated as 4.262 × $5,000, or $21,311. At $8,000 per cycle in the Progressive state the total cost in this state is $21,043. Thus, in this tutorial example, the cohort can expect to survive 6.892 cycles, or 6.103 quality-adjusted cycles, for a total cost of over $42,000. These values would substitute for the outcomes at the terminal node of a decision tree model, and could be used for decision or cost-utility analysis.

An alternative way to use a Markov model is to simulate the behavior of a cohort of patients, one at a time. This approach is known as a Monte Carlo analysis. Each patient begins in the starting state (Well, in this example) and, at the end of each cycle, the patient is randomly allocated to a new state based on the transition probability matrix. Life expectancy and quality adjustments are

TABLE 4.7

Markov Cohort Costs and Expected Utilities

	Well ($Q = 1.0$)	Progressive ($Q = 0.7$)	Total
Expected cycles	4.262	2.630	6.892
Quality-adjusted	4.262	1.841	6.103
Cost/cycle	$5,000	$8,000	
Total costs	$21,311	$21,043	$42,354

handled as in the cohort solution. When the patient enters the Dead state, the simulation terminates and a new patient is queued. This process is repeated a large number of times, and a distribution of survival, quality-adjusted survival, and costs results. Modern approaches to Monte Carlo analysis incorporate probability distributions on the transition probabilities, to enable statistical measures like mean and variance to be determined [8].

Two enhancements to the Markov model render the formalism more realistic for clinical studies; both involve adding a time element. First, although the Markov property requires no memory of prior states, it is possible to superimpose a time function on a transition probability. The most obvious example of this is the risk of death, which rises over time regardless of other clinical conditions. This can be handled in a Markov model by modifying the transition probability to death using a function: in the tutorial example, time could be incorporated as p (Well->Dead) = 0.05 + G(age), where G represents the Gompertz mortality function [9] or another well-characterized actuarial model.

Second, standard practice in decision modeling discounts future costs and benefits to incorporate risk aversion and the decreasing value of assets and events in the future. Discounting (see Chapter 11) may be incorporated in Markov models as simply another function that can modify (i.e., reduce) the state-dependent incremental utilities.

4.3 MARKOV MODEL EXAMPLE: ADVANCED PROSTATE CANCER

Figure 4.3 depicts a simplified model of the treatment of hormone-naive advanced prostate cancer with abiraterone acetate (AA). This model and its attendant data are drawn from Ramamurthy et al.'s study of the costs and projected benefits of AA versus docetaxel in the treatment of this malignancy, to which the reader is referred for the complete model and cost-effectiveness analysis [5]. For this chapter, the model and data are simplified in favor of didactic value.

In Figure 4.3, states are represented for Stable on AA (denoted AA-Stable in the figure), AA with the side effect of fatigue (AA-Fatigue), progressive disease (PD), and Death (Dead). For clarity, arrows from states to themselves have not been drawn. The figure thus depicts the principal transitions in the model. The largest state-to-state transition is from progressive disease to death. Table 4.8 contains the initial monthly cycle transition probability matrix for a 68-year-old man (the median age in the clinical trials on which the model is based). This table is calculated from baseline estimates given by Ramamurthy et al.

Note that from AA-Stable, the most likely result after one month is to stay in AA-Stable, but there is a little greater than 2% chance of transitioning to PD. Additionally, there is a 0.3% chance of developing fatigue within the first six months of treatment, which would decrease quality of life for up to a year. A time-dependent general population risk of death must also be added to the model. At 68 years of age, the annual risk of death is 1.83%, rising over time according to the Gompertz exponential function. At 84, the risk of death is 10%. Table 4.9 shows the experience over 12 monthly cycles of 10,000 men aged

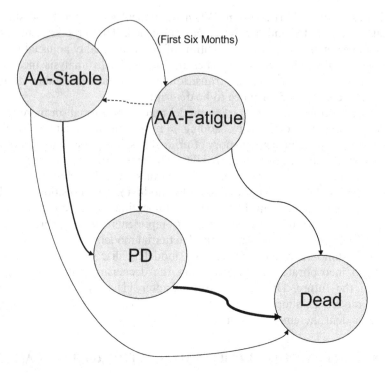

FIGURE 4.3 Principal transitions in prostate cancer model. Transitions to same state (e.g., Well–Well) are not shown.

TABLE 4.8

Transition Probability Matrix for the Prostate Cancer Model

	AA-Stable	AA-Fatigue	PD	Dead
AA-Stable	0.9746	0.0030	0.0208	0.0016
AA-Fatigue	0	0.9776	0.0208	0.0016
PD		0	0.9795	0.0205
Dead			0	1

68, treated with AA, according to the Markov model with the rising general death rate. In one month, 254 men have transitioned out of the AA-Stable state, with the greatest fraction to PD. The number of men in AA-Fatigue rises over the first six months of treatment, and then decreases as no more are added to this state and patients recover from treatment-induced fatigue. The number of men in PD rises each month, but as fewer men are on AA treatment with each passing month, the increase lessens with each month. In fact, after 32 monthly

TABLE 4.9

Expected State Membership of Markov Cohort Over 12 Monthly Cycles

Month	AA-Stable	AA-Fatigue	PD	Dead
0	10,000	0	0	0
1	9,746	30	208	16
2	9,498	59	407	36
3	9,257	86	598	60
4	9,022	112	780	87
5	8,793	136	954	117
6	8,570	159	1,120	151
7	8,393	140	1,278	188
8	8,219	123	1,430	228
9	8,047	109	1,574	271
10	7,877	96	1,711	316
11	7,710	84	1,842	364
12	7,546	74	1,966	414

cycles (not shown), the number of men in the PD state peaks, then begins to decline as death due to progressive cancer and the general population mortality takes a greater toll.

Over an expected lifetime, the Markov model yields a membership of each state as shown in Figure 4.4. The AA-Stable cohort declines steadily as men transition to one of the other model states, and back transitions from AA-Fatigue are never significant. AA-Fatigue rises over the first six months of the model, then declines to zero by Month 18. PD rises steadily to Month 32, and then falls slowly as patients die from their disease. The Dead state shows a typical sigmoid function, as initially few die, then the rate increases as more men reach PD, and then the rate slows as fewer men remain alive.

Baseline results from this model are presented in Table 4.10. Averaged over a cohort, the patient with advanced prostate cancer treated with AA can expect to live 32.9 months with stable disease. The overall 2% risk of fatigue, averaged across the entire cohort, adds 0.2 months per man in AA-Fatigue. A further 19.5 months are expected in PD, for an overall life expectancy of 52.6 months. Of course, no single patient has precisely this experience.

Sensitivity analysis (see Chapter 13) can be conducted on Markov transition probabilities, and modern software easily supports this. An Appendix to this chapter provides R code developed by the authors that can be used to replicate the model over the initial five years, and can be adapted to change parameters for sensitivity analysis or extend the model time [10].

Ramamurthy et al.'s more complete Markov formulation incorporates quality adjustments and a cost model, and is truncated to five years based on the

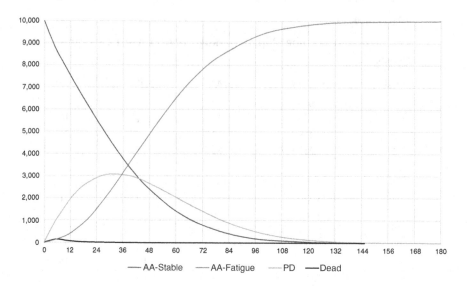

FIGURE 4.4   Natural history of prostate cancer example.

TABLE 4.10

Expected Results of Abiraterone Treatment Model

	AA-Stable	AA-Fatigue	PD	Total
Expected months	32.9	0.2	19.5	52.6

---

clinical trial results. Later chapters in this book will illustrate how costs and structural interventions can modify Markov and other stochastic models to generate sophisticated analyses of pharmacoeconomic problems.

4.3.1   SOFTWARE IMPLEMENTATION

The modeler has a choice of different types of software to run a Markov model. TreeAge Pro is a specialized program for decision analysis with a full graphical user interface, where models are set up via "point-and-click" options. This interface makes it easy to work with, but the proprietary software limits transparency. It also may be challenging to set up especially complex models via a graphical interface, and model specifications are limited to the options available in the software [11]. Alternatively, the modeler could use a general purpose programming language to implement the model. Here we focus on R (R Foundation for Statistical Computing), but many other programming languages could be used, including MATLAB (The Math Works Inc.), Python, and SAS

(SAS Software). R is a freely available, open source statistical programming language, with a large library of user-contributed packages written for many types of analyses. If models are implemented with clear and well-documented code, using open source programming languages can improve reproducibility and transparency, making it easier for modelers to share and fully understand one another's work [11–13]. Modelers can also borrow functionality from other packages, giving greater flexibility than what is available from specialized software. These advantages have led to an increase in the popularity of R for health economic evaluations [13]. One drawback of R is the learning curve for users unfamiliar with the language, especially for those with limited programming experience. Also, due to the nature of the user-contributed code libraries, there may be syntax differences between packages, and the amount of detail in the documentation and example code can vary, making some libraries easier to use than others.

Several R libraries contain useful implementations of Markov models, and more may be added in the future. The heemod (Health Economics Evaluation Modelling) package is particularly convenient, as it was specifically designed for cost-effectiveness analysis. We used this library to run our example (code available online at https://github.com/BethHandorf/Pharmacoeconomics-Mar kovModels). Other libraries for discrete-time Markov models are CTMCPack and markovchain. For a more thorough discussion on using R software for health economic decision modeling, see Jalal et al. [13].

ACKNOWLEDGMENT

Some of the didactic material concerning regular and absorbing Markov chains has been adapted from "Markov Models (Introduction, Markov Property, Absorbing States)," an entry in Kattan MW, Cowen ME (eds.) *Encyclopedia of Medical Decision Making*, Sage Publications, Thousand Oaks CA, 2009; DOI: http://dx.doi.org/10.4135/9781412971980.n209

REFERENCES

[1] J.R. Beck, J.P. Kassirer, S.G. Pauker, A convenient approximation of life expectancy (the "DEALE"). I. Evaluation of the method. *The American Journal of Medicine* 73(6) (1982) 883–888.

[2] J.R. Beck, S.G. Pauker, J.E. Gottlieb, K. Klein, J.P. Kassirer, A convenient approximation of life expectancy (the "DEALE"). II. Use in medical decision making.. *The American Journal of Medicine* 73(6) (1982) 889–897.

[3] J.R. Beck, S.G. Pauker, The Markov Process in medical prognosis. *Medical Decision Making* 3(4) (1983) 419–458.

[4] F.A. Sonnenberg, J.R. Beck, Markov models in medical decision making. *Medical Decision Making* 13(4) (1993) 322–338.

[5] C. Ramamurthy, E.A. Handorf, A.F. Correa, J.R. Beck, D.M. Geynisman, Cost-effectiveness of abiraterone versus docetaxel in the treatment of metastatic hormone naïve prostate cancer. *Urologic Oncology: Seminars and Original Investigations* 37 (10) (2019) 688–695.

[6] J. Bernoulli, Ars conjectandi, opus posthumum: Accedit tractatus de seriebus infinitis, et epistola Gallice scripta de ludo pilæ reticularis, Basileae, 1713, Ch. 1–4 trans.

Bu Sung B. Technical Report No. 2, Dept. of Statistics, Harvard University, 1966, The Hong Kong University of Science and Technology Library, 1966.

[7] G.P. Basharin, A.N. Langville, V.A. Naumov, The life and work of A.A. *Markov, Linear Algebra and Its Applications* 386 (2004) 3–26.

[8] A. Briggs, M. Sculpher, An introduction to Markov modelling for economic evaluation. *PharmacoEconomics* 13(4) (1998) 397–409.

[9] B. Gompertz, XXIV. On the nature of the function expressive of the law of human mortality, and on a new mode of determining the value of life contingencies. In a letter to Francis Baily, Esq. F. R. S. &c. *Philosophical Transactions of the Royal Society of London* 115 (1825) 513–583.

[10] A. Filipovic-Pierucci, K. Zarca, I. Durand-Zaleski, Markov models for health economic evaluation modelling in R with the Heemod Package. *Value in Health* 19(7) (2016) A369.

[11] C. Hollman, M. Paulden, P. Pechlivanoglou, C. McCabe, A comparison of four software programs for implementing decision analytic cost-effectiveness models. *PharmacoEconomics* 35(8) (2017) 817–830.

[12] F. Alarid-Escudero, E.M. Krijkamp, P. Pechlivanoglou, H. Jalal, S.-Y.Z. Kao, A. Yang, E.A. Enns, A need for change! A coding framework for improving transparency in decision modeling. *PharmacoEconomics* 37(11) (2019) 1329–1339.

[13] H. Jalal, P. Pechlivanoglou, E. Krijkamp, F. Alarid-Escudero, E. Enns, M.G. M. Hunink, An overview of R in health decision sciences. *Medical Decision Making* 37(7) (2017) 735–746.

APPENDIX   SAMPLE R CODE FOR PROSTATE CANCER PROBLEM.

```
#################################################
# Example Markov model for first-line treatment of metastatic prostate cancer
# Adapted from Abiraterone Acetate (AA) strategy described in:
#   Ramamurthy C, Handorf EA, Correa AF, Beck JR, Geynisman DM.
#   Cost-effectiveness of abiraterone versus docetaxel in the treatment of metastatic
#   hormone naïve prostate cancer. Urologic Oncology: Seminars and Original
Investigations
# 2019 Oct 1 (Vol. 37, No. 10, pp. 688–695). Elsevier.

library(heemod)

###### Set probabilities
par_mod <- define_parameters(
  Pr_SD_to_PD = 0.0208, # Monthly probability of progression from stable disease
            # (estimated from LATITUDE trial results)
  Pr_SD_to_Death = 0.00164, # Monthly probability of death from progression
                  # (SSA actuarial life tables - 68 y/o male probability of death 2016)
  Pr_PD_to_Death = 0.0205, # Monthly probability of death from progression
                  # (estimated from MAINSAIL trial results)
  Pr_FAT = 0.003, # Probability of fatigue in first 6 months
            # (estimated from LATITUDE trial results)
  Pr_SD_to_SDFAT = ifelse(model_time≤6, 0.003, 0),
            # After 6 months, assume zero probability of fatigue
```

```
  Pr_SDFat_to_SD = ifelse(model_time>6, .1, 0)
          # After 6 months, 10% per month back transition to SD
)


###### Define transition matrix

#Possible states:
#1) SD: M1 disease (no progression)
#2) SD_FAT: No progression, fatigue
#3) PD: Progressed disease
#4) Death

matAA<-define_transition(
  state_names=c("SD","SD_FAT","PD","Death"),
  C, Pr_SD_to_SDFAT, Pr_SD_to_PD, Pr_SD_to_Death, #SD
  PR_SDFAT_to_SD, C,        Pr_SD_to_PD, Pr_SD_to_Death, #SD_FAT
  0, 0,             C, Pr_PD_to_Death, #PD
  0, 0,             0, C        #Death
)


###### Define states, assign value

    # Costs, QALYs accrued per cycle in each state would be added here
    # for full cost-effectiveness analysis

state_SD<-define_state(
  SurvMo = 1
)
state_SD_FAT<-define_state(
  SurvMo = 1
)
state_PD<-define_state(
  SurvMo = 1
)
state_Death<-define_state(
  SurvMo = 0
)


###### Set up AA stragegy

strat_AA <-define_strategy(
  transition=matAA,

  SD = state_SD,
  SD_FAT = state_SD_FAT,
  PD = state_PD,
  Death = state_Death
)
```

```
###### Run the model
res_mod <- run_model(
 parameters=par_mod,
 AA=strat_AA, # Only 1 strategy considered here
 cycles=60,    # 5 years, 1 month cycles
 effect=SurvMo, # Effect in months of life
 method="life-table"
)

#Plots of state counts by markov cycle
plot1<-plot(res_mod, type="counts", panel="by_state",free_y=TRUE)
#Re-order the facets of the graph
plot1[["data"]]$state_names<-factor(plot1[["data"]]$state_names,levels=c
("SD","SD_FAT","PD","Death"))
print(plot1)
```

5 Retrospective Database Analysis

Renée J.G. Arnold, PharmD, RPh
Icahn School of Medicine at Mount Sinai
Arnold Consultancy & Technology, LLC
New York, NY, USA

Sanjeev Balu, PhD
Novartis Pharmaceuticals Corporation
East Hanover, NJ, USA

TABLE OF CONTENTS

5.1 INTRODUCTION

Retrospective databases, whether created de novo from pre-existing sources, such as patients' written charts, or from pre-existing electronic data sets, such as medical and pharmacy claims databases, electronic medical records (EMRs), national insurance administrative data, hospital medical records, disease-specific patient registries, or via patient and provider survey data, are a rich source of data for pharmacoeconomic analyses [1–5]. A listing of some population-based data sources (Table 5.1) and data sources available commercially or from the US government (Table 5.2) is provided. In addition to health economic analyses, the data collected from these

TABLE 5.1

Databases Available for Retrospective Analyses

Database Name	Inpatient Data	Outpatient Data	Advantage(s)	Limitation(s)
			Claims	
IQVIA Real-World Data Adjudicated Claims (PharMetrics Plus) and Hospital Charge data Master Databases	√ (limited)	√	Large database. Potentially more generalizable. Single-record layout (rather than multiple databases), multiple linkages (including to lab data for a portion of the data set)	Limited hospital drug data, cost
General Practice Research Database (GPRD)/Clinical Practice Research Datalink[1]	√ (very limited)	√ (in UK)	Comprehensive outpatient data, available online	UK only. Limited inpatient, only available to academic institutions
THIN	√ (very limited)	√ (in UK)	Extension of GPRD/CPRD, available commercially	UK only. Extension of GPRD/CPRD
			Claims + Hospital	
Geisinger	√	√	Comprehensive inpatient and outpatient/lab data. Information on all payer types	Regional (rural Pennsylvania). takes approximately 16–20 weeks to obtain data
Medicare 5% data sets	√	√	Inpatient and outpatient data	Patients ≥65 years old, Limited Data Sets (LDS) files available quarterly to qualified researchers (does not include medications); Research identifiable files or RIFs (include medications) only available to academic institutions; more costly recently
IBM MarketScan Hospital/drug	√	√	Hospital drug information	Unsure about viability of linking inpatient and outpatient data. Limited data licensing to independent third party.
Premier	√	√	Comprehensive	Cost/exclusivity
			Hospital only	
Cerner	√	√ (limited)	Comprehensive inpatient/ICU LOS/labs	Limited outpatient

(Continued)

TABLE 5.1 (Cont.)

Database Name	Inpatient Data	Outpatient Data	Advantage(s)	Limitation(s)
Premier	√	√ (very limited)	Comprehensive inpatient/ICU LOS	Very limited outpatient
Optum Research Data	√	√ (limited)	Large cohort of Medicare beneficiaries	Standardized financials, high cost

[1] Not really claims, since payer is NHS, but outpatient data.

data sets can be used for outcomes research (such as analysis of healthcare practice patterns, epidemiologic analysis of disease progression, prevalence, and characteristics of patient populations), evaluation of populations for prediction of future events, for formulary evaluation and to supplement prospective data sets, among other activities. When evidence is not available for a decision that is imminent, analyses utilizing retrospective databases can provide decision support that is real-time, relevant, and comprehensive, provided that precautions are taken to address statistical considerations that may be inherent in these data sources. Indeed, several studies have found that treatment effects in observational studies were neither quantitatively nor qualitatively different from those obtained in "well-designed" randomized controlled trials (RCTs) [6, 7]. Advantages of retrospective analyses in comparison to, for example, RCTs, include the fact that they are relatively inexpensive, quickly done, reflective of different populations, encompass a realistic time frame, organizationally specific, can be used for benchmarking purposes, include large sample sizes, and can capture real-world prescribing patterns [1–4, 8].

5.2 CLAIMS AND MEDICATION DATABASES

Healthcare administrative claims data, generally developed and maintained by third-party payers, offer a convenient and unique approach to studying healthcare resource utilization and associated cost. These databases represent a convenient alternative because data already are collected and stored electronically by health insurance companies. Claims data include outpatient, inpatient, and emergency room services, along with cost of outpatient prescription drugs. Computerized health insurance claims databases are maintained largely for billing and administrative purposes. Unlike studies with primary data collection, claims data are not collected to meet specific research objectives. Nevertheless, these databases are useful for describing healthcare utilization, patterns of care, disease prevalence, drug and disease outcomes, medication adherence, and cost of care. Administrative claims data are thus an important source of information about major processes of care.

Administrative claims databases tend to be highly representative of a large, defined population. Large sample sizes permit enhanced precision and are particularly useful for studying rare events. As the data already are collected and computerized, data analysis is inexpensive, particularly in relation to prospective studies. Claims data also include outpatient drug information for patients younger than 65 years and, in some instances, for patients aged 65 years or

TABLE 5.2

US Survey Databases

Data Set	Description	Comment	Patient-level data	Cost Data	Source	Media	Most Recent Year Available	Basis for Release of Data
		National Center for Health Statistics						
National Health Care Survey (NHCS)	• National Ambulatory Medical Care Survey (NAMCS)	Statistical support re: adequate sample size; extrapolation to US	No - encounter data	No	Providers	Internet for NAMCS, NHAMCS	2014	Annual
	• National Hospital Ambulatory Medical Care Survey (NHAMCS)						2014	
	• National Hospital Discharge Survey (NHDS[1])					CD and down-load-able (FTP) for NHDS	2010	
	• National Nursing Home Survey (NNHS)	listing of nursing homes, residen-tial care facilities,					2004	
	• National Health Provider Inventory[2]	hospices, and home health					2004	
	• National Home and Hospice Care Survey	agencies					2007	
National Health Interview Survey (NHIS)	• Nationwide survey by US Bureau of Census	• Productivity data • Modified ICD-9/ICD-10	Yes	No	Patients	CD	2020	Annual

Agency for Healthcare Research and Quality (AHRQ[3])

Medical Expenditure Panel Survey[4] (MEPS)	• Series of surveys of healthcare utilization and costs last conducted in 2019	• Modified ICD-9 codes (CCS[5])/ICD-10	Yes	Yes	Patients	CD, diskette, Internet	2020	Longitudinal, roughly every 2 yrs
Healthcare Cost & Utilization Project (HCUP)	• 20% sample of US community hospitals • 1997-2016	• Inpatient data only • Uses nonspecific CCS codes	Yes	Yes	Hospitals	CD	2016	Periodically

[1] Now also includes National Survey of Ambulatory Surgery (NSAS).
[2] Also includes National Employer Health Insurance Survey (NEHIS).
[3] Formerly Agency for Health Care Policy and Research (AHCPR).
[4] Formerly National Medical Expenditure Survey (NMES).
[5] Clinical Classification Software; condenses >12,000 ICD-9-CM codes into 260 categories.

older. This is very useful for studying drug outcomes and drug safety. An added benefit of using claims data is that it precludes any imposition on the patient, physician, or other provider.

As previously stated, the most important benefit of using claims databases to analyze clinical and economic outcomes is ease and convenience. The need to examine clinical, economic, and humanistic outcomes usually is limited by practical considerations, such as financial and time constraints, as well as concerns about patient privacy. Given these practical realities, the use of a claims database for some or all data collection offers an attractive alternative. Claims databases offer many important advantages for conducting health outcomes research. As mentioned, unlike RCTs, they reflect routine clinical "real world" practice. RCTs include carefully selected populations of particular ages and disease severities with few or no comorbidities. In addition, the procedures and protocols in RCTs are not often representative of routine clinical care. Moreover, patient compliance typically is greater in RCTs than in the "real world" because of the support services available to treat adverse effects and the tendency of RCT participants to be more compliant than the population at large. For example, although guideline-recommended therapies reduce major adverse cardiovascular events (MACE) in patients after myocardial infarction (MI) or those with atherosclerotic disease (ATH), adherence is poor. Bansilal and colleagues used a large managed care organization (MCO) database to determine the association between medication adherence levels and long-term MACE in these patients [9]. The primary outcome measure was a composite of all-cause death, MI, stroke, or coronary revascularization. Using proportion of days covered for statins and angiotensin-converting enzyme inhibitors, patients were stratified as fully adherent ($\geq 80\%$), partially adherent ($\geq 40\%$ to $\leq 79\%$), or nonadherent ($<40\%$). Per-patient annual direct medical (ADM) costs were estimated by using unit costs from two national files. Data were analyzed for 4,015 post-MI patients and 12,976 patients with ATH. In the post-MI cohort, the fully adherent group had a significantly lower rate of MACE than the nonadherent (18.9% vs. 26.3%; hazard ratio [HR]: 0.73; $p = 0.0004$) and partially adherent (18.9% vs. 24.7%; HR: 0.81; $p = 0.02$) groups at 2 years. The fully adherent group had reduced per-patient ADM costs for MI hospitalizations of $369 and $440 compared with the partially adherent and non-adherent groups, respectively. In the ATH cohort, the fully adherent group had a significantly lower rate of MACE than the nonadherent (8.42% vs. 17.17%; HR: 0.56; $p < 0.0001$) and the partially adherent (8.42% vs. 12.18%; HR: 0.76; $p < 0.0001$) groups at 2 years. The fully adherent group had reduced per-patient ADM costs for MI hospitalizations of $371 and $907 compared with the partially adherent and nonadherent groups, respectively.

Claims databases allow for the measurement of clinical and economic outcomes (e.g., hospital and emergency room visits) and provide a timely means of analyzing a problem. Answers can be found in days or weeks, rather than months or years. Finally, databases offer a great deal of flexibility. Rare diseases or specific subpopulations can be researched or a problem can be approached in a number of different ways.

Beyond such high-level outcome measures, the availability of the diagnosis, procedure, and revenue codes allow for further specification of a patient's outcome. ICD-10-CM codes provide diagnostic information allowing for identification of patients with a particular diagnosis or combination of diagnoses. *Physicians' Current Procedural Terminology*, 4th Edition (CPT-4 codes) identifies procedures that are used to bill physician and other professional services. For example, CPT-4 codes could be used to determine whether a depressed patient received hypnotherapy. The Healthcare Common Procedure Coding System (HCPCS) [10] can be used to provide further information on physician and nonphysician services that are not included in the CPT-4, such as whether a patient obtaining care in a physician's office for asthma received an injection of epinephrine.

The processes of care also can be assessed from a claims database. For example, the number of outpatient physician visits might be considered a good measure of the quality of care received by hypertension patients. Procedure codes allow for the measurement of additional processes of care such as whether atrial fibrillation patients are receiving annual electrocardiograms or electrical cardioversion. A typical example of using medical databases for human papillomavirus (HPV) vaccine-associated studies would be to obtain a preliminary estimate of the burden of cervical cancer within a particular region. One such study by Watson et al. [11] used multiple databases to estimate the burden of cervical cancer in the United States. This study used data from two federal cancer surveillance programs, the Centers for Disease Control and Prevention (CDC)'s National Program of Cancer Registries and the National Cancer Institute's Surveillance, Epidemiology, and End Results (SEER) Program to estimate cervical cancer incidence among different subpopulations. Identification of the study patients through diagnosis codes obtained in medical databases, incidence and prevalence rates among different age populations, race and gender mix, and across various geographical regions [12] can be easily accomplished through such databases. Another example would be a study examining the cervical cancer incidence before the HPV vaccine was introduced in the United States market [13]. Patients who are or are not provided HPV vaccines for prevention of certain cancers could also be studied to evaluate the incidence of future complications and associated total healthcare costs through most medical databases that provide clinical and economic data. Important examples include co-payment amount, formulary coverage of specific drugs, prescription quantity limits, and limits on mental health benefits. However, most measures of the structure of care are not found in the database itself but within the patient benefit manual or other records held by the MCO.

Although databases offer many advantages for conducting outcomes management, they have some limitations. They may be affected by certain biases that may compromise the internal validity and, thereby, the robustness of the data (see Section 5.7). It is widely recognized that the diagnosis found in databases is not always valid or reliable. While some overcoding or upcoding does occur, in most cases undercoding of actual diagnoses is more common. Undercoding is an even bigger problem with chronic diseases, which are notoriously underreported [14, 15]. The principal finding in the Kern study was that identification of veteran diabetes patients with comorbid chronic kidney disease with a low glomerular filtration rate was severely underreported in Medicare administrative records [15]. Similarly, the Icen study found misclassification of patients diagnosed with psoriasis [14]. Several potential reasons for this misclassification would include the psoriasis diagnosis being differential (rather than actual) in initial and follow-up physician visits, incorrect initial diagnosis followed by actual psoriasis treatment, and the use of a psoriasis code that does not specify the type of psoriasis [14]. Given these limitations, it is helpful to know for which disease states the coding is insufficient, calling for a review of the medical record. Unfortunately, there is no published research to provide guidance on this issue.

Another important consideration is the severity of illness in patients. The goal often is to compare the outcomes of care for persons receiving different treatments or receiving care from different types of providers. Zhao et al. [16] used a claims database to analyze the prevalence of diabetes-associated complications and comorbidities and its impact on healthcare costs among patients with diabetic neuropathy. This study identified the various complications and comorbidities through diagnosis codes and healthcare costs in the claims data. However, there may be important differences in the patients being compared that cannot be measured or controlled when using the information in the database. Other significant indicators of a patient's disease severity, including smoking or alcohol consumption status, laboratory values, and results of other diagnostic tests, are sometimes not available for analysis in the database. Pharmacy use described in the claims databases usually provides information about prescription medications. However, over-the-counter medications that are being used are generally not captured in such databases.

5.2.1 Description of Claims Database Files

Medication or claims databases usually have several files that characterize different patient settings where care is provided. These include, among others, inpatient, outpatient, emergency room, and pharmacy (medication) files. The outpatient file, for example, contains final action claims data submitted by institutional outpatient providers. Outpatient claims provide detailed information on the date of service, site of service (e.g., home care, physician office), provider specialty, type of service, and reimbursed charges. These variables allow us to calculate the frequency of healthcare utilization and its respective cost. Among several variables listed in outpatient files are date of service, amount billed, amount paid, and provider information. Each outpatient visit record in the outpatient file usually includes the following information: date of visit, whether the respondent/patient saw a physician, type of care received, type of services received, medicines prescribed, flat-fee information, imputed sources of payment, total payment, and total charge, among others.

Similarly, claims data for hospitalizations can be an extremely valuable source for evaluating health outcomes in terms of incidence and frequency of hospitalization episodes, severity of the hospitalization episode in terms of length of stay, and hospitalization costs. Inpatient claims data are also useful to assess the hospitalization costs associated with a condition or disease in a population. For each claim during a hospitalization episode, the file contains fields such as patient identification number, provider number, ICD-10 diagnosis code for which service was provided, CPT code for procedures and services provided, Diagnosis-Related Group (DRG) codes, date of hospital admission, date of discharge, location of service (outpatient, emergency room, or inpatient), total amount billed, and total amount paid.

The prescription drug file in a claims data set contains useful information on medications prescribed and taken by patients. Information is captured when the patient fills the prescription and a claim is then filed by the pharmacy. Importantly, the primary focus of the claim is the fill transaction; claims will show the activity of when the fills occur, but they will not show whether the patient actually took the medications. Thus, while claims serve as a proxy for compliance and adherence due to their ability to show fills, primary research may be used as an adjunct to determine if the patient actually used the medications when at home. Each record in the prescription drug file represents one reported prescribed medicine that was purchased for a particular episode. Only prescribed medicines that were purchased for a particular episode are usually represented in this file. Medication refills are also usually captured in this file, which allows for tracking medication usage by the patient longitudinally. The typical descriptors for medications on record include an identifier for each unique prescribed medicine; detailed characteristics associated with the event (e.g., national drug code (NDC), medicine name, etc.); conditions, if any, associated with the medicine; the date on which the person first used the medicine; total expenditure and sources of payments; and the types of pharmacies that filled the household's prescriptions.

Similarly, information provided by the emergency room visits file includes date of the visit, whether the patient saw a doctor, type of care received, type of services (i.e., lab test, sonogram or ultrasound, X-rays, etc.) received, medicines prescribed during the visit, cost information, imputed sources of payment, total payment, and total charge.

5.3 EMRS AND MEDICAL CHARTS

5.3.1 Medical Chart/Medical Record in General

A medical chart or record is a confidential document that contains detailed, comprehensive, and current information about a patient's healthcare experience, including diagnoses, treatment, tests, and treatment responses, in addition to other factors that might play a significant role in his or her health condition. This document summarizes the overall collected information of an individual related to health status. Once a patient enters a healthcare setting, be it a hospital or a clinic, documentation in a medical chart or record begins. Different medical settings follow different types of such documentation practices; however, there are certain aspects of such a document that remain universal.

Some of the most common entries in a medical chart or record include the following: admission information (if to an inpatient facility), medical history and physical information, medication and treatment orders, medications and other treatments received, procedures, diagnostic and other tests, insurance, consultations, patient consents, and discharge information [17]. Documentation in the chart or record is usually done by the physician or the nurse.

5.3.2 EMRs or Charts

With recent advances in technology, written medical charts or records are gradually being converted to computerized or electronic versions. The electronic version (EMR or electronic health record [EHR]), similar to the paper version of the medical record or chart, serves the same purpose of communication and documentation of an individual's contact with a healthcare provider and the decisions made by the provider regarding the patient, including diagnoses and treatments provided.

5.3.2.1 Advantages/Disadvantages

Several advantages of EMRs over print medical records or charts recommend their use by a medical institution. These include ease of chart or record accessibility, reduction of medical errors and task automation, legible medical notes, continuity of care and accountability, availability of an organized chart, and increased security [18]. Other advantages include patient report generation for certain screening methods, including mammography and cholesterol screening, patients taking medications that have been recalled, computerized practice or treatment guidelines that can be easily accessible, adequate alert systems that would notify the healthcare provider about certain adverse results that require prompt action, improved documentation and care management, and potential cost savings [19–22]. However, certain disadvantages of EMRs also should be noted. There have been instances where a patient's laboratory and other clinical data have not been integrated with the computerized system. This affects the comprehensiveness of the medical record, as key elements pertaining to a patient's health are missing. Efforts must be made to integrate all detailed and pertinent patient information. Another significant disadvantage would be system crashes during a patient visit that render unavailability of patient information during that period. Appropriate measures should ensure adequate backup in the event of such crashes or system malfunction [18]. Cybersecurity of EMRs has become a major concern for health systems and patients alike, as theft of patient-protected health information and wide-scale sequestering of medical records by ransomware (malware that encrypts records that cannot be decoded by the health systems) may occur unless a ransom is paid [23].

5.3.2.2 Current Use of EMRs

EMRs show potential benefits for healthcare organizations to adopt them into their systems and seem to be relatively ubiquitous. In contrast to a 2008 report that only 4% of US physicians had access to an EMR system, a 2016 publication from a 2016 survey of 6,375 responding physicians in active practice, 5,389 (84.5%) reported that they used EMRs [24, 25]. Moreover, primary care physicians and those working in large groups are more likely to use EMRs than physicians in other medical specialties and smaller size practices, respectively. Practices report use of EMRs to facilitate computerized prescription order entry, record clinical notes, patient's medications, allergies, and problem lists, and view laboratory results [26]. Prominent reasons for nonuse include, among others, the significant direct and indirect cost for licensing the EMR software. Indirect costs include staff training to use the software and system maintenance. In addition, large physician practices have greater financial and technological resources than smaller practices and solo physician practices and, thus, the higher adoption rate of technological advances, including EMRs, in large practices. Other factors include data entry obstacles, lack of trained staff, lack of uniformity, legal issues, and patient confidentiality and security concerns [27]. Similarly, another study found a higher adoption rate of EMRs among physicians owned by HMOs [28].

Some specific examples of how EMRs have been used as databases to provide insights into various therapeutic areas are provided below. The main advantages of using EMRs as databases to conduct pharmacoeconomic analyses include the richness and comprehensiveness of the data to estimate prevalence, incidence, physician treatment patterns, and cost of various prevention and treatment strategies available to medical practitioners. One example would be a study that estimated the tobacco-use prevalence using EMRs [29]. The availability of data needed to achieve the study objective eliminates the need to do expensive multiple surveys of different subpopulations to get the needed answer. This particular study used the EMR database of a large medical group in Minnesota. The study showed that out of the overall included population, 19.7% were tobacco users during the year March 2006 to February 2007, of which 24.2% were aged 18–24 years, 16% were pregnant women, 34.3% were Medicaid enrollees, 40% were American Indians, and 9.5% were Asians.

Another study used an EMR to analyze associations between cardiometabolic risk factors and body mass index based on diagnosis and treatment codes [30]. This particular study used the General Electric (GE) Centricity research database, which is a rich source of data used by more than 20,000 physicians to manage about 30 million patient records in 49 states. The availability of data, including clinical data captured in the practice setting, such as diagnoses, patient complaints, medication orders, medication lists, laboratory orders and results, and biometric readings, was a significant factor in the appropriateness of this data set for the particular study. The Kaiser Permanente EMR was used to evaluate the complications associated with dysglycemia and medical costs associated with nondiabetic hyperglycemia [31]. The EMR database used for this study provided information on all inpatient admissions, outpatient visits, pharmacy medication dispenses, and results of laboratory tests. As the study was based on diabetes patients, clinical information on isolated impaired fasting glucose (available in the database) was the primary factor used in classifying those patients. The study found that more than half of the studied dysglycemia patients had at least one associated complication as compared with only 34% of normoglycemic patients ($p < 0.001$). The study also found that macrovascular and microvascular complications had an incremental annual cost of \$3,863 ($p < 0.0001$) and \$1,874 ($p < 0.0001$) for dysglycemic patients and normoglycemic patients, respectively.

Another example of use of a practice-based EHR in diabetes assessed the relationship between diabetes treatment intensification and quality measure performance [32]. The value of timely treatment intensification for diabetes patients with above-target HbA1C levels has been well documented, and treatment guidelines from the American Diabetes Association (ADA) and American Association of Clinical Endocrinologists (AACE) recommend treatment intensification for patients not at treatment goal after 3 months of therapy [33, 34]. Even with abundant evidence of the value of treatment adjustment, failure of treatment intensification among patients with above-target HbA1C is commonly observed. This study aimed to assess the relationship between diabetes treatment intensification and HbA1C control quality-of-care measures among patients with uncontrolled type 2 diabetes. Index date for each included patient was defined as the date of the first above-target HbA1C test (i.e., ≥8.0%) within the index identification period. The baseline period was defined as the 6 months prior to the index and the follow-up period was 1 year following the index. Within the follow-up period, the treatment intensification window was defined as the first 120 days following the study index date. The presence or absence of timely adjustments to treatment for each uncontrolled diabetes patient was assessed based on the patient's treatment intensification status, and practice quality performance status was assessed based on patients' HbA1C control categories (HbA1C levels <8.0%, between 8.0% and 9.0%, or >9.0% were defined as the cohort with superior, moderate, or poor HbA1C control, respectively) during the follow-up period. Patients' diabetes treatment intensification statuses were evaluated using the post-index medication history for each included patient. Following the above-target index HbA1C level (≥8.0%), treatment intensification was defined as at least one medication treatment change that satisfied one or more of the following conditions: (1) adding one or more oral antidiabetic (OAD) agents to the existing treatment; (2) adding or switching to an injectable antidiabetes medication; or (3) increasing the dosage of existing OADs. Lack of treatment intensification within the 120-day window after index date was considered treatment inertia. A total of 547 patients with type 2 diabetes were identified after applying all inclusion and exclusion criteria; of those, 480 patients had at least one HbA1C test after the treatment intensification window and were included for statistical analyses that incorporated an HbA1C test result. Evaluations of patient baseline characteristics by treatment intensification status demonstrated that a greater proportion of patients in the cohort with poor HbA1C control at the index test received treatment intensification than patients in the cohort with superior HbA1C control ($p = 0.0016$). The odds of receiving treatment intensification were about 1.8 times higher among the cohort with poor HbA1C control in comparison to the cohort with moderate HbA1C control, $p = 0.0027$. The more types of OADs used at baseline, the less likely patients received treatment intensification, with p values of 0.0058, 0.0102, and 0.0119 for 4, 3, and 2 OAD types, respectively. Patients with higher BMI were more likely to receive treatment intensification ($p = 0.0159$). Timely treatment intensification was significantly associated with superior HbA1C control but not with poor HbA1C control. Hispanic patients were approximately three-fold more likely than White patients to still have poor HbA1C control after treatment intensification, and male patients were approximately half as likely as female patients to experience poor HbA1C control after treatment intensification. The study showed that after an above-target HbA1C level ($\geq 8.0\%$), more than 60% of patients with type 2 diabetes still did not receive treatment intensification, an outcome not discernibly different from previous studies. Although researchers typically rely on large data sets available commercially, the current research showed results consistent with previous publications using a data set available to practicing clinicians on a daily basis in their practices. Importantly, the use of a practice's patient data for important research such as this demonstrates that these types of analyses are not restricted to researchers with large data sets, but can also be used to evaluate outcomes for individual clinicians and practices.

A final example would be a study evaluating the acceptance of HPV vaccine by gynecologists in an urban setting [35]. This study found that the overall vaccination rate was 28% (6–55.8%) for the initial 3-month period when the vaccine became available to the health plan. Unfortunately, vaccination rates for HPV remain suboptimal to this day [36], more than 10 years later.

5.4   PATIENT-REPORTED OUTCOMES

A patient-reported outcome (PRO), as discussed at length in Chapter 12, is a measurement and assessment of a patient's health status coming directly from the patient rather than from a physician or any other healthcare provider [37, 38]. The Food and Drug Administration refers to a PRO as any report coming from patients about a health condition and its treatment [37, 38]. An important feature that differentiates a PRO from any other measurement is that the measurement is done directly from the patient. A PRO thus provides a patient's perspective on treatment effectiveness [39, 40], adverse events, and so on. Health-related quality of life (HRQoL), a term closely related to PRO, specifically refers to measures that are not only patient reported, but also include the impact of the disease and its treatment on the patient's well-being and functioning (see Chapter 12 on PROs) [39, 40]. A PRO measure includes various facets of disease treatment and its effectiveness as reported directly by the patient. These include, among others, reports of symptoms such as pain, fatigue, physical functioning, and well-being in the physical, mental, and social domains of life [41]. Many health behaviors, including use of tobacco and alcohol, participation in exercise programs, and so on, are also included in a typical PRO. Other end points captured in a PRO include patient preferences for a particular treatment and treatment satisfaction [41]. A PRO measure can include patient satisfaction with treatment, medication adherence, and other aspects of disease treatment, functional status, psychological well-being, and health status in addition to HRQoL [42, 43].

5.4.1   USE OF PRO INSTRUMENTS IN PHARMACOECONOMIC STUDIES: FOCUS ON HPV VACCINE STUDIES

Although PROs usually consist of specific health-related questionnaires or instruments, providing a simple survey questionnaire for patient response also makes up a simpler form of PRO. This section provides examples of how such PRO questionnaires have been used in HPV vaccine-related issues and studies. Gerend and Magloire assessed the awareness, knowledge, and beliefs about HPV in a racially diverse sample of young adults [44]. The authors used a survey to obtain respondent-reported responses among 124 students aged 18–26 years from two southeastern universities. The survey assessed demographics, sexual history, awareness and knowledge of HPV, HPV-related beliefs, and interest in the HPV vaccine (women only). This study reported some interesting findings that could be used for further economic studies on HPV vaccine, including great knowledge of HPV, greater awareness among women of HPV as compared with men, and a greater interest in HPV education among blacks and sexually active respondents. Another study examined the stage of adoption of the HPV vaccine among college women aged 18–22 years at a New England University [45]. This study used an online survey as a means to complete the PRO instrument. The survey examined knowledge of HPV, perceived susceptibility, severity, vaccine benefits or barriers, and stage of vaccine adoption. The use of such PRO measures provides a useful means to obtain responses directly from patients (in this case, women) who have had HPV vaccines or have potential to have one in the future. The analyzed results indicated that the acceptance of the vaccine was high among the study respondents and that the importance of Pap smears was also high [45]. Yet another study analyzed the acceptance of HPV vaccine among mid-adult women [46]. This particular study used a convenience sample of 472 mid-adult women who completed a survey that examined the demographic, knowledge, and behavioral variables associated with HPV vaccine acceptance. The study assumed clinical significance, as some of the variables that were found to be associated with vaccination among the study respondents could be useful to clinicians to identify potential female patients who might be more receptive to the vaccine. These variables included women who were younger than 55 years, had had an abnormal Pap test, understood the association of HPV and cervical cancer, and those who felt at risk for HPV infection.

Though HPV-related diseases are more common among women, men are also exposed to the virus in varying forms and severity. A study similar to the previous study based on women and by the same authors examined the variables associated with HPV vaccine acceptance among men [47]. Similar results were obtained from this study in that the (male) respondents with a higher education and knowledge about HPV were more likely to accept HPV vaccination than others.

5.5 ALTERNATIVE POPULATION-BASED DATA SOURCES

As mentioned in Table 5.1, numerous data sets are available either commercially or from the US government. These include:

1. IBM MarketScan® Research Data Sets (formerly Truven MarketScan® Commercial Claims and Medicare Supplemental databases)

The MarketScan database is a private sector health data resource that reflects the healthcare experience of employees and their dependents, as well as Medicare-eligible retirees with employer-provided Medicare Supplemental plans covered by the health benefit programs of large employers. It contains medical and pharmacy claims of over 150 employers, including more than 100 health plans (payers), representing approximately 43 million covered lives, and encounters data representing commercially-insured, Medicare supplemental, and Medicaid patients. Longitudinal tracking, across health plans and across payers, is possible. Health care for the individuals in the commercial database is provided under several fee-for-service and fully/partially capitated health plans that include PPOs, EPOs (exclusive provider organizations), indemnity plans, and HMOs. Medical claims are linked to outpatient prescription drug claims and person-level enrollment information.

The Medicare Supplemental database includes the Medicare-covered portion of payment, the employer-paid portion, and out-of-pocket patient expenses. This database provides detailed information on cost, use, and outcomes data in both the inpatient and the outpatient settings. For the majority of the population, the medical claims are linked to outpatient prescription drug claims and person-level enrollment data through use of unique patient identifiers.

In addition to the commercial claims and Medicare supplemental data sets, other data sets within the MarketScan network include the multi-state Medicaid database (provides information on medical-surgical, and prescription drugs of more than 47 million Medicaid enrollees from multiple states), Health and Productivity Management database (providing information on workplace absence, short and long-term disability, and worker's compensation data), the Lab Results database (a claims-linked database providing information on inpatient, outpatient drug data, as well as laboratory and enrollment data), and the Dental database.

2. IQVIA Real-World Data Adjudicated Claims (PharMetrics Plus) and Hospital Charge Data Master Databases

The IQVIA PharMetrics Plus database comprises information on pharmacy, provider, and facility claims for more than 150 million patients enrolled in approximately 60 US health plans, with data from 90% of US hospitals and 80% of all US doctors. Due to the broad reach of these data, records in the database are representative of the national, commercially-insured population based on age and gender for individuals aged 65 and under. The database includes standard fields such as inpatient and outpatient diagnoses and procedures, and retail and mail-order prescription records and payments. The database also includes information on demographic variables, product type, payer type, and start and stop dates of health plan enrollment.

In addition to the claims database, the IQVIA hospital charge data master (CDM) comprises records from hospital charge data master files, the service order records drawn from hospital operational files and other reference sources that roll up to the UB-04 claim form (also known as the CMS-1450 form; the standard claim form that can be used by institutional facilities for the billing of medical claims). This data set comprises data from more than 450 hospitals within the United States. Data elements include, among others, all inpatient and outpatient encounters within a facility, linked to individual departments, with detailed drug, procedure, diagnosis, and applied charge data for the entire stay.

3. Medicare Data Sets

Available from the Centers for Medicare and Medicaid Services (CMS), a benefit of using the Medicare databases is that they include inpatient and outpatient data for most US hospitals, with the exception of VA (Veterans Affairs) and military hospitals. These data are readily available for transformation to a usable form for comparative purposes. A limitation is that they are primarily constituted by an elderly sector of the population (approximately 44 million patients), so are not generalizable to younger populations.

There are several types of encrypted general-use Medicare data sets, available in 5% or 100% segments, which are described below:

- LDS (Limited Data Set) Standard Analytical Files (SAFs): contain payment information for each institutional (inpatient, outpatient, skilled nursing facility, hospice, or home health agency) and noninstitutional (physician and durable medical equipment providers) claim type.
- LDS MEDPAR (Medicare Provider Analysis and Review) Files: contain inpatient hospital "final action stay" records, summarizing all services received by a patient from admission through discharge.
- LDS Denominator File: contains demographic and enrollment data about each beneficiary in the Medicare and Medicare Managed Care Organizations.
- LDS Outpatient Hospital Prospective Payment System (PPS): contains select claim level data from the Hospital Outpatient PPS claims.

In contrast to LDS files, Research Identifiable Files (RIFs) may include medications, which may be necessary for some types of studies. However, RIFs are only available to academic institutions or the rare commercial institution that has a data use agreement from CMS.

4. Geisinger Electronic Health Records

Geisinger Health System is a regional healthcare provider to central, south-central, and northeastern Pennsylvania and southern New Jersey. The EHR databases from Geisinger provide information on more than three million patients on inpatient and outpatient clinic records, with integrated electronic scheduling, clinical lab, and radiology system data. The data include an associated reason code for every prescription. Being from hospitals and community-based physicians throughout rural Pennsylvania, the data may not be generalizable to all US patients.

5. Cerner

Cerner Health Facts™ contains inpatient and hospital outpatient data on over 12 million patients; the Cerner data set also contains lab results data. However, no longitudinal (claims) data are available from community-based outpatient settings.

6. Premier Healthcare Database

Premier's Healthcare Database (PHD) is a large, US hospital-based, service-level, all-payer database that includes information on inpatient discharges, primarily from geographically diverse nonprofit, nongovernmental and community and teaching hospitals and health systems from rural and urban areas. Hospitals/healthcare systems submit administrative, healthcare utilization, and financial data from patient encounters. Inpatient admissions include over 108 million visits since 2012, representing approximately 25% of annual US inpatient admissions. Outpatient encounters include over 765 million outpatient visits, with more than 71 million visits per year since 2012. The PHD contains data from over 208 million unique patients, who can be tracked within the same hospital across the inpatient and hospital-based outpatient settings within the database using a unique masked identifier.

7. Optum Research (formerly Ingenix) Data (data)

Comprehensive real-world data from Optum (a part of UnitedHealth group) include 180+ million patients with administrative claims records, 80+ million patients with electronic health records, and 12+ million patients with integrated claims and electronic health records data. The Optum De-identified Clinformatics extended data mart database, within the Optum Research Data, is an adjudicated administrative health claims database for members with private health insurance who are fully insured in commercial plans or in administrative services only, legacy Medicare Choice lives (prior to January 2006), and Medicare Advantage (Medicare Advantage Prescription drug coverage starting January 2006).

8. General Practice Research Database (GPRD)/Clinical Practice Research Datalink (CPRD)

The General Practice Research Database, or GPRD is a computerized database of anonymized data from patient records. Diagnoses and prescribing data have been collected continuously since 1987, and data on approximately 4.8 million patients in the United Kingdom (England and Wales), equivalent to about 7% of the population, were collected from nearly 600 general practices nationwide. This data set provides valuable information on side effects of medicines, causes of disease and medical disorders and associated risk factors, outcomes of treatments, unmet medical need, improvement of screening or diagnosis, and comparative effectiveness of treatments. In 2012, the GPRD was incorporated into the CPRD (cprd.com), resulting in a linkage of UK primary care practitioner data with other data sets, currently comprising 45 million patients, including 13 million currently registered patients [48]. The GPRD/CPRD is maintained by the UK Medicines and Healthcare Products Regulatory Agency (MHRA) in London. Unlike THIN (described below), CPRD does not extract data from a particular proprietary clinical system, is available only non-commercially, and is the only database accessible online [48].

9. THIN (The Health Improvement Network)

The Health Improvement Network, or THIN, is a large UK primary care database providing data collected from over 550 general practitioners across the United Kingdom, for research in cardiovascular disease, mental health, pharmacoepidemiology, and other fields of primary care research. Data collection commenced in January 2003, using information extracted from Vision, a widely used general practice management software package developed by In Practice Systems. The database is regularly updated and currently contains data on over 10 million individuals living in the United Kingdom and is available for commercial use via third-party vendors [48]. THIN was developed as a replacement for the GPRD, because the EPIC version of the GPRD was discontinued from April 2002. THIN's pluses and minuses are the same as GPRD.

10. Framingham Heart Study (FHS) Database

The Framingham Study is a longitudinal, population-based observational study that began in 1948 in Framingham, Massachusetts, USA. The original cohort, founded in 1948, consisted of 5,209 men and women. In 1971, a second-generation cohort was recruited into the Framingham Offspring/Spouse (FOS) study [49], for which children of the original cohort were eligible. Spouses were also eligible if they had become pregnant with or sired two or more children by a participant in the Offspring cohort. Cohort members are examined in the clinic every 4 years, on average, where they undergo a standardized protocol for data collection approved by the Boston University Institutional Review Board. This database provides a rich source of information related to cardiovascular disease, including coronary heart disease, stroke, hypertension, peripheral arterial disease, and congestive heart failure.

11. Atherosclerosis Risk in Communities (ARIC) Database

The ARIC Study, sponsored by the US National Heart, Lung, and Blood Institute (NHLBI) of the National Institutes of Health, is a prospective, observational biracial follow-up of 15,792 men and women between the ages of 45 and 64, recruited from Forsyth County, North Carolina; Jackson, Mississippi; suburbs of Minneapolis, Minnesota; and Washington County, Maryland. This database provides key clinical information on the etiology and risk factors associated with atherosclerosis, along with differences in medical care obtained by patients of different races and genders, as well as those residing in different locations.

5.6 ISSUES AND CHALLENGES

Although numerous advantages exist with use of retrospective databases over RCTs, considerations of internal validity (reproducibility of results) and external validity (generalizability of results) must be addressed. For example, with RCTs, because they are protocol-based, it is relatively easy to reproduce the results of a trial of a hypertension drug using an identical protocol in a patient population following the same inclusion and exclusion criteria. With retrospective databases, however, confounding factors (see Section 5.7), such as a center effect or regional variation in the prevalence of hypertension, may limit the ability to duplicate these results between different populations, such as between two MCOs or even between two locations of the same MCO. However, the very measure that helps to ensure reproducibility, namely, the protocol, may reduce the study's usefulness in the real world, as any analysis would have to consider protocol-induced (artificial) resource use and costs. Generalizability refers to the ability to extrapolate results across healthcare settings or even countries. A pharmacoeconomic analysis must provide segregated healthcare resource units (e.g., numbers of MRIs) and costs per unit (e.g., cost of an individual MRI), so that if a resource is not used the same way in the United States and Canada or the costs are very dissimilar, each country can use the resource data, but customize it to its own cost structure. The caveat here, of course, is to determine whether the resource utilization itself is similar across the two countries.

To determine whether a data set is appropriate to answer a pharmacoeconomic question, key attributes of the population (such as demographics), covered services, benefit design (e.g., nationalized or private insurance, deductibles, patient co-payments), formulary design (e.g., open [allowing any drug], closed [allowing only specific drugs]), and any special programs (e.g., physician detailing, disease management initiatives) that might affect its generalizability should be enumerated. Johnson outlines a six-step process for conducting outcomes analyses using administrative databases, as seen in Table 5.3 [50]. Since practice, including available treatments and procedures, changes over time, it is essential to use retrospective data to continuously inform health policy decisions [51]. An example of use of data from a pharmacy benefits management claims database to evaluate two decision-analytic models regarding the cost-effectiveness of therapeutic regimens to eradicate

TABLE 5.3

Steps to Designing a Database Study

Define the study objective

Extract key data elements

Apply inclusion, exclusion criteria

Perform initial data analyses

Create "calculated" analysis variables

Compare groups

Helicobacter pylori in ulcer patients is a case in point [52]. The authors found that model results overstated the cost-effectiveness of the previously more cost-effective regimen and underestimated the cost-effectiveness of the other regimen such that the model assumptions and, ultimately, the outcomes, were not supported by the data.

Regardless of how the data are used, issues of data quality must be addressed. A checklist detailing many of these issues was published as a result of an International Society for Pharmacoeconomics and Outcomes Research (ISPOR) Task Force's being convened to examine the quality of published studies using retrospective databases [4]. It is important to have plans to examine a representative number or percentage of source documents (e.g., patient charts) to determine that diagnosis and procedure codes are reasonably accurate. For example, Fivenson, Arnold, and colleagues determined that approximately 10% of diagnosis codes in an atopic dermatitis study utilizing a claims data set were inaccurate [3]. Moreover, coding may change over time, such as use of different versions of the ICD-9-CM/ICD-10-CM coding set, differing frequencies of use of codes according to reimbursement policies, or varying regional codes (e.g., HCPCS codes) [10]. In a study to evaluate the coding data quality of the Healthcare Cost & Utilization Project (HCUP) National Inpatient Sample, claims data failed to identify more than 50% of patients with prognostically important conditions, and miscoding of diagnoses resulted in nonspecific disease identification or coexisting conditions [53]. Coding error rates were found to vary widely among states, hospitals within states, geographic location, and hospital characteristics. Coding errors were significantly different among patient demographic groups and whether the state used billing versus abstract data.

In addition, services may not be captured in the database because they are administered elsewhere (e.g., carved out, such as mental health services) [4]. It is important to minimize missing and out-of-range values, ensure consistency of data (e.g., no menopausal men), control duplication of records, assure continuous enrollment, ascertain the availability of the continuum of care, and make certain that data have been recorded uniformly because if there is inconsistency in coding, there is inconsistency in the resulting judgments derived from that data [54]. Sax [55] mentions the pharmacy field "days supply" as potentially problematic as an indicator of patient adherence to a medication regimen due to dose titrations (e.g., gradual reductions in prednisone "burst" during asthma exacerbation [56–58]) unknown actual use, as-needed medications, and possible unknown sources of additional medication, such as from an unrelated pharmacy. As with prospective data collection, benchmarking values against established norms, such as the SF-36 for quality of life, will assure researchers that the data are representative of the population at large [59].

It is also important that data links across relational databases be consistent. For example, there should be unique identifiers for each family member. Many times, data must be concatenated (or joined) from several fields in a database to make sure that this is the case [22]. Moreover, events may not be recorded at the same time when they actually occurred for the patient, as with provider charges occurring perhaps 6 months to a year after a procedure for a Medicare patient, so it is essential that this lag time is considered when evaluating an episode of care [60].

In addition, temporal factors may play a role in analyses using preexisting data, either in terms of hypothesis testing or as a confounder. For example, Arnold et al. [61] used clinical trials, published literature, and a modified Delphi panel to establish the effect of timing of administration of a thrombin inhibitor, argatroban, on its cost-effectiveness in patients with heparin-induced thrombocytopenia (that is, heparin hypersensitivity). It is also necessary to define and identify disease-related costs. For example, in patients with asthma, should claims be related only to the various ICD-9/10 diagnosis codes for the various types of asthma [62, 63] or should there be the added requirement of an asthma medication or diagnostic testing sometime during the index or eligibility period? It is useful to be able to "tease out" costs during a hospitalization related specifically to the diagnosis of interest; however, this is often not possible because of potential overlap between the diagnosis of interest and concomitant illness, for example, pneumonia in the case of asthma. In addition, especially with the changeover from ICD-9 to ICD-10 and other "advances" in coding, inclusion or exclusion of certain diagnoses or inadequate/inappropriate characterization of a disease state may cause selection bias in a study. For example, in a study of FeNO use in asthma discussed at length in Chapter 3 (Cost of Illness), in recent years, patients with an ICD-9 code of 493.2 (asthmatic bronchitis) have been noted to have characteristics more similar to patients with chronic obstructive pulmonary disease (COPD) than those with only asthma [64, 65]. Since 39% of the patients in that study had a diagnosis code of 493.2 at their index date and FeNO is less predictive of responsiveness in patients with COPD [66–68], this would bias the study against FeNO. It is also important to account for natural history of disease progression and medical and technological advances that may have impacted on the course of the disease in terms of the index date (beginning of data collection) and duration of data inclusion. Indeed, Motheral et al. [4] discuss the idea of censoring or the time limits placed at the beginning (left censoring, period prior to initiation of therapy of interest) or end (right censoring, follow-up time) of the study period.

5.7   STATISTICAL ISSUES

Bias is a significant problem that must be addressed. The types of biases include selection bias, measurement bias, length of measurement bias, misspecification bias, interdependence [69] of observations, diagnostic ascertainment bias, auto-correlation, omitted variables, quasi-omitted variables, investigator bias, obsolescence bias, vintage bias (human and physical capital), claims versus encounter bias and recall bias. The reader is referred to a lengthy review of these types of bias by Sackett et al. [69].

The previously discussed ISPOR checklist has categorized many of the statistical issues faced by users of retrospective databases in general [4]. These are reviewed below. The first is control variables. It is important to account for the effects of all variables so that biased estimates of treatment effects, or confounding bias, do not occur. For example, it is important to control for the likelihood of prescribing certain compounds given a patient's history of comorbid conditions. Common approaches to adjust for confounding bias include stratification of the cohort by different levels of the confounding variables with comparison of the treatments within potential confounders, such as demographic variables; the use of multivariate statistical techniques; cohort matching and propensity adjustment [4, 70]. Multivariate regression can be used to estimate the association among the intervention, confounders, and the outcome of interest [70, 71]. Stratification divides the study population into subgroups on the basis of confounding characteristics to reduce confounding. With cohort matching, a comparator cohort is generated based on the characteristics associated with confounding bias [72]. A Chronic Disease Score or the Charlson Index can be used to control for comorbidities [73] or disease severity [74], respectively. Moreover, instrumental variable techniques can be used to group patients by choice of treatment, but without unmeasured confounders.

Selection bias may be introduced by the inclusion and exclusion criteria used in the study design, especially considering that missing data, such as a diagnosis code, may cause records not to be chosen for analysis. Thus, the population selected may not be representative of all patients that should be included [54]. A method that is frequently used to account for potential inherent differences in treatment assignment due to selection bias in retrospective databases is propensity scoring [75]. The propensity score, defined as the conditional probability of being treated given the covariates, or the probability that a patient would have been treated, can be used to balance the covariates in the groups, thereby adjusting the estimate of the treatment effect. To estimate the propensity score, one models the distribution of the treatment indicator variables, considering the observed covariates. The propensity score is then estimated using logistic regression or discriminant analysis. Once estimated, the propensity score can be used to reduce bias through matching, stratification (sub-classification), regression adjustment, or some combination of all three. All of these methods are an attempt to affect a "quasi-randomized" treatment allocation.

Since much data in retrospective databases are expected to be skewed in its distribution, techniques such as log-transformation and two-part models should be considered. Methods such as hierarchical linear modeling may be appropriate when using pooled data from several different health plans or multiple sites from a single health plan to account for center (i.e., facility) effects [4].

Outliers are another issue that must be addressed in economic analyses using retrospective databases. As mentioned earlier and particularly true when using costs rather than the quantity of units, such as hospital days or physician office visits, to measure resource use, just a small number of outliers can greatly skew the analysis. Logarithmic transformations that have been used previously to reduce skewness can create difficulties with non-log-transformed costs. For this reason, it is often prudent to record unit costs and quantities separately and, if a high degree of skewness is present, use the quantities for the statistical calculation, then multiply by a set dollar amount from a fee schedule.

5.8   NON-US COUNTRIES

As with US data sources, international retrospective databases encompass such sources as national insurance administrative data, hospital medical records, disease-specific patient registries, and provider survey data [5]. Table 5.1 contains two (UK) sources of such data from a study that qualitatively reviewed the methodological challenges of using non-US databases to conduct retrospective economic and outcomes research studies. The researchers conducted a MEDLINE search to obtain a sample of literature published after the year 2000 on retrospective analyses incorporating non-US databases using the ISPOR checklist and found that few economic studies included information on indirect cost components because of the lack of relevant data. Moreover, they found that the quality of non-US retrospective database analyses varied, leading to problems of internal validity, that is, study design errors that could compromise conclusions. The economic data sets were from Italy, Australia, United Kingdom, Switzerland, Singapore, seven other European countries, Canada, Japan, and France. Only 2 of the 12 studies reviewed included indirect costs. Ten of the 12 economic studies reviewed made adjustments for confounders or sampling schemes (i.e., to reduce selection bias), typically with some form of regression model. The authors thought that five studies did not sufficiently address external validity. Sensitivity analysis was the most common approach to dealing with uncertainty in the studies. Five studies extensively discussed study limitations; however, all of the study authors, as well as the review author, advised caution regarding the external validity of the studies.

5.9   THE FUTURE IN USE OF RETROSPECTIVE DATABASES

What is the future for use of retrospective databases to inform pharmacoeconomic analyses? Stallings et al. [76] developed a decision-analytic model to test the likely cost impact of a hypothetical pharmacogenomic test to determine a preferred initial therapy in patients with asthma. They compared annualized per patient cost distributions using a "test all" strategy for a nonresponse genotype prior to treating versus "test none." They found that the cost savings per patient of the testing strategy simulation ranged from US$200 to US$767 (95% confidence interval) and concluded that upfront testing costs were likely to be offset by avoided nonresponse costs. This shows the potential use of retrospective database studies in analytic data mining and improved hypothesis testing.

Indeed, there is an increasing likelihood that genomics will play a role in decisions about drug use. For example, a theoretical Markov model showed pharmacogenomic-guided dosing for anticoagulation with warfarin not to be cost-effective in patients with nonvalvular atrial fibrillation [77]. Interestingly, another algorithm using logistic regression from international retrospective databases published around the same time as the Markov model showed that incorporating pharmacogenetic information was more likely to result in a therapeutic international normalized ratio (INR), the major method of determining anticoagulation, than use of clinical data alone [78]. However, the data used to inform the Markov model were published studies that did not include the latter study and the algorithm did not indicate the clinical diagnoses, or the clinical outcomes, of the patients who were more or less likely to be within a therapeutic INR. Indeed, over the past 10 years, research has still not demonstrated definitive results on the subject [79]. Therefore, more research is needed to coordinate these conflicting results. Indeed, another potential for the use of such easily available databases is to increase their use in validation studies. Testing the same hypothesis in several databases increases the validity of the study results, thereby increasing the credibility of the findings. However, in the near future, retrospective databases are more likely to continue being used for quick identification of treatment patterns, prevalence, and incidence of a medical condition, medication adherence, and persistence, and healthcare resource utilization and associated costs related to a particular medical condition. With clinical trials becoming more and more time consuming and expensive, retrospective databases offer an attractive alternative to provide this "real-life" medical information.

REFERENCES

[1] R.G. Arnold, J.G. Kotsanos, Panel 3: Methodological issues in conducting pharmacoeconomic evaluations–retrospective and claims database studies, *Value Health* 2 (2) (1999) 82–87.

[2] R.J.G. Arnold, Use of interactive software in medical decision making, in: S. Ekins (Ed.), *Computer Applications in Pharmaceutical Research and Development*, John Wiley & Sons, Inc., Hoboken, NJ, 2006, pp. 571–590.

[3] D. Fivenson, R.J. Arnold, D.J. Kaniecki, J.L. Cohen, F. Frech, A.Y. Finlay, The effect of atopic dermatitis on total burden of illness and quality of life on adults and children in a large managed care organization, *J Manag Care Pharm* 8(5) (2002) 333–342.

[4] B. Motheral, J. Brooks, M.A. Clark, W.H. Crown, P. Davey, D. Hutchins, B. C. Martin, P. Stang, A checklist for retrospective database studies–report of the ISPOR Task Force on Retrospective Databases, *Value Health* 6(2) (2003) 90–97.

[5] L. Shi, E.Q. Wu, M. Hodges, A. Yu, H. Birnbaum, Retrospective economic and outcomes analyses using non-US databases: A review, *Pharmacoeconomics* 25(7) (2007) 563–576.

[6] K. Benson, A.J. Hartz, A comparison of observational studies and randomized, controlled trials, *New England Journal of Medicine* 342(25) (2000) 1878–1886.

[7] J. Concato, N. Shah, R.I. Horwitz, Randomized, controlled trials, observational studies, and the hierarchy of research designs, *N Engl J Med* 342(25) (2000) 1887–1892.

[8] R. Goldberg Arnold, Applications of large databases to evaluate cost-effective therapy, *Clinical Therapeutics* 18 (1996) 15–16.

[9] S. Bansilal, J.M. Castellano, E. Garrido, H.G. Wei, A. Freeman, C. Spettell, F. Garcia-Alonso, I. Lizano, R.J. Arnold, J. Rajda, et al, Assessing the impact of medication adherence on long-term cardiovascular outcomes, *J Am Coll Cardiol* 68 (8) (2016) 789–801.

[10] Centers for Medicare and Medicaid Services, HCPCS general information, 2019. www.cms.gov/Medicare/Coding/HCPCSReleaseCodeSets/index. (Accessed January 7 2020).

[11] M. Watson, M. Saraiya, V. Benard, S.S. Coughlin, L. Flowers, V. Cokkinides, M. Schwenn, Y. Huang, A. Giuliano, Burden of cervical cancer in the United States, 1998-2003, *Cancer* 113(S10) (2008) 2855–2864.

[12] T.M. Becker, D.K. Espey, H.W. Lawson, M. Saraiya, M.A. Jim, A.G. Waxman, Regional differences in cervical cancer incidence among American Indians and Alaska Natives, 1999-2004, *Cancer* 113(S5) (2008) 1234–1243.

[13] M. Saraiya, F. Ahmed, S. Krishnan, T.B. Richards, E.R. Unger, H.W. Lawson, Cervical cancer incidence in a prevaccine era in the United States, 1998-2002, *Obstet Gynecol* 109(2Pt 1) (2007) 360–370.

[14] M. Icen, C.S. Crowson, M.T. McEvoy, S.E. Gabriel, H. Maradit Kremers, Potential misclassification of patients with psoriasis in electronic databases, *J Am Acad Dermatol* 59(6) (2008) 981–985.

[15] E.F.O. Kern, M. Maney, D.R. Miller, C.-L. Tseng, A. Tiwari, M. Rajan, D. Aron, L. Pogach, Failure of ICD-9-CM codes to identify patients with comorbid chronic kidney disease in diabetes, *Health Serv Res* 41(2) (2006) 564–580.

[16] Y. Zhao, W. Ye, K.S. Boye, J.H. Holcombe, J.A. Hall, R. Swindle, Prevalence of other diabetes-associated complications and comorbidities and its impact on health care charges among patients with diabetic neuropathy, *Journal of Diabetes and Its Complications* 24(1) (2010) 9–19.

[17] Encyclopedia of Surgery. Medical charts, At www.surgeryencyclopedia.com/La-Pa/Medical-Charts.html. Accessed January 7, 2020.

[18] F.A. Tahil, Hello electronic medical records, farewell paper charts, *Psychiatric News* 38(9) (2003) 34–51.

[19] R. Hillestad, J. Bigelow, A. Bower, F. Girosi, R. Meili, R. Scoville, R. Taylor, Can electronic medical record systems transform health care? Potential health benefits, savings, and costs, *Health Aff (Millwood)* 24(5) (2005) 1103–1117.

[20] R.H. Miller, I. Sim, Physicians' use of electronic medical records: Barriers and solutions, *Health Aff (Millwood)* 23(2) (2004) 116–126.

[21] W.V. Sujansky, The benefits and challenges of an electronic medical record: Much more than a "word-processed" patient chart, *West J Med* 169(3) (1998) 176–183.

[22] R.R. Zaid, Electronic medical records: What are you waiting for?, *J Am Osteopath Assoc* 108(2) (2008) 81–82.

[23] M.P. Jarrett, Cybersecurity—A Serious Patient Care Concern, *JAMA* 318(14) (2017) 1319–1320.

[24] T.D. Shanafelt, L.N. Dyrbye, C. Sinsky, O. Hasan, D. Satele, J. Sloan, C.P. West, Relationship between Clerical Burden and characteristics of the electronic environment with physician burnout and professional satisfaction, *Mayo Clinic Proceedings* 91(7) (2016) 836–848.

[25] C.M. DesRoches, E.G. Campbell, S.R. Rao, K. Donelan, T.G. Ferris, A. Jha, R. Kaushal, D.E. Levy, S. Rosenbaum, A.E. Shields, et al, Electronic health records in ambulatory care — A national survey of physicians, *New England Journal of Medicine* 359(1) (2008) 50–60.

[26] B. Monegain, More than 80% of docs use EHRs, 2015. www.healthcareitnews.com/news/more-80-percent-docs-use-ehrs. (Accessed January 7 2020).

[27] K.A. Wager, F.W. Lee, A.W. White, D.M. Ward, S.M. Ornstein, Impact of an electronic medical record system on community-based primary care practices, *J Am Board Fam Pract* 13(5) (2000) 338–348.

[28] C.W. Burt, J.E. Sisk, Which physicians and practices are using electronic medical records?, *Health Affairs* 24(5) (2005) 1334–1343.

[29] L.I. Solberg, T.J. Flottemesch, S.S. Foldes, B.A. Molitor, P.F. Walker, A.L. Crain, Tobacco-use prevalence in special populations taking advantage of electronic medical records, *Am J Prev Med* 35(6 Suppl) (2008) S501–7.

[30] D. Brixner, S.R. Ghate, C. McAdam-Marx, R. Ben-Joseph, Q. Said, Association between cardiometabolic risk factors and body mass index based on diagnosis and treatment codes in an electronic medical record database, *Journal of Managed Care Pharmacy* 14(8) (2008) 756–767.

[31] G.A. Nichols, B. Arondekar, W.H. Herman, Medical care costs one year after identification of hyperglycemia below the threshold for diabetes, *Med Care* 46(3) (2008) 287–292.

[32] R.J.G. Arnold, S. Yang, E.J. Gold, S. Farahbakhshian, J.J. Sheehan, Assessment of the relationship between diabetes treatment intensification and quality measure performance using electronic medical records, *PLoS One* 13(6) (2018) e0199011.

[33] American Association of Clincal Endocrinologists, American College of Endocrinology, Clinical practice guidelines for developing a diabetes mellitus comprehensive care plan, 2015.

[34] American Diabetes Association, Standards of medical care in diabetes, *Diabetes Care* 40 (2017) S1–S135.

[35] D.M. Jaspan, C.J. Dunton, T.L. Cook, Acceptance of Human Papillomavirus Vaccine by Gynecologists in an Urban Setting, *Journal of Lower Genital Tract Disease* 12(2) (2008) 118–121.

[36] M. Bowden, J. Yaun, B. Bagga, Improving human papilloma virus vaccination rates: Quality improvement, *Pediatr Qual Saf* 2(6) (2017) e048.

[37] M.L. Rothman, P. Beltran, J.C. Cappelleri, J. Lipscomb, B. Teschendorf, Patient-Reported Outcomes: Conceptual issues, *Value in Health* 10 (November/December (Suppl 2)) (2007) S66–S75.

[38] U.S. Department of Health and Human Services, Food and Drug Administration, Center for Drug Evaluation and Research (CDER), Center for Biologics Evaluation and Research (CBER), Center for Devices and Radiological Health (CDRH), Guidance for industry patient-reported outcome measures: Use in medical product development to support labeling claims, 2009.

[39] D.A. Revicki, D. Osoba, D. Fairclough, I. Barofsky, R. Berzon, N.K. Leidy, M. Rothman, Recommendations on health-related quality of life research to support labeling and promotional claims in the United States, *Quality of Life Research* 9(8) (2000) 887–900.

[40] R.J. Willke, L.B. Burke, P. Erickson, Measuring treatment impact: A review of patient-reported outcomes and other efficacy endpoints in approved product labels, *Controlled Clinical Trials* 25(6) (2004) 535–552.

[41] C.H. Fung, R.D. Hays, Prospects and challenges in using patient-reported outcomes in clinical practice, *Qual Life Res* 17(10) (2008) 1297–1302.

[42] C. Acquadro, R. Berzon, D. Dubois, N.K. Leidy, P. Marquis, D. Revicki, M. Rothman, Incorporating the patient's perspective into drug development and communication: An ad hoc task force report of the Patient-Reported Outcomes (PRO) Harmonization group meeting at the food and drug administration, February 16, 2001 *Value in Health* 6(5) (2003) 522–531.

[43] K.N. Lohr, B.J. Zebrack, Using patient-reported outcomes in clinical practice: Challenges and opportunities, *Quality of Life Research* 18(1) (2008) 99–107.

[44] M.A. Gerend, Z.F. Magloire, Awareness, knowledge, and beliefs about human papillomavirus in a racially diverse sample of young adults, *J Adolesc Health* 42(3) (2008) 237–242.

[45] J.D. Allen, A.P. Mohllajee, R.C. Shelton, M.K.D. Othus, H.B. Fontenot, R. Hanna, Stage of adoption of the human papillomavirus vaccine among college women, *Preventive Medicine* 48(5) (2009) 420–425.

[46] D.G. Ferris, J.L. Waller, A. Owen, J. Smith, HPV vaccine acceptance among mid-adult women, *J Am Board Fam Med* 21(1) (2008) 31–37.

[47] D.G. Ferris, J.L. Waller, J. Miller, P. Patel, G.A. Price, L. Jackson, C. Wilson, Variables associated with human papillomavirus (HPV) vaccine acceptance by men, *J Am Board Fam Med* 22(1) (2009) 34–42.

[48] P. Vezyridis, S. Timmons, Evolution of primary care databases in UK: A scientometric analysis of research output, *BMJ Open* 6(10) (2016) e012785.

[49] W.B. Kannel, M. Feinleib, P.M. McNamara, R.J. Garrison, W.P. Castelli, An investigation of coronary heart disease in families. The Framingham offspring study, *Am J Epidemiol* 110(3) (1979) 281–290.

[50] N. Johnson, The six-step process for conducting outcomes analyses using administrative databases, *Formulary* 37 (2002) 362–364.

[51] R.J.G. Arnold, Cost-effectiveness analysis: Should it be required for drug registration and beyond?, *Drug Discovery Today* 12(21–22) (2007) 960–965.

[52] K.A. Fairman, B.R. Motheral, Do decision-analytic models identify cost-effective treatments? A retrospective look at helicobacter pylori eradication, *J Manag Care Pharm* 9(5) (2003) 430–440.

[53] C.L. Berthelsen, Evaluation of coding data quality of the HCUP National Inpatient Sample, *Top Health Inf Manage* 21(2) (2000) 10–23.

[54] M.J. Sax, Benchmarking as a management tool in decision making, *Journal of Managed Care Pharmacy* 11(1 Supp A) (2005) S3–S4.

[55] M.J. Sax, Essential steps and practical applications for database studies, *J Manag Care Pharm* 11(1 Suppl A) (2005) S5–8.

[56] E.D. Bateman, H.A. Boushey, J. Bousquet, W.W. Busse, T.J.H. Clark, R. A. Pauwels, S.E. Pedersen, Can guideline-defined asthma control be achieved?, *American Journal of Respiratory and Critical Care Medicine* 170(8) (2004) 836–844.

[57] C.M. Dolan, K.E. Fraher, E.R. Bleecker, L. Borish, B. Chipps, M.L. Hayden, S. Weiss, B. Zheng, C. Johnson, S. Wenzel, Design and baseline characteristics of the epidemiology and natural history of Asthma: Outcomes and treatment regimens (TENOR) study: A large cohort of patients with severe or difficult-to-treat asthma, *Annals of Allergy, Asthma & Immunology* 92(1) (2004) 32–39.

[58] Z.K. Ballas, Asthma clinical practice guidelines: Time for an update, *Journal of Allergy and Clinical Immunology* 142(3) (2018) 787.

[59] R.J. Arnold, A. Donnelly, L. Altieri, K.W. Wong, J.C. Sung, Assessment of outcomes and parental effect on quality-of-life endpoints in the management of atopic dermatitis, *Manag Care Interface* 20(2) (2007) 18–23.

[60] R.L. Lewis, D.M. Canafax, K.G. Pettit, J. DiCesare, D.J. Kaniecki, R.J. Arnold, M.S. Roberts, Use of Markov modeling for evaluating the cost-effectiveness of

immunosuppressive therapies in renal transplant recipients, *Transplant Proc* 28(4) (1996) 2214–2217.

[61] R.J. Arnold, R. Kim, B. Tang, The cost-effectiveness of argatroban treatment in heparin-induced thrombocytopenia: The effect of early versus delayed treatment, *Cardiol Rev* 14(1) (2006) 7–13.

[62] P. Marcus, R.J.G. Arnold, S. Ekins, P. Sacco, M. Massanari, S. Stanley Young, J. Donohue, D. Bukstein, A retrospective randomized study of asthma control in the US: Results of the CHARIOT study, *Current Medical Research and Opinion* 24 (12) (2008) 3443–3452.

[63] M. Massanari, A. Layton, R. Arnold, Comparative cost analysis of monitoring exhaled nitric oxide (FeNO) in asthma management, *J Allergy Clin Immunol* 141(2) (2018) Abstracts AB221.

[64] R.G. Arnold, K. Pettit, J. DiCesare, D. Canafax, R. Lewis, D. Kaniecki, Application of medicare databases to a theoretical renal transplant markov model, *Clinical Therapeutics* 18 (1996) 28.

[65] D. Cher, M. Frasco, R. Arnold, D. Polly, Cost-effectiveness of minimally invasive sacroiliac joint fusion, *ClinicoEconomics and Outcomes Research* 8 (2015) 1.

[66] M.F.S. Beg, M.A. Alzoghaibi, A.A. Abba, S.S. Habib, Exhaled nitric oxide in stable chronic obstructive pulmonary disease, *Annals of Thoracic Medicine* 4(2) (2009) 65–70.

[67] L. Bjermer, K. Alving, Z. Diamant, H. Magnussen, I. Pavord, G. Piacentini, D. Price, N. Roche, J. Sastre, M. Thomas, et al, Current evidence and future research needs for FeNO measurement in respiratory diseases, *Respiratory Medicine* 108(6) (2014) 830–841.

[68] F.-J. Chen, X.-Y. Huang, Y.-L. Liu, G.-P. Lin, C.-M. Xie, Importance of fractional exhaled nitric oxide in the differentiation of asthma–COPD overlap syndrome, asthma, and COPD, *International Journal of Chronic Obstructive Pulmonary Disease* 11 (2016) 2385–2390.

[69] D.L. Sackett, Bias in analytic research, *Journal of Chronic Diseases* 32(1–2) (1979) 51–63.

[70] S.K. Takemoto, W. Arns, S. Bunnapradist, L.P. Garrison, L. Guirado, Z. Kalo, G. Oniscu, G. Opelz, M.P. Scolari, S. Stefoni, et al, Expanding the evidence base in transplantation: The complementary roles of randomized controlled trials and outcomes research, *Transplantation* 86(1) (2008) 18–25.

[71] S.-L.T. Normand, K. Sykora, P. Li, M. Mamdani, P.A. Rochon, G.M. Anderson, Readers guide to critical appraisal of cohort studies: 3. Analytical strategies to reduce confounding, *BMJ* 330(7498) (2005) 1021–1023.

[72] T. Kurth, A.M. Walker, R.J. Glynn, K.A. Chan, J.M. Gaziano, K. Berger, J. M. Robins, Results of multivariable logistic regression, propensity matching, propensity adjustment, and propensity-based weighting under conditions of nonuniform effect, *Am J Epidemiol* 163(3) (2006) 262–270.

[73] D.O. Clark, M.V. Korff, K. Saunders, W.M. Balugh, G.E. Simon, A chronic disease score with empirically derived weights, *Medical Care* 33(8) (1995) 783–795.

[74] R. Deyo, Adapting a clinical comorbidity index for use with ICD-9-CM administrative databases, *Journal of Clinical Epidemiology* 45(6) (1992) 613–619.

[75] R.B. D'Agostino, Propensity score methods for bias reduction in the comparison of a treatment to a non-randomized control group, *Statistics in Medicine* 17(19) (1998) 2265–2281.

[76] S.C. Stallings, D. Huse, S.N. Finkelstein, W.H. Crown, W.P. Witt, J. Maguire, A. J. Hiller, A.J. Sinskey, G.S. Ginsburg, A framework to evaluate the economic impact of pharmacogenomics, *Pharmacogenomics* 7(6) (2006) 853–862.

[77] M.H. Eckman, J. Rosand, S.M. Greenberg, B.F. Gage, Cost-effectiveness of using pharmacogenetic information in warfarin dosing for patients with nonvalvular atrial fibrillation, *Ann Intern Med* 150(2) (2009) 73–83.

[78] International Warfarin Pharmacogenetics Consortium, T.E. Klein, R.B. Altman, N. Eriksson, B.F. Gage, S.E. Kimmel, M.T.M. Lee, N.A. Limdi, D. Page, D. M. Roden, M.J. Wagner, et al, Estimation of the warfarin dose with clinical and pharmacogenetic data, *N Engl J Med* 360(8) (2009) 753–764.

[79] L.C. Tavares, L.R. Marcatto, P. Santos, Genotype-guided warfarin therapy: Current status, *Pharmacogenomics* 19(7) (2018) 667–685.

6 What Is Cost-Minimisation Analysis?

Alan Haycox, MD
University of Liverpool
Liverpool, UK

TABLE OF CONTENTS

6.1   INTRODUCTION

The principal issues that are addressed in this chapter are:

1. In what circumstances is cost-minimisation analysis (CMA) an appropriate methodology to undertake health economic evaluations?
2. What steps can be taken to improve the quality of CMAs and, hence, their reliability as a basis for healthcare decision-making?

The appropriateness of any economic methodology depends on the nature and quality of the underlying clinical evidence, with evaluations based on inappropriate or poor-quality clinical data failing to provide a reliable basis for healthcare decision-making. The primacy of clinical data is particularly evident in the case of CMA in which, depending on the health benefits between two equivalent competing options, the least expensive option is preferred. Perhaps as a consequence of this apparent simplicity, scant attention has been previously paid to the theoretical and practical methods used to obtain the analysis or to establish the appropriateness of this choice of methodology.

Many sources of clinical evidence can be used to support economic analyses; however, the 'gold standard' is normally considered to be the randomised controlled trial (RCT), which holds everything constant except the drug being evaluated. Given that, by definition, the results of clinical trials cannot be known in advance, it is impossible to plan to undertake a CMA alongside an RCT because it is not certain that the health outcomes being compared will be equivalent [1]. Therefore, no prospective economic evaluation starts out as a CMA; only when the health outcomes generated are empirically demonstrated to be 'identical or similar' will the CMA be adopted as an appropriate methodology by the Health Economist.

CMA is frequently portrayed as being the 'poor relation' amongst health economic methodologies, with its apparent simplicity making it 'unworthy' of being considered alongside more theoretically rigorous health economic methodologies. However, it is important that Health Economists recognise and acknowledge that the theoretical underpinnings of CMA are just as rigorous as those underpinning other methods of economic evaluation. Perhaps as a consequence of the comparative disdain in which CMA has been held, its use to date appears to have been poorly conceived and frequently inappropriate. In this regard, CMA has been frequently employed as an evaluative tool to support and justify the introduction of cheaper, but potentially less effective, treatments. The 'normal' procedure is for the analyst to simply assume that the benefits of a new health technology are equivalent to the existing 'gold standard' therapy without having sufficient evidence to justify such a claim. For example, by assuming a 'class effect' for similar types of drugs (each drug in a class having equivalent outcomes), it then becomes possible to base subsequent analysis solely on a comparison of costs—an attractive strategy if you are introducing a cheaper but less effective drug.

The methods currently used to justify equivalence in outcomes in a CMA therefore appear to be inherently flawed and indicate an urgent need to improve the theoretical rigour underlying this aspect of CMAs if they are to be taken seriously as a method of economic evaluation. The current haphazard approach leads to a situation in which CMA is typically described in health economics textbooks as a form of economic evaluation where:

> ... the decision simply revolves around the costs. [2]

This interpretation ignores the extreme rigour that should be required to ensure equivalence in health benefits prior to deciding on the appropriateness of employing CMA as an economic methodology. The crucial decision relates to the fact that CMA has been defined as being an appropriate methodology. Underpinning this decision is a detailed analysis of clinical data that convince the analyst that the interventions being compared lead to equivalent health outcomes. Only in these strictly controlled circumstances is it legitimate for CMA to concentrate on costs alone. As such, a crucial and indispensable element underpinning the decision to use CMA as an economic methodology is the need to unambiguously determine the therapeutic equivalence of competing interventions [3]. In practice, therefore, the extent to which CMA represents an appropriate methodological structure is entirely determined by the interpretation that can be placed on the available clinical evidence.

6.2   WHAT IS MEANT BY 'THERAPEUTIC EQUIVALENCE'?

The extent to which alternative healthcare technologies are sufficiently similar to justify the use of CMA is an area of theoretical uncertainty and, thus, still open to subjective interpretation, with the majority of published CMAs appearing to be based on assumptions rather than evidence of clinical equivalence. This primacy of 'hope' over 'experience' may lead to misleading recommendations being made for healthcare resource allocation.

Given this fact, it is perhaps surprising that the exact nature of the evidence base required to support therapeutic equivalence and, hence, the appropriateness of CMA as an economic methodology, has not been subjected to more intense scrutiny. CMAs are frequently based on the results of clinical trials that have attempted but failed to identify the superiority of a new drug over the existing 'gold standard' therapy. This occurs despite the obvious fact that the inability of a health intervention to prove superiority in a superiority trial (ST) in no way indicates that this necessarily implies clinical equivalence. Advances in clinical trial design have made it easier to directly compare clinical equivalence in a more meaningful manner with the development of non-inferiority (NI) trials allowing this issue to be directly addressed. Alternatively, when a trial is initially designed as an ST but such superiority remains unproven, the analysis can then be switched from superiority to NI in appropriate cases. The use of such improvements in trial design should enable CMAs to be more effectively targeted in a manner that ensures that they are only undertaken in appropriate circumstances using rigorous sources of evidence. In this manner, only CMAs that meet minimum standards with regard to clinical equivalence will be accepted; CMAs that fail to meet such criteria will be dismissed. Such an approach would enable Health Economics to gain enhanced credibility from the use of this potentially valuable economic methodology.

6.3   OPTIMIZING EVIDENCE FROM CLINICAL TRIALS

If CMAs are to form a reliable basis for healthcare decision-making, then due consideration must be given to the claims of clinical equivalence that are crucial to the adoption of the CMA methodology. The implications of adopting an inappropriate clinical trial design or misinterpreting the results of a clinical trial are often considerable:

> ... wrongly discounting treatments as ineffective will deprive patients of better care. Wrongly accepting treatments as effective exposes patients to needless risks and wastes. [4]

RCTs typically compare the gold standard existing treatment with a new intervention [5]. RCTs can be structured to evaluate superiority (ST), therapeutic equivalence (equivalence trial or ET) or therapeutic non-inferiority (NI). The trial designs differ in terms of their objectives and these differences have significant implications for the use of the CMA methodology. The greatest support for the use of CMA occurs when an ET proves that two healthcare technologies are clinically equivalent; however, there exists a myriad of 'grey' areas that may be indicative of therapeutic equivalence and, hence, require more careful analytical consideration and judgement. Such 'grey' areas are analysed in detail in the remainder of this chapter.

6.4   SOURCES OF CLINICAL TRIAL EVIDENCE

6.4.1   SUPERIORITY TRIALS

The extent to which clinical evidence can be used to inform CMAs is dependent on the design of the RCT. STs are specifically designed to show a difference in health benefits between two healthcare technologies. Typically, the primary objective of the research is to determine whether an experimental intervention is more efficacious than the established gold standard treatment. In order to identify whether or not there is a difference in health benefits between two healthcare technologies it is necessary to begin with a null hypothesis that treatment X yields the same health benefits as treatment Y.

The ST estimates the probability that the effect exists when the null hypothesis is true using the test statistic (p-value). The smaller the size of the p-value, the more likely it is that the null hypothesis is false and that a difference *does* exist between the health benefits generated by the treatments. p-Values, therefore, can statistically identify whether an effect is likely by conveying information about the probability of an incorrect inference given the observed effect but can say nothing about the size of the effect or its clinical relevance.

Newby and Hill [3] emphasize the inadequacy of using p-values obtained in STs to interpret the results of clinical trials and recommend the use of confidence intervals (CIs) and personal judgement when determining clinical equivalence before accepting or rejecting an equivalence claim.

> leaving it up to the reader to decide whether the confidence interval includes or excludes potentially clinically important differences between two treatments. If it does not exclude differences ... assume that the two drugs are not the same. [3]

When the original objective of an ST is not achieved, there is an obvious incentive to refocus the analysis to support more restricted claims of clinical equivalence. However, STs are specifically designed to demonstrate that there is, indeed, a difference and, thus, to reject the null hypothesis in favour of the alternative hypothesis (i.e., that there is a difference). In STs, it is impossible to prove that the null hypothesis is true, as the aim is to reject it by proving that the observed difference is unlikely to be commensurate with equivalent health outcomes of the competing healthcare interventions.

In CMAs, the clinical evidence from failed STs is often misinterpreted as proving that the healthcare interventions being compared are clinically equivalent. Such methodological flaws resulting from the misinterpretation of clinical trial results can also '... lead to false claims, inconsistencies and harm to patients' [6].

However, if appropriately planned for, it is possible to switch the focus of the analysis from superiority to NI in a single trial if the ST is well designed and has adequate sample size to provide evidence of health equivalence for use in CMAs.

6.4.2 Equivalence Trials

6.4.2.1 Characteristics of ETs

ETs are intended to demonstrate that the effect of a new treatment is not worse than the effect of the current treatment by more than a specified equivalence margin. The aim of an ET is, therefore, to specifically rule out significant clinical differences between the treatments by directly evaluating the extent to which two healthcare interventions have equivalent therapeutic effects. Briggs and O'Brien [7] argue that CMA should only be used when clinical evidence has been obtained from an ET. They argue that it is inappropriate to use the results of a failed ST to demonstrate clinical equivalence '... unless a study has been specifically designed to show the equivalence of treatments it would be inappropriate to conduct cost-minimisation analysis' [7].

However, even where an ET indicates clinical equivalence in primary outcomes, scrutiny of secondary outcomes may reveal significant differences in safety, cost or convenience.

> ... one therapy may offer clinical benefits such as a more convenient administration schedule, less potential for drug interaction or lower cost. [8]

Reliance on a single clinical measure of effectiveness may potentially be misleading, as it may fail to capture an important difference in health outcome between two alternatives. Thus, ideally, clinical equivalence should be established for a range of health outcomes before the use of CMA can be supported. In addition, in evaluating claims of clinical equivalence it is important to acknowledge that:

> It is never correct to claim that ... there is no difference in effects of treatments ... There will always be some uncertainty surrounding estimates of treatment effects, and a small difference can never be excluded. [9]

Even if one compared a drug with itself, there may be a difference; therefore, it cannot be unequivocally claimed that two healthcare technologies are clinically equivalent. Thus, even where the results of ETs indicate no difference, this may simply indicate that the true difference exists outside of the specified probabilities of error.

If clinical equivalence is demonstrated in a good-quality ET, there remain two other issues that must be addressed prior to unambiguously supporting the use of the cost-minimisation approach. Firstly, the primary health outcome must encompass the main benefit(s) of the treatments being compared. Secondly, any differences in other health outcomes, for example, secondary health outcomes, must be sufficiently small so as not to attain clinical significance. If these assumptions cannot be substantiated, then it would not be appropriate to adopt the CMA approach despite the availability of equivalence obtained in an ET.

6.4.3   EQUIVALENCE RANGE/MARGIN

A crucial step in the design of an ET is the definition of clinical equivalence. The equivalence margin attempts to incorporate all values that represent unimportant clinical differences in treatment and must be stipulated in advance of the clinical trial. The equivalence range, therefore, includes the largest difference between treatments that is clinically acceptable before treatments become defined as providing significantly different benefits. The first step in any ET is, therefore, to define the smallest unacceptable degree of inferiority/superiority to ensure that the ET can be appropriately powered. For example:

> ... if the difference between the two groups in respect of change in pulmonary function was within ± 1.5 units, then the treatments would be considered clinically equivalent. [11]

This means that if treatment A is better or worse than treatment B by more than a 1.5 unit change in pulmonary function, then the two treatments cannot be considered to be clinically equivalent. Clinical equivalence can be claimed if the 95% CI around the difference in treatments is found to lie entirely within the pre-determined clinical equivalence margin. The setting of the equivalence margin communicates a judgement about what is and what is not clinically and statistically acceptable [12].

Clearly, different clinical situations require different equivalence margins and analysts must justify their chosen range with regard to clinician's opinion and previous trials comparing active controls with placebo. An equivalence margin that is too wide could mean that significantly different treatments are considered to be clinically equivalent; conversely an equivalence margin that is too narrow could mean that clinically equivalent treatments are mislabelled as being significantly different. It is important that good clinical judgement be combined with sound clinical and statistical reasoning to ensure that the chosen margin is clinically relevant and statistically feasible.

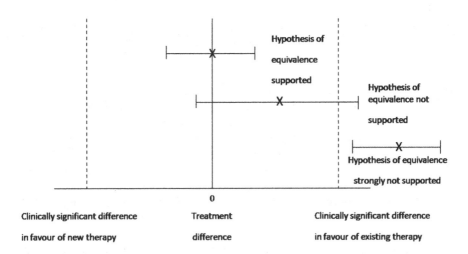

FIGURE 6.1 Interpretation of equivalence trials.

A negative study result from an ET can take two forms. The CI around the treatment difference may lie partially within the equivalence margin or it can lie entirely outside, leading to the conclusion that the probability of a difference between the two treatments has not been rejected (see Figure 6.1).

6.5 NI TRIALS

6.5.1 CHARACTERISTICS OF AN NI TRIAL

The rationale behind an NI trial is to demonstrate that the new healthcare technology is not worse than the current healthcare technology by a pre-stated clinical margin. This type of trial is useful when the clinical issue relates to the extent to which the new healthcare technology is as good as the current therapy. In NI trials, analysis is focussed entirely in one direction—typically the new treatment is not worse than the established therapy by more than the specified non-inferiority margin. An improvement of any size fits within the definition of non-inferiority. Span et al. published the first paper that acknowledged the link between CMA and NI trials:

> ... the most efficient analysis of the clinical effect in a cost minimisation study is the non-inferiority analysis. [13]

They conclude that: '... to obtain valid results from a cost-minimisation study, care has to be taken to adapt the correct methodology for non-inferiority testing in clinical outcomes'.

To ensure a robust interpretation of trial results, some analysts call for both per protocol and intention to treat analyses to be conducted, and only if both types of analyses support the hypothesis should non-inferiority be claimed [14]. Therefore, the extent and nature of the evidence of non-inferiority that is required to provide an acceptable platform on which to base a CMA is still open to debate.

6.5.2   NON-INFERIORITY RANGE/MARGIN

The non-inferiority range should be set in relation to the clinical notion of a minimally important effect, a notion akin to the minimally important difference in clinical studies (see Chapter 12). An acceptable non-inferiority margin depends on defining a difference that has previously been identified as being not clinically significant. To do this, two additional conditions must be met. Firstly, the smallest expected effect of the active control over placebo must exceed this margin to ensure that no positively harmful treatments can be introduced and, secondly, the margin must be no greater than the difference between active treatments judged clinically important.

In an NI trial, non-inferiority is demonstrated when the CI around the treatment difference lies entirely to the right of the lower bound of the non-inferiority margin. Non-inferiority is not demonstrated if the lower bound of the CI lies to the left of the non-inferiority margin (see Figure 6.2).

6.6   OTHER ISSUES TO BE ADDRESSED IN EVALUATING 'EQUIVALENCE'

6.6.1   STATISTICAL VERSUS CLINICAL SIGNIFICANCE

One of the failings of statistical analyses undertaken in the context of an ST is that statistical significance may differ from clinical significance. Variables that

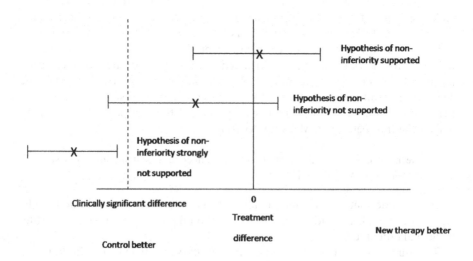

FIGURE 6.2 Interpreting NI trials using CIs.

are identified as exhibiting statistically significant differences may be entirely unimportant from a clinical perspective, whereas clinically crucial differences remain crucial even if they fail to achieve statistical significance. In contrast, in ETs and NI trials, statistical and clinical significance are inextricably linked via the setting of equivalence and non-inferiority margins.

6.6.2 EQUIVALENCE IN SINGLE OR MULTIPLE OUTCOMES?

In any clinical trial it is necessary to identify a primary health outcome that is common to the competing alternative interventions. Choice and measurement of such an outcome measure is a crucial step in determining the appropriateness of the trial as an evidence source on which to undertake CMAs. To be of value, the primary health outcome must be the dominant outcome from the perspective of both patients and clinicians and capture the most clinically relevant benefits of the competing treatments. If not, then the claims of clinical equivalence, even when based on ETs, are not sufficient to support the use of CMA.

In clinical practice it is highly unlikely that two healthcare interventions will yield exactly the same health benefits in all dimensions of clinical and patient outcomes. Typically, the design of ETs and NI trials identifies a single endpoint for comparison despite the perception that one of the treatments is likely to offer significant advantages in another area. For example, where two treatments have equal efficacy, yet one is more convenient to patients, the extent to which CMA can be appropriately utilized depends largely on the perspective adopted by the analysis. Where equivalence is not demonstrated for all important outcomes, the analyst must provide explicit justification for using the cost-minimisation approach in light of the study question and perspective. In large part, the interpretation of clinical equivalence will depend on the specific circumstances of the clinical trial, the range of outcomes being measured and the judgement of the analyst. In such cases it is difficult to provide specific guidance that would be appropriate in all cases.

6.6.3 WHOSE VIEWS OF CLINICAL EQUIVALENCE SHOULD BE PRE-EMINENT?

Definitions of clinical equivalence will depend on whose views we consider to be the most important (patients, clinicians or society). Generally, lead investigators in clinical trials specify the primary and secondary health outcomes to be measured, with the identification of the primary outcome measure being based on relevant clinical experience, published clinical evidence and knowledge of patient needs. The crucial factor is to ensure that the choice of health outcome measures used to determine clinical equivalence is clinically meaningful to the patient.

6.6.4 OVER WHAT PERIOD SHOULD WE EVALUATE CLINICAL EQUIVALENCE?

The benefits of healthcare technologies will vary in relation to the time point at which they are measured. In a clinical trial, the primary health outcome measure might exhibit statistically significant differences at three months but not at six or twelve months. In such circumstances, do we interpret the therapeutic interventions as being equivalent and, hence, appropriate for analysis in the context of a CMA? It is important to acknowledge that clinical equivalence is a dynamic rather than a static concept and that any demonstration of clinical equivalence is likely to be sustained over time.

6.7   EFFECTIVELY TARGETING THE USE OF CMA

The current use of RCT evidence to support statements of clinical equivalence is inadequate, and clear and appropriate decision rules are required in the future to ensure that unambiguous evidence of clinical equivalence is a feature of future CMAs. In the absence of such evidence it would be potentially misleading to use flawed analyses as the basis for healthcare decision-making. While it is comparatively simplistic to identify circumstances in which the use of CMA as an economic methodology is clearly inappropriate, it is more difficult to specify unambiguous decision rules that identify circumstances in which clinical evidence clearly supports the use of CMA. The appropriateness of using CMA must be judged in the light of the totality of the clinical evidence supporting or refuting the hypothesis of therapeutic equivalence between two competing interventions, combined with the specialist knowledge and expertise required to place such evidence in context. However, certain limited guidance can be provided with regard to effectively targeting CMAs.

Firstly, clinical evidence from a well-designed ET represents the gold standard in supporting claims of clinical equivalence in support of the use of CMA. However, even where data are available from an ET, it still remains important to consider the extent to which the primary health outcome fully captures the benefits being derived from the healthcare treatments being compared. If other benefits are clinically meaningful to patients and clinicians, additional comparisons of clinical equivalence may be required.

Secondly, failure to prove clinical superiority should not be interpreted as providing evidence of clinical equivalence. In certain circumstances, and if planned into trial design, trial data may be reanalysed to assess clinical equivalence, but such reinterpretation of the data set requires further analysis if the use of CMA is to be justified. In particular, a non-inferiority statement should be stipulated in the clinical trial protocol to ensure that valuable information can still be derived even if superiority is not proven.

Thirdly, the extent to which data from NI trials can be used to justify CMAs is currently subject to a great amount of uncertainty. In particular, to what extent proof of non-inferiority represents an acceptable approximation of 'therapeutic equivalence' and, hence, justifies the use of CMAs, is still open to debate.

Finally, where CMAs are based on valid claims of clinical equivalence derived from appropriate sources of RCT evidence it represents an appropriate and powerful method of economic evaluation. However, it is crucial that in interpreting the results of CMAs, the informed decision-maker uses his/her clinical judgement to assess the quality and quantity of the evidence in support of therapeutic equivalence and, hence, identifies the theoretical justification for the use of CMA. In cases where the decision maker does not accept claims of clinical equivalence, the results of the CMA should clearly not be used as the basis for their decision-making.

6.8 CONCLUSIONS

The cost-minimisation method of economic evaluation has always been employed in a more haphazard manner than other methods of economic evaluation. It is crucial to rectify this situation to ensure that only techniques that prove to be robust and reliable in improving healthcare decision-making are incorporated into the toolkit employed by the Health Economist. However, exactly how 'similar' do outcomes have to be to support the application of this powerful economic methodology? The most appropriate design for a clinical trial to generate evidence that two healthcare technologies are 'identical or similar' is the ET. Such trials are specifically designed for this purpose and, therefore, any differences that are identified between the health interventions being compared are neither clinically nor statistically significant.

It is essential that Health Economists and decision makers are clear on what is meant by the concept of clinical equivalence and to acknowledge that, given the heterogeneous nature of patient populations and treatment outcomes, it is likely to prove impossible to achieve exact equivalence between competing healthcare interventions. Ultimately, it is up to the Health Economist to justify the use of CMA just as it is up to the decision maker to judge the extent to which the results obtained should be influential in determining their decision-making.

REFERENCES

[1] C. Donaldson, V. Hundley, E. McIntosh, Using economics alongside clinical trials: Why we cannot choose the evaluation technique in advance, *Health Economics Letters* 5 (1996) 267–9.

[2] M. Gold, J. Siegel, L. Russell, M. Weinstein, *Cost-effectiveness in health and medicine*, Oxford University Press, New York, 1996.

[3] D. Newby, S. Hill, Use of pharmacoeconomics in prescribing research. Part 2: Cost-minimization analysis–when are two therapies equal?, *Journal of Clinical Pharmacy & Therapeutics* 28 (2) (2003) 145–50.

[4] W. Tarnow-Mordi, M. Healy, Distinguishing between 'no evidence of effect' and 'evidence of no effect' in randomised controlled trials and other comparisons, *Archives of Disease in Childhood* 80 (1999) 210–11.

[5] M. Tramer, R. Reynolds, A. Moore, H. McQuay, When placebo controlled trials are essential and equivalence trials are inadequate, *British Medical Journal* 317 (1998) 875–80.

[6] W.L. Greene, J. Concato, A.R. Feinstein, Claims on equivalence in medical research: Are they supported by the evidence?, *Annals of Internal Medicine* 132 (2000) 715–22.

[7] A.H. Briggs, B.J. O'Brien, The death of cost-minimization analysis?, *Health Economics* 10 (2) (2001) 179–84.

[8] R. Hatala, A. Holbrook, C.H. Goldsmith, Therapeutic equivalence: All studies are not created equal, *The Canadian Journal of Clinical Pharmacology* 6 (1) (1999) 9–11.

[9] P. Alderson, I. Chalmers, Survey of claims of no effect in abstracts of Cochrane reviews, *British Medical Journal* 326 (2003) 475.

[11] L. Huson, Statistical assessment of superiority, equivalence and non-inferiority in clinical trials, *CR Focus* 12 (5) (2004) 1–4.

[12] C. Pater, Equivalence and non-inferiority trials – Are they viable alternatives for the registration of new drugs? (III), *Current Controlled Trials in Cardiovascular Medicine* 5 (8) (2004) 1–7.

[13] M. Span, E. TenVergert, S. van der Hilst, R. Stolk, Noninferiority testing in cost-minimization studies: Practical issues concerning power analysis, *International Journal of Technology Assessment in Healthcare* 22 (2) (2006) 261-6.

[14] S. Snappinn, Noninferiority trials, *Current Controlled Trials in Cardiovascular Medicine* 1 (2000) 19–21.

7 Cost-Effectiveness Analysis

Ken Smith, MD, MS
University of Pittsburgh
Pittsburgh, PA, USA

Mark S. Roberts, MD, MPP
University of Pittsburgh
Pittsburgh, PA, USA

TABLE OF CONTENTS

7.1 THE RATIONALE FOR COST-EFFECTIVENESS ANALYSIS

As noted in prior chapters, the economic evaluation of pharmacotherapies and other healthcare interventions is growing in importance as the resources directed toward health care account for progressively larger portions of the budgets of governments, employers, and individuals. Making rational decisions under conditions of resource constraints requires a method for comparing alternatives across a range of outcomes that allow a direct ranking of the costs and benefits of specific strategies for preventing or treating a particular illness.

Cost-effectiveness analysis (CEA) provides a framework to compare two or more decision options by examining the ratio of the differences in costs and the differences in health effectiveness between options. The overall goal of CEA is to provide a single measure, the *incremental cost-effectiveness ratio (ICER)*, which relates the amount of benefit derived by making an alternative treatment choice to the differential cost of that option. When two options are being compared, the ICER is calculated by the formula:

$$\frac{C_{Option\ 2} - C_{Option\ 1}}{Effectiveness_{Option\ 2} - Effectiveness_{Option\ 1}}$$

In medical or pharmacoeconomic CEA, health resource costs (the numerator) are in monetary terms, representing the difference in costs between choosing option 1 or option 2. In CEA, the differential benefits of the various options (the denominator) are nonmonetary terms and represent the change in health effectiveness values implied by choosing option 1 over option 2. Typically, these health outcomes are measured as lives saved, life years gained, illness events avoided, or a variety of other clinical or health outcomes. Unlike CEA, cost-benefit analysis values both the costs and benefits of interventions in monetary terms. Cost-utility analysis, a subset of CEA where intervention effectiveness is adjusted based on the desirability (or utility) of the resulting health states, is discussed in Chapter 4.

7.2   THE COST-EFFECTIVENESS PLANE

A pharmacoeconomic analysis is often interested in how much more of a health outcome can be obtained for a given financial expenditure. Limited resources may, many times, constrain choices between medical options. The cost-effectiveness plane serves to clarify when these choices may be easy or difficult [1]. It is typically drawn with the differences in cost (or the incremental cost) on the *y*-axis and the differences in effectiveness (or incremental effectiveness) between the two options on the *x*-axis (Figure 7.1). In this example, we will compare an existing program to a new program. The existing program, acting as the comparator, will be at the origin of both the cost and effectiveness axes, depicting the current level of expenditure and benefit to which a new therapy is compared. The new therapy can be more expensive, less expensive, or equivalent in costs to the current option. Similarly, the new

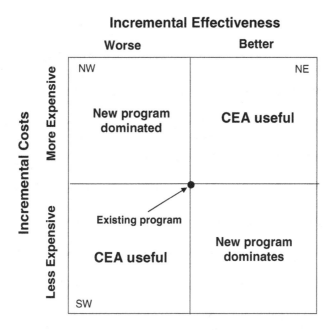

FIGURE 7.1   The cost-effectiveness plane.

option can be more effective, less effective, or equivalent in clinical effectiveness as compared with the existing strategy or therapy.

This produces four possible options for the results of the analysis of a new strategy compared to an existing one. If the new program is less expensive and more effective than the existing program, then the point representing the new program falls into the southeast (SE) quadrant of the cost-effectiveness plane. Points in this quadrant are called *dominant*, and strategies that have such a characteristic should be chosen over the existing strategy due to their superior outcome at diminished costs. These strategies are "cheaper and better" than current therapy and should be adopted. Examples of strategies in this quadrant are laparoscopic cholecystectomy compared to other therapies for symptomatic gallstones [2, 3] or interventions to decrease cigarette smoking [4, 5].

If, in contrast, the new program is more expensive and less effective than the existing one, this program falls into the northwest quadrant (NW) of the plane. Strategies in this quadrant are considered to be *dominated* by the current strategy and should not be chosen due to poorer outcomes at greater cost. Although existing strategies in this quadrant are perhaps relatively rare, there are examples of strategies that do not appear to derive a benefit, yet incur substantially more healthcare costs than other options. Examples include amoxicillin prophylaxis compared to no antibiotic for dental procedures in patients at moderate risk for infective endocarditis [6], and magnetic resonance imaging vs. endocrinologic follow-up of patients with asymptomatic pituitary microadenomas [7].

If the new program is either dominant or dominated (i.e., in the SE or NW quadrants), a formal CEA is not needed to assist the decision – the decision is (or should be) obvious. However, if the new program is both more effective and more costly, falling in the northeast (NE) quadrant, then a CEA would be useful to define the trade-off between increases in costs and effectiveness and to calculate the cost per unit of effectiveness gained. Similarly, a CEA would also be useful if the new strategy fell into the SW quadrant as being both less costly and less effective than the existing program, once again to define the trade-offs between programs and to ascertain the cost-effectiveness ratio. This graphical display emphasizes one of the most fundamental and important concepts of CEA: it is only useful when there is a trade-off between the cost of a strategy and the benefit derived from that strategy.

7.3   BASIC COMPONENTS OF A CEA

Several factors should be considered in the construction of a CEA (Table 7.1) A high-quality analysis will include and describe the relevant options, clearly state the perspective of the analysis, choose a relevant time horizon over which to track costs and effects, consider the appropriate population, accurately measure the costs and effectiveness of the competing options, account for the differential value of costs and outcomes that occur at different times in the future, and account for uncertainties of assumptions and values in the context of an appropriately constructed analytic model. These concepts are described in more detail later.

7.3.1   ENUMERATION OF THE OPTIONS

A CEA requires a comparison between two or more options. A single option cannot be cost-effective in isolation – an option can be considered cost-effective

---

TABLE 7.1

Basic Components of a CEA

Component	Examples
Options/comparisons	Existing program compared to new program
Perspective of the analysis	Societal, health system, patient
Time horizon	1 month, 5 years, lifetime
Scope of the analysis	Population affected, inclusion (or not) of secondary or collateral effects
Measuring and valuing costs	Cost categories included in the analysis are determined by the perspective taken
Measuring and valuing outcomes	Life years saved, illnesses avoided, cases found
Time preference	Discounting future costs and effectiveness
Analytic models	Clinical trial data, decision analysis model
Accounting for uncertainty	Sensitivity analysis

or not cost-effective only in comparison to other options. Additionally, the cost-effectiveness of a strategy is highly dependent upon the specific choice of comparators included in the analysis and care must be taken to include all clinically reasonable options. At a minimum, the comparators include the current standard of care and a range of typically utilized options. A CEA of a new therapy compared to a strategy that is not typically used, or is only used in atypical circumstances, is not useful for clinicians or policy makers. It is often reasonable to include a "do nothing" option, especially if doing nothing is a legitimate clinical strategy, but also as a baseline comparator to assess the clinical realism of the model and analysis. In all cases, the strategies should be described in sufficient detail such that the reader could replicate or implement the strategy in their own setting.

7.3.2 Perspective of the Analysis

Choosing the perspective or set of perspectives to be considered in a CEA is essential, since this choice determines the cost values to be contained in the analysis. For example, an analysis from the societal perspective considers all costs, while an analysis from the patient perspective would only consider costs borne by the patient. Other possible perspectives include the third-party payer (insurance) or health system perspective where costs for which these entities are responsible are considered in the analysis; the hospital or health agency perspective includes the costs of providing various health services. Whenever possible, the societal perspective should be included in the set of perspectives to be considered in analysis, since it is the broadest and is recommended for the reference case analysis by the Panel on Cost-Effectiveness in Health and Medicine, although the most recent edition of the book developed based on this panel recommends also including the third-party perspective [8–10].

7.3.3 Time Horizon

The analyst must decide *a priori* how long the costs and effects of the various interventions in the analysis will be tracked. This is usually determined by the clinical features of the illness or its treatment. For example, a CEA of a new antibiotic for acute dysuria treatment in otherwise healthy women might appropriately have a very short time horizon of only a month, as there are virtually no long-term effects of either the disease or its treatments. On the other hand, CEAs designed to value the effects of cardiovascular risk reduction need to assess the outcomes for much longer time periods; typically, such an analysis would follow treatments and effects until death. In any case, all strategies must be followed and/or modeled for the same time horizon. Methods for modeling costs and effects, even in situations where this modeling extends beyond the existence of specific data, are provided in Chapters 2, 4, 6, 7, 9, and 10.

7.3.4 Scope of the Analysis

An analysis might be relevant for an entire population or for only a relatively small population subgroup; the analyst will need to appropriately choose the cohort to be considered in the analysis. For example, if an intervention is to be directed toward elderly patients with diabetes in order to prevent diabetes complications, limiting the scope of the analysis to an elderly, diabetic population is a logical choice, while if the question is regarding diabetes prevention in adults, a broader population scope is required. The scope of outcomes to be considered is another important consideration. In the example above, a broad or narrow range of diabetes outcomes could be considered in an analysis of elderly diabetics. If a small number of complications is modeled, the data requirements of the model would be less but the conclusions might be limited compared to a model with a broader range of complications considered. However, a more comprehensive model would have greater data needs and require more complex model construction. Choosing the scope of an analysis often means finding a balance between simplicity and complexity, frequently determined by the clinical situation modeled and the question to be examined.

7.3.5   Measuring and Valuing Costs

Data sources for costs must be found and incorporated into the analysis. Cost data can be obtained from clinical trials, but more often other sources will need to be utilized. In addition, the analyst will need to choose between micro-costing or macro-costing methodologies or some mix of the two, often based on the perspective taken in the analysis [8, 9]. Micro-costing enumerates and identifies each item that is incorporated into a particular service, requiring detailed data on supplies used, personnel, room, and instrument costs, and often needing time-and-motion studies to accurately capture medical service costs. Macro-costing (or gross costing) uses data, often from large government databases, to estimate average costs for a care episode, for example, the average cost of coronary artery bypass grafting or of a hospital stay for pneumonia. In the United States, Medicare reimbursement data or the Healthcare Cost and Utilization Project (HCUP) database are often used for this purpose. Further detail on cost estimation can be found in Chapter 3.

7.3.6   Measuring and Valuing Outcomes

The effectiveness outcome for the analysis must be chosen and outcomes data found, often based on data availability. Randomized trials are excellent data sources on the effects of therapies, but study entrance criteria frequently limit applicability to a more general patient population (see Chapter 5 for more on this). Cohort studies are useful for risk factor determination and for determining the natural history of an illness. Administrative databases are excellent sources for broad population-based estimates of disease and for the effectiveness of therapies, unlike randomized trials which, in general, estimate efficacy. However, administrative databases often pose difficulties in accounting for possible confounding variables in the data set (see Chapter 5). Meta-analyses provide summary measures for parameters, but studies considered are generally limited to randomized trials, thus limiting generalizability. The perspective of the analysis may also influence the effectiveness outcome chosen. Life years or quality-adjusted life years (QALYs) gained are certainly relevant for analyses using the relatively broad-based societal or health system perspectives, but may not be as important when a narrower perspective is chosen, such as that of an individual hospital, when effectiveness measures such as bed day saved or drug administration error avoided might be more relevant.

7.3.7 TIME PREFERENCE

The differential timing of costs and outcomes should be considered in the analysis. This is typically accomplished through the use of discount rates, where costs and outcomes that occur in the present have higher values than those in the future (see Chapter 11).

7.3.8 CHOICE OF ANALYTIC MODELING METHOD

The analytic model must also be selected. Cost data from clinical trials can allow relatively straightforward calculation of ICERs between management options, often the intervention arms of the clinical trial. More often, data for the analysis must come from a variety of sources (see Chapter 5) and may require a decision analysis model as a framework for data synthesis.

7.3.9 ACCOUNTING FOR UNCERTAINTY

Finally, a sensitivity analysis to elucidate the effects of uncertainty on model results should be performed. There are many goals of sensitivity analysis, and methods for conducting such analyses are detailed in Chapter 13. During model construction and validation, sensitivity analysis is useful as a "debugging tool" to assure that the model behaves as it was designed to behave. After the model is finished, sensitivity analysis is useful to determine which variables have a large impact on the outcomes. Sensitivity analyses can be used to determine the cost-effectiveness ratio in specified subgroups of an analysis, as well as to determine how much a change in one variable will alter the cost-effectiveness ratio. Finally, probabilistic sensitivity analyses (described in Chapter 13) can be used to produce a version of a confidence limit or probability range around the cost-effectiveness ratio.

7.4 CALCULATION OF ICERS

The ICER requires a detailed enumeration of the costs and benefits of the strategies being compared. Methods for measuring and estimating the costs and benefits of strategies and interventions are often quite complicated, and are detailed in Chapters 3 and 4. In this section, we use the results of two existing pharmacoeconomic studies to illustrate the calculation and use of the ICER. Details of the enumeration of costs and outcomes in these studies are detailed in the studies themselves [11, 12].

TABLE 7.2

Cost-effectiveness of LMWH Compared to Warfarin for the Secondary Prevention of Venous Thromboembolism

Strategy	Cost	Life Expectancy (yrs)	Incremental Cost	Incremental Effectiveness	Incremental Cost-Effectiveness Ratio
Warfarin	$7,720	1.377	—	—	—
LMWH	$15,329	1.442	$7,609	0.066	$115,847

The following example considers low-molecular-weight heparin (LMWH) compared to warfarin for the secondary prevention of venous thromboembolism in patients with cancer. Aujesky [11] used a decision analysis model and data from a variety of sources to estimate the incremental cost-effectiveness of two anticoagulant regimens. Analysis results, with effectiveness in life years, are outlined in Table 7.2.

Typically, the first step in calculation of ICERs among mutually exclusive options is to order the options by cost. LMWH is both more costly and more effective than warfarin, thus, neither strategy is dominant or dominated, and a CEA would be useful. Subtracting the cost of the warfarin strategy from that of the LMWH strategy produces the incremental cost; the difference in life expectancy between strategies is the incremental effectiveness. Dividing the incremental cost by the incremental effectiveness produces the ICER, $115,847 per life year gained, the unit cost of an additional life year occurring as a result of LMWH rather than warfarin use.

7.4.1 Dominance and Extended Dominance

Calculation of the ICER can be more complicated when more than two strategies are being considered. One of the complicating characteristics of the analysis of many options is that some strategies may be dominated by others and should be removed from further analysis. As noted above in the description of the cost-effectiveness plane, any strategy that is more expensive and less effective than an existing option for the same illness (e.g., as in the left upper quadrant compared to the existing strategy) is said to be strictly dominated: one would never choose such a strategy when an alternative would produce a better outcome at a cheaper price. Strict dominance is also termed strong dominance by some authors. A second type of dominance occurs when a particular strategy is more expensive and less effective than a linear *combination* of two other strategies. This is called *extended dominance*, and represents a situation where one could achieve a better outcome at less cost by treating a proportion of the population with a combination of two alternative strategies. Extended dominance can also be referred to as weak dominance. We illustrate both types of dominance in the following example.

Using a decision analysis model, the authors [12] performed a CEA of testing and antiviral treatment strategies for adult influenza, using days of influenza illness avoided as an effectiveness term in the analysis. Cost and effectiveness values estimated by this analysis are shown in Table 7.3. (Please note that in a separate analysis the other neuraminidase inhibitor, oseltamivir, was substituted for zanamivir, with similar cost-effectiveness results.) Once again, the first step in calculation of ICERs among mutually exclusive options is to order the options by cost. Doing so with these data will result in Table 7.4. Next, options of lesser effectiveness and of equal or greater cost than another option are removed due to strict, or strong, dominance. These strictly dominated options, which are inferior both in terms of cost and effectiveness, do not need to be considered further in the analysis [13]. In this example, "Testing, then amantadine" costs more and is less effective than "Amantadine (without testing)." Thus "Testing, then amantadine" is strictly dominated and can be removed from consideration. Similarly, "Testing, then rimantadine" also costs more and is less effective than the "Amantadine" strategy and the "rimantadine (without testing)" strategy and, thus, can be eliminated due to strict dominance. The results after the removal of these two strategies are shown in Table 7.5.

TABLE 7.3
Cost and Effectiveness Values for Influenza Management Strategies

Strategy	Cost	Illness Days Avoided
No testing or treatment	$92.70	0
Amantadine	$97.50	0.54
Rimantadine	$119.10	0.59
Zanamivir	$137.10	0.74
Testing, then amantadine	$115.00	0.44
Testing, then rimantadine	$125.50	0.48
Testing, then zanamivir	$134.30	0.60

TABLE 7.4
Strategies Ordered by Cost

Strategy	Cost	Illness Days Avoided
No testing or treatment	$92.70	0
Amantadine	$97.50	0.54
Testing, then amantadine	$115.00	0.44
Rimantadine	$119.10	0.59
Testing, then rimantadine	$125.50	0.48
Testing, then zanamivir	$134.30	0.60
Zanamivir	$137.10	0.74

TABLE 7.5

Remaining Strategies When Strictly Dominated Strategies Are Removed

Strategy	Cost	Illness Days Avoided
No testing or treatment	$92.70	0
Amantadine	$97.50	0.54
Rimantadine	$119.10	0.59
Testing, then zanamivir	$134.30	0.60
Zanamivir	$137.10	0.74

Then, starting with the second row, the differences in cost and effectiveness between that row and the preceding row are calculated. These results are the incremental cost and incremental effectiveness between the two adjacent strategies. The incremental cost divided by the incremental effectiveness produces the ICER, the cost per illness day prevented. This same procedure is then followed for the remaining rows in Table 7.6.

Next, the calculated ICERs are examined for extended, or weak, dominance of strategies [14]. This occurs when the ICER of a strategy is greater than the strategy below it, signifying that the subsequent strategy would be preferred. In this case, both "rimantadine" and "Test/zanamivir" have higher ICERs than zanamivir; thus, these strategies would not be preferred over zanamivir due to extended dominance and can be removed from consideration. Removing these strategies from the table and recalculating the ICER of zanamivir compared to Amantadine results in Table 7.7.

This same procedure can be performed graphically using the cost-effectiveness plane [8]. Figure 7.2 depicts all the testing and treatment strategies on the cost-effectiveness plane. Starting with "No testing or treatment," the least costly option, a line is drawn to the strategy that produces the shallowest slope (i.e., the smallest ICER), which is "Amantadine." From Amantadine, the shallowest

TABLE 7.6

Calculation of the ICER

Strategy	Cost	Illness Days Avoided	Incremental Cost	Incremental Effectiveness	ICER
No testing or treatment	$92.70	0	—	—	—
Amantadine	$97.50	0.54	$4.90	0.54	$9.06
Rimantadine	$119.10	0.59	$21.50	0.05	$430.00
Test/zanamivir	$134.30	0.60	$15.20	0.01	$1520.00
Zanamivir	$137.10	0.74	$2.80	0.14	$20.00

TABLE 7.7

Removal of Strategies Due to Extended Dominance

Strategy	Cost	Illness Days Avoided	Incremental Cost	Incremental Effectiveness	ICER
No testing or treatment	$92.70	0	—	—	—
Amantadine	$97.50	0.54	$4.90	0.54	$9.06
Zanamivir	$137.10	0.74	$39.60	0.20	$198.00

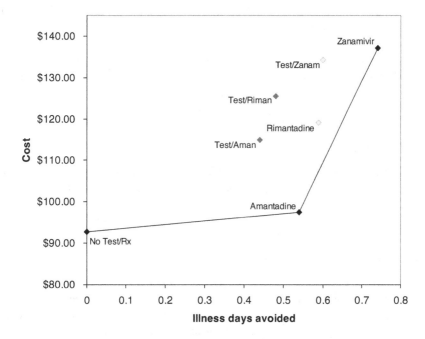

FIGURE 7.2 Cost and effectiveness values for influenza management strategies plotted on the cost-effectiveness plane. The line represents the cost-effectiveness efficient frontier, red points denote strategies that are strictly dominated, and open points show strategies that are eliminated from consideration by extended dominance.

positive slope is to zanamivir. The resulting line is the cost-effectiveness efficient frontier; any point not on this frontier is dominated, either by strict dominance or extended dominance, as illustrated by the "Testing" strategies and by the "rimantadine" strategy.

All reasonable strategies should be included in CEAs so that true ICERs can be calculated. For example, if the Amantadine strategy was omitted from the analysis above, the ICER of zanamivir would be $60 per illness day avoided when compared to "No testing or treatment" rather than $198 when compared to Amantadine. Omitting Amantadine would not give a true picture of the incremental value of zanamivir, that is, it would not tell us how much more would be paid for the gains in effectiveness seen with zanamivir compared to all other reasonable strategies [8].

Similar considerations apply to the average cost-effectiveness ratio, here the cost divided by the illness days avoided; for example, the average cost-effectiveness ratio for zanamivir is $137.1/0.74 or $185.27 per illness day avoided. When comparing mutually exclusive strategies, as we are in this example, the absence of incremental comparisons between strategies in the average cost-effectiveness calculation does not allow for elimination of dominated strategies or for calculation of incremental gains and costs between strategies [8]. The average cost-effectiveness ratio is useful, however, in the evaluation of mutually compatible programs that are subject to a budget constraint, where programs are ranked, lowest to highest, by average cost-effectiveness ratio, then funded in that order until the budget is exhausted (see Chapter 8 on Budgetary Impact Analysis). Use of the average cost-effectiveness ratio in this fashion would maximize the health benefits for a given monetary expenditure; however, its use for this purpose has been largely theoretical to this point.

7.4.2 SENSITIVITY ANALYSIS

The next step in a CEA is the performance of sensitivity analyses. Typically, univariate, or one-way, sensitivity analyses are performed on parameter values, and further multiple parameter sensitivity analyses may also be performed. Further consideration of sensitivity analysis issues can be found in Chapter 13.

7.4.3 INTERPRETATION OF CEA RESULTS

To reiterate a prior point, CEA hinges on comparisons between strategies. A single option alone cannot be cost-effective; options can only be cost-effective compared to other options. The relative cost-effectiveness of one option compared to another is subject to interpretation and, perhaps as a result, the term "cost-effective" has been misused (although perhaps less so now than in the past, due to increasing familiarity with the true meaning of the term) [15]. Cost-effective does not necessarily mean cost saving. New health programs that are less costly and more effective than existing programs are clearly good buys, but a new program that costs more and is more effective than the existing program can be cost-effective without costs being saved, depending on how much is willing to be paid for a given health benefit. Cost-effective has also been incorrectly used to mean cost saving when no determination of effectiveness differences between options has been performed: buying health insurance from one carrier that costs less than insurance from another carrier is not making a cost-effective decision when there is no comparison of health benefits between insurance plans; this would be a cost-minimisation evaluation (see Chapter 6). Similarly, "cost-effective" has been misused to mean "effective" when there is no cost comparison. The correct meaning of "cost-effective" is that a program or a strategy is worth the added cost because of the benefit it adds compared to other interventions. The application of the method requires a determination of the value of healthcare benefits as well as costs.

Returning to our influenza example, how can one interpret the ICERs of the amantadine and zanamivir strategies? One of the first steps in interpreting CEAs is to understand what cost-effectiveness cannot do. It cannot make the "correct" choice; instead, it provides an analysis of the consequences of each choice. CEA is not designed to address the social, political, or legal issues that might arise from a medical decision. Thus, if differing strategies involve questions of equity, social justice, legal responsibilities, or public opinion that need to be weighed in making a medical decision, consideration of cost-effectiveness, more than strategy, is necessary. Cost-effectiveness is one of many aspects of a decision to be considered and interpreted by decision makers, be they physicians in the care of an individual patient or health policy makers in a broader population-based medical care context [8].

Let us assume for now that sociopolitical issues are similar between our example strategies, allowing us to concentrate on the cost-effectiveness results as a major basis for the decision. In this case the question is: which strategy should we choose based on the ICERs calculated for each strategy? Or more bluntly, which strategy is the most "cost-effective?" The answer depends on the willingness-to-pay per unit health outcome (here, per illness day avoided). If the willingness-to-pay is less than $9 per illness day avoided, then "No testing or treatment" would be chosen, since the ICERs of the other strategies are greater than or equal to $9 per illness day. If willingness-to-pay thresholds are higher, other strategies would be chosen: amantadine is chosen if the willingness-to-pay is $9–$197, and zanamivir is chosen if the willingness-to-pay is greater than or equal to $198 per illness day avoided.

How, then, is a reasonable cost-effectiveness willingness-to-pay threshold determined? This is a difficult question with no clear answer at this point, complicated by the many possible effectiveness values (life years gained, lives saved, illness days avoided, etc.) that could be considered. Cost-effectiveness comparisons between interventions using a common effectiveness measure can be useful in gaining a sense of an intervention's relative value. For example, if Treatment x for Disease X costs $100 per illness day prevented and is considered economically reasonable while Treatment y for Disease Y costs $500 per illness day avoided and is considered too expensive, then Treatment z for Disease Z costing $550 per illness day prevented might also be considered too expensive. However, the usefulness of this comparison depends upon the similarity of illness days between Diseases X, Y, and Z. If Disease Z is worse than X or Y, then there might be a higher willingness-to-pay threshold to avoid a more severe illness day from Disease Z than to avoid a more moderate illness day due to X or Y.

Sensitivity analysis may also be useful in the interpretation of results. If variation of analysis parameter values does not change the conclusion drawn from the base case analysis results, the analysis is said to be "robust," and increases the confidence in analysis results. Analyses that are not robust, where conclusions may change with variation of one or more parameter values, are termed "sensitive to variation," and their results are viewed with less confidence. Depending on the data used in the analysis, this confidence or uncertainty can be quantified through the development of confidence intervals for cost-effectiveness ratios in empiric data sets or the use of probabilistic sensitivity analysis and acceptability curves when empiric data sets are not available. These issues are covered in greater detail in Chapter 13.

A number of other factors can make interpretation of CEAs challenging. Differences in analysis results can be due to methodologic differences between analyses. CEA results are often dependent on the perspective, time horizon, and assumptions used in the analysis and, unless these factors are well aligned between analyses, discordant results can arise based solely on these technical differences. Analyses using effectiveness values that are very specific to the medical scenario being examined, such as deep venous thrombosis prevented or lumbar discectomies avoided, may have few similar analyses available for comparison, making interpretation of their results challenging. Even if analyses with similar effectiveness values are available, their results could be difficult to compare to those of interventions for other disease processes using other effectiveness measures, thus limiting their comparability and interpretability. In these cases, a common effectiveness measure would facilitate cost-effectiveness comparisons over a broad spectrum of medical interventions. The use of quality of life utilities and QALYs in cost-utility analysis (as discussed in Chapter 4), along with methodologic recommendations to standardize analysis practices, such as those of the US Panel on Cost-Effectiveness in Health and Medicine [8, 10], is largely motivated by the need to facilitate such comparisons, and has resulted in resources, such as the online CEA Registry from Tufts University [16], to make direct comparisons possible .

7.5 SUMMARY

CEAs compare medical intervention strategies through the calculation of the ICER, a measure of the cost of changes in health outcomes. These analyses can be performed on clinical trial data when information on both costs and effectiveness is available or, more commonly, using decision analysis models to synthesize data from many sources. Interpretation of CEA results can be challenging due to the variety of health outcomes that can be used as the effectiveness term in these analyses and due to the absence of a definitive criterion for "cost-effective." A subset of CEA, cost-utility analysis, attempts to make interpretation of results less difficult using a common effectiveness term, the QALY.

REFERENCES

[1] Black WC. The CE plane: A graphic representation of cost-effectiveness. *Med Decis Making.* 1990;10(3):212–14.
[2] Bass EB, Pitt HA, Lillemoe KD. Cost-effectiveness of laparoscopic cholecystectomy versus open cholecystectomy. *Am J Surg.* 1993;165(4):466–71.

[3] Cook J, Richardson J, Street A. A cost utility analysis of treatment options for gallstone disease: Methodological issues and results. *Health Econ.* 1994;3(3):157–68.

[4] Ahmad S. The cost-effectiveness of raising the legal smoking age in California. *Med Decis Making.* 2005;25(3):330–40.

[5] Johansson PM, Tillgren PE, Guldbrandsson KA, Lindholm LA. A model for cost-effectiveness analyses of smoking cessation interventions applied to a Quit-and-Win contest for mothers of small children. *Scand J Public Health.* 2005;33(5):343–52.

[6] Agha Z, Lofgren RP, VanRuiswyk JV. Is antibiotic prophylaxis for bacterial endocarditis cost-effective? *Med Decis Making.* 2005;25(3):308–20.

[7] King JT, Jr.,, Justice AC, Aron DC. Management of incidental pituitary microadenomas: A cost-effectiveness analysis. *J Clin Endocrinol Metab.* 1997;82(11):3625–32.

[8] Gold MR, Siegel JE, Russell LB, Weinstein MC, **eds.**, *Cost-effectiveness in Health and Medicine.* New York: Oxford University Press; 1996.

[9] Drummond M, Sculpher M, Torrance G, O'Brien B, Stoddart G. *Methods for the Economic Evaluation of Health Care Programmes,* 3rd edition. Oxford: Oxford University Press; 2005.

[10] *Cost-effectiveness in Health and Medicine.,* 2nd *edition.* Neumann, P, Sanders, G, Russell, L, Siegel, J, TG, G eds., New York: Oxford University Press; 2016.

[11] Aujesky D, Smith KJ, Cornuz J, Roberts MS. Cost-effectiveness of low-molecular-weight heparin for secondary prophylaxis of cancer-related venous thromboembolism. *Thromb Haemost.* 2005;93(3):592–99.

[12] Smith KJ, Roberts MS. Cost-effectiveness of newer treatment strategies for influenza. *American Journal of Medicine.* 2002;113(4):300–07.

[13] Weinstein MC. Principles of cost-effective resource allocation in health care organizations. *Int J Technol Assess Health Care.* 1990;6(1):93–103.

[14] Cantor SB. Cost-effectiveness analysis, extended dominance, and ethics: A quantitative assessment. *Med Decis Making.* 1994;14(3):259–65.

[15] Doubilet P, Weinstein MC, McNeil BJ. Use and misuse of the term "cost effective" in medicine. *N Engl J Med.* 1986;314(4):253–56.

[16] Center for the Evaluation of Value and Risk in Health. The cost-effectiveness analysis registry [Internet]. (Boston), Institute for Clinical Research and Health Policy Studies, Tufts Medical Center. Available from: www.cearegistry.org.

8 Budget Impact Analysis

Josephine Mauskopf, MA, MHA, PhD
RTI International
Research Triangle Park, NC, USA

Lieven Annemans, MSc, MMan, PhD
Ghent University, Brussels University
Brussels, Belgium

TABLE OF CONTENTS

8.1   INTRODUCTION

A comprehensive economic evaluation for a new medicine or technology should include a cost-effectiveness analysis (CEA), estimated for the duration of the condition, whose purpose is to determine the efficiency of the new intervention for an individual or a disease cohort. The evaluation should also include a budget impact analysis (BIA), sometimes referred to as a budget impact model (BIM). The purpose of a BIA is to determine the impact of the decision to use a new intervention on annual healthcare costs for a health plan or a country population for each year after the introduction of the intervention. Both CEAs and BIAs must include information about the condition for which the new intervention is indicated, the types of patients likely to use the new intervention, how the use of the new intervention will affect the use of alternative interventions, and how the new intervention will change other condition-related costs. Specifically, a CEA takes an incidence perspective and estimates the changes in lifetime costs and health outcomes for a representative individual or a cohort of individuals who initiate treatment with the new intervention and compares these costs and outcomes to a similar individual or cohort initiating treatment with an alternative intervention. In contrast, a BIA takes a prevalence perspective and estimates the total changes in annual healthcare costs for the entire population of individuals who have the condition of interest; total changes are reported for each year that the new intervention is introduced into the treatment mix, typically 3–5 years. The BIA is the topic of this chapter.

8.2 GUIDELINES FOR BUDGET IMPACT ANALYSES

In 2007, Mauskopf et al. presented the first international guidelines for BIAs [1]. In 2014, Sullivan et al. updated these guidelines [2]. Although both sets of guidelines provide a detailed insight into all issues related to the conduct and reporting of BIAs, local implementation is not straightforward, and the guidelines leave room for several interpretations and methodological options regarding the different aspects of BIA. In addition, reviews of published BIAs in Europe [3] and in the United States (US) [4] have shown that these guidelines are often not followed. Furthermore, recent studies that reviewed estimated budget impacts before adoption of a new intervention showed that these estimates both underestimated and overestimated the observed budget impact after adoption of the intervention [5–7]. In this chapter, we attempt to establish a set of clear standards for improving the consistency of analyses and the usefulness of the results to the budget holder. This chapter aims to serve both those developing BIAs as well as those reviewing and making decisions based on these BIAs. A BIA is defined here as the best possible estimation each year of the financial consequences to the budget holder as a result of the adoption and diffusion of a new pharmaceutical drug or medical device over a well-defined time period. In the remainder of the chapter, we often refer to drugs, but the same principles apply to devices.

8.2.1 PERSPECTIVE AND TARGET AUDIENCE

A budget impact of a new pharmaceutical drug or medical device should consider the perspective of the budget holder. This could be a national health insurer, a national health service, a private insurer, a hospital manager, and so on (see Chapter 1 for further details about the perspective).

8.2.2 OUTCOME

Given the BIA's perspective, all estimated increased expenses and cost savings must relate to the annual total expenditures on healthcare services for the condition of interest. A narrower perspective, related to changes in spending on individual drugs or to the total pharmaceutical spending for the condition of interest, can also be shown; however, for all BIAs the impact on total spending for all healthcare services for the condition of interest is the primary outcome, provided sufficient data are available to show the impact on all condition-related costs. It is also recommended that the BIA contain information on the annual health impacts for the eligible population, if available, since these impacts will be needed to estimate changes in condition-related costs, as recommended in the guidelines from the International Society for Pharmacoeconomics and Outcomes Research [2]. Health impacts may be complications avoided, cured patients, deaths avoided, or other "hard" endpoints occurring each year after the introduction of the new intervention. The use of this information gives the decision maker not only an estimate of the financial impact but also an estimate of how many units of health, either condition-specific or generic, can be obtained in the eligible population each year during the BIM's time horizon. If health impacts from the new intervention are observed only after the end of the BIM's time horizon, these interventions can still be included in the results summary but should be presented without estimates of their financial impacts and without applying these financial impacts to expenditures observed during the model time horizon.

8.2.3   HEALTH CONDITION AND TARGET POPULATION

The BIA addresses the impact of the use of a new drug in a well-defined health condition and population eligible for the new intervention. Therefore, a complete and detailed description of the health condition, its current treatment, and related outcomes is essential. The eligible population should include *all* patients who are diagnosed with the condition of interest and who are indicated for the new drug and, hence, who might be given this new intervention in the time horizon of interest (see Section 8.2.5 for further guidance for the time horizon).

The eligible population must be defined starting from the approved marketing indication and, possibly, narrowed down to the population for which reimbursement is approved. Note that this eligible population should include patients newly diagnosed and/or newly eligible for the new intervention. Patients in the prevalent population must also be included in a BIA for the treatment of a chronic disease if these patients are currently being treated and are eligible to switch to the new intervention. For example, if a new treatment is introduced for depression, two populations must be included in the BIA: (1) incident populations, that is, those whose diagnosis or treatment history makes them newly eligible for the new treatment each year of the model time horizon, and (2) a prevalent population, that is, patients diagnosed and currently being treated who would have become eligible for the new intervention in previous years and who may consider switching to the new intervention, especially if they are not being successfully treated with the current interventions.

Moreover, in some disease areas, there may be patients with a condition who currently have no adequate treatment option and therefore are not receiving any treatment. The introduction of a new drug enables them to be successfully treated (for instance, patients whose rheumatoid arthritis has been insufficiently controlled for several months or years). This is called induced demand, which means that the new drug may lead to additional patients entering the treated population when a new drug is approved; therefore, this population should be considered in estimating the eligible population size.

Regardless of induced demand, the eligible population may evolve over time for conditions with an increasing or a decreasing temporal incidence and/ or prevalence; an evolving population can occur because of changes in mortality or morbidity rates with the new intervention or because of changes in the age distribution or size of the population of interest. These changes must also be considered in estimating eligible population size.

Within the eligible population, it is recommended that subpopulations, determined by patient characteristics or condition severity, be considered if there is evidence that such subpopulations are associated with different levels of effectiveness of the new drug or with different cost consequences.

Finally, possible off-label use of the new drug must be discussed, and its magnitude estimated and considered in the BIA.

8.2.4   THE INTERVENTION

The new drug must be fully described in terms of its efficacy, effectiveness, adverse events, and convenience of use. This description must focus on a comparison of these measures to those of the drugs and nondrug treatments that may be replaced by the new drug (see Section 8.2.6 for further guidance about comparators).

8.2.5   TIME HORIZON

The time horizon must meet the needs of the decision maker. Therefore, it is recommended that a time horizon of 3–5 years be applied as a base case. Further, it is mandatory to show a flow of financial consequences on a yearly basis, that is, the year-by-year impact, as well as the total budget impact, over 3–5 years must be shown. It is possible to have longer time horizons in BIAs, for example, for treatments of chronic diseases, but we recommend using a time horizon that allows outcomes to be validated by clinical trial or credible observational data.

8.2.6   INTERVENTION MIX

A BIA must predict how a change in the current mix of drugs and other therapies used to treat a particular health condition will impact the flow of spending on that condition. Hence, the comparison must be made between the current intervention mix and the new intervention mix (i.e., a mix with the new drug included) that can be used in the population eligible for treatment with the new intervention. The current intervention mix consists of those drugs (and possibly other treatments, such as surgery) that are currently used in the population eligible for the new treatment and that may be replaced by the new drug. In case there are numerous current drugs and other treatments currently being used, it is possible to consider only a subset of the current interventions, focusing on those most likely to be replaced by the new intervention.

In order to estimate the new intervention mix, the market penetration of the new drug must first be estimated. Market penetration should be based on evidence such as experience in other countries (if the drug was already approved there) or experience with a similar drug in the same disease area that was launched earlier in the same setting. Evidence from market research studies can also be used. If market penetration is based on market research, the study's report, with methods and results of the study, must be added to the appendix of the budget impact report. In addition to the expected market penetration of the new drug over the model time horizon, the extent to which the new drug will be added to the mix or replace each of the current drugs and other treatments must be estimated. Thus, the new intervention mix should consist of the new drug plus the remix of the current drugs and treatments.

The model must also allow for evolution of both the current and new intervention mixes as the penetration of the new treatment changes, as well as any expected changes in the current intervention mix that may occur over the model time horizon. For example, the expected entry of generic products for currently branded products may cause changes over time in the evolution of the intervention mix without and with the new intervention and should be accounted for in the BIM. Finally, note that off-label use (mentioned in Section 8.2.3) may occur in both the current treatment mix and the new treatment mix.

8.2.7 MODEL STRUCTURE AND STRUCTURAL ASSUMPTIONS

A BIA requires a combination of data from many different data sources into a cost-calculator or decision-analytic model structure. For example, if the available clinical trials do not describe the economic and health consequences of reaching an endpoint, other data sources must be consulted in order to obtain this type of information. In a BIM, information and data from these different sources should be combined in a manner that is similar to that used in a CEA (see Chapters 4 and 7 for further guidance). The BIM should be as simple as possible but must be a credible reflection of the health condition, its natural history, and its consequences (as far as these consequences are affected by the new drug) for each year after the new drug is introduced to the market. The BIM's clinical and economic assumptions should be consistent with the CEA, if there is one.

It is important to note, however, that the complexity of the BIM, and its alignment with the CEA, will depend on the type of health condition (acute health conditions and self-limiting health conditions may be associated with simpler models than chronic conditions or acute conditions with sequelae) and the type of intervention (preventive, curative, palliative, one time, ongoing, or periodic). The final model structure must consider these aspects and be justified accordingly. A BIM must be an open cohort model, that is, the BIM should be constructed so that individuals can enter the model as they become eligible for the new treatment or leave the population as they are cured, lose eligibility for the treatment, or die.

Figures 8.1–8.4 show examples of model structures for different types of health conditions. Figure 8.1 shows a model structure for a new antiviral drug treatment for influenza, an acute condition; the structure is based on data from clinical trials

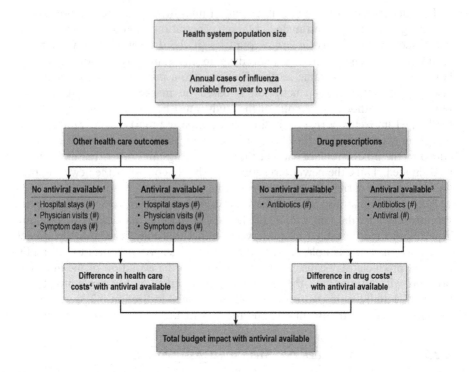

FIGURE 8.1 Budget impact model: influenza.

[1] Hospital stays, physician visits, and symptom days were estimated as rates without new antiviral drug from clinical trial data.

[2] The number of health outcomes with antiviral available can change over the model time horizon as uptake of the antiviral increases.

[3] The number of antiviral prescriptions can vary over the model time horizon with uptake; the number of antibiotic prescriptions with and without antiviral was estimated using percentages from the clinical trial.

[4] Healthcare and drug costs were calculated by applying unit costs for each resource to the units of the resource used; the difference in symptom days can also be calculated and presented.

Source: Based on unpublished study.

on the reduction in the number of symptom days and a reduction in hospitalization rates. Figure 8.2 shows a model structure for a new drug treatment for relapsing–remitting multiple sclerosis, a chronic condition; in this model, the treatment is assumed not to impact either mortality or disease progression within the model time horizon. However, the model includes a reduction in annual relapse rates based on data from clinical trials [8]. Figure 8.3 shows a model structure for systolic congestive heart failure for which add-on drug treatment has been shown in a clinical trial to reduce both hospitalization and mortality rates [9]. These three models can be programmed as simple cost-calculator models, which is the preferred

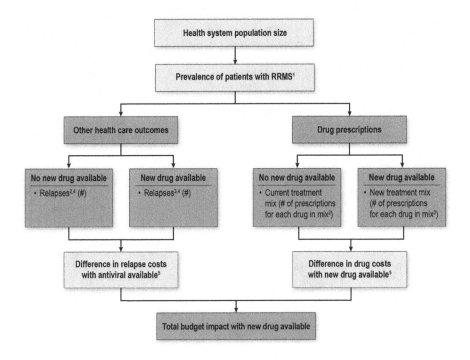

FIGURE 8.2   Budget impact model: multiple sclerosis.

[1]Assume no impact of new drug on mortality during model time horizon

[2]Treatment mix and relapses might change over model time horizon, for example with generic entry

[3]Treatment mix and relapses will change over model time horizon as uptake of new drug increases

[4]Number of relapses estimated as a weighted average of relapse rates for each drug in the treatment mix derived using a mixed treatment comparison analysis

[5]Health care and drug costs calculated by applying unit costs for each resource to the units of the resource used; difference in number of relapses can also be presented

Source: Based on Dorman et al. [8].

approach when the condition and intervention impact allow for this approach. However, simplifying assumptions may be needed, such as assuming that the impact of the new drug on disease progression is similar to the drugs in the current treatment mix and/or the new drug does not affect disease-stage treatment costs during the model time horizon (e.g., see Figure 8.2).

Figure 8.4 shows a Markov model structure for a new drug regimen for individuals with highly drug-resistant human immunodeficiency virus infection who are failing current antiviral combination regimens and for whom the new drug regimen has been shown to reduce mortality rates and to slow disease progression within the model time horizon. The Markov model structure used for the CEA of such new

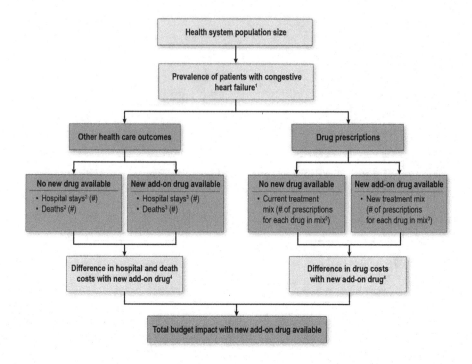

FIGURE 8.3 Budget impact model: congestive heart failure.

[1] Prevalence of patients with congestive heart failure will increase over model time horizon with new add-on drug treatment because the clinical trial of add-on therapy showed reduced mortality rate.

[2] Hospital stay and death estimates were taken from clinical trial current treatment arm; treatment mix without new drug assumed to remain constant over the model time horizon.

[3] Hospital stays and deaths will change over model time horizon as uptake of the new add-on drug increases.

[4] Healthcare and drug costs were calculated by applying unit costs for each resource to the units of the resource used; the difference in the number of hospital stays and deaths can also be presented.

Source: Based on Borer et al. [9].

regimens was converted to a BIM by running the Markov model with the starting prevalent population size and CD4 cell-count distribution and allowing a new incident cohort to enter the model each year with a different CD4 cell-count distribution [10]. The model can be run both with and without the new drug regimen included in the treatment mix, and the uptake of the new drug regimen can be allowed to change each year for the incident populations. In the case of HIV infection, the efficacy of the new drug regimen in the prevalent population should be allowed to differ from the efficacy of the new drug regimen in the incident cohorts because of greater drug resistance in the prevalent population. Once the model has been run with and without the new drug regimen included in the

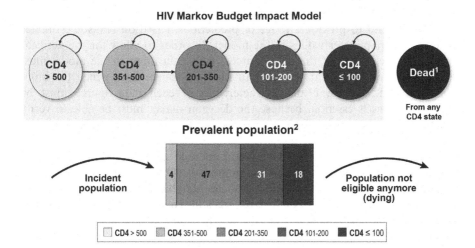

FIGURE 8.4   Markov budget impact model: HIV.

HIV = human immunodeficiency virus. [1] Patients can transition from any health state to death at any time but at higher rates, depending on the CD4 cell-count range.

[2] Assumed the distribution among the CD4 health states of the prevalent population with highly resistant HIV1 infection remained constant over model time horizon without the new intervention at the distribution observed for those individuals entering the clinical trial for the new intervention. Distribution among the CD4 health states of the prevalent population with highly resistant HIV1 infection will change over the model time horizon with new, more effective interventions. The size of the prevalent population with highly resistant HIV1 infection with the new intervention will increase over the model time horizon with the decrease in mortality rates. To estimate the change in drug costs, subtract the estimated costs of the mix of drugs used without the new interventions from the estimated costs of the mix of drugs used with the new intervention, accounting for both changes in drug costs per person and changes in the size of the prevalent population. To estimate the impact on other healthcare costs of the new intervention, compute the costs for the prevalent and incident populations with and without the new interventions by multiplying the number of individuals in each CD4 range with and without the new intervention by the average annual healthcare costs (not including drug costs) in that range.

Source: Based on Mauskopf [10].

treatment mix, the difference in annual population costs can be presented for each year after the introduction of the new drug regimen.

The BIM must be fully transparent. This means that, along with a model flow diagram, all the data inputs must be clearly presented, together with their sources and their ranges of uncertainty (see Section 8.3 for further guidance about reporting and Chapter 13 about sensitivity analysis). In addition, the model should be developed in a readily accessible software program; an electronic copy of the model, where possible, should be delivered to the decision maker to allow him or her to run scenarios that reflect their population's characteristics, health plan practices, and costs.

8.2.8 DATA SOURCES

A BIA is meant to provide a range of predictions, based on realistic estimates
of the input parameter values in the model. In order to allow for the verification of the reliability of the data sources, each data input in the model must
be documented by a clear reference to the data source from which the input
was obtained. Moreover, the characteristics of each data source must be
described. This is essential because the decision maker must be able to verify
whether the information in the data source is relevant to the considered eligible
population.

The primary data sources should be published clinical trial estimates and
studies of efficacy and safety for comparators. Other data sources include
population statistical information; healthcare databases; patient chart reviews;
observational data; and, if data gaps are still present despite all the above
sources, expert opinion (see Chapter 5 for further guidance about data
sources). The BIA's developers can build a more credible BIA if they are able
to access the budget-holder's data on patient characteristics and condition
severity, current treatment patterns, and costs.

If assumptions about input data values are needed (which is often the
case), the assumptions must be realistic and justifiable, and their impact
should be tested in the sensitivity analysis (see Section 8.2.11 for further guidance and Chapter 13 for guidance about sensitivity analysis results).

8.2.9 CALCULATIONS

As mentioned previously, the budget impact must be calculated on an annual
basis. For each year, the expenses associated with the current intervention mix
and the new intervention mix, as well as condition-related medical resource
use and costs associated with the current intervention mix and the new intervention mix, must be calculated. From this information, the additional treatment expenses due to the new intervention mix, the possible changes in
medical resource use, and the net budget impact can be calculated. These
should be reported for different scenarios (see Section 8.2.11 for further
guidance).

As the BIA deals with financial streams over time, it is not necessary to discount
the costs.

Note that costs and savings need to be condition- and treatment-related and
must be calculated by multiplying resource use (induced or avoided) by the unit
cost per resource item, which should reflect the cost or price paid from the perspective of the decision maker and should include discounts from the suppliers
and any co-pays made by the patients. The calculations should address the
impact of adherence and persistence with therapy on the cost and outcomes of
treatments to the extent that these data are available. It may be, however, that the
payer will bear the cost regardless (e.g., even if poorly adherent, the patient still
pays for the prescription).

8.2.10   MODEL VALIDATION

The validity of the model (Eddy et al., 2012) must be assessed and the result of this assessment must be reported. The validation involves the following steps.

8.2.10.1   Face Validity

It is important to confirm with budget holders that the model structure, assumptions, and input parameter values that have been used for the base case and alternative scenarios are a good representation of the changes in condition outcomes and budget-holder costs.

8.2.10.2   Internal Validity

A peer reviewer should have the chance to examine the data input, sources, and calculations of the model, to ensure that there are no transcription or calculation errors. This can be facilitated by providing the peer reviewer with an electronic version of the model.

8.2.10.3   External Validity

The closer the model's clinical predictions approach reality, the greater the validity of the results. Obviously, this cannot yet be examined for the branch of the model with the new intervention, but the model results can be compared to budget-holder data for the current treatment mix.

8.2.11   REPORTING OF THE RESULTS

The BIA model report should follow the CHEERS guidelines for reporting economic models [11] and should have the following elements: a complete and transparent description of the model structure, including a flow diagram and details of all model calculations; a listing of all model structural assumptions and their rationale; and a table presenting all input parameter values, data sources, and derivations, if required, for the model. The main results of the BIA can be presented for a base-case estimate, using a credible set of input parameter values, but should also include a comprehensive set of sensitivity analyses based on plausible alternative scenarios. The following are examples of such alternative scenarios and assumptions: different patient age distributions or disease or condition severity mixes that may be expected in various health plans; market penetration for the new intervention; changes in current interventions when the new intervention is introduced; change in efficacy and adverse events with the new intervention in the mix; and drug and other resource costs. In addition, the model should be designed to be interactive so that the user can run scenarios that reflect the budget holder's own decision context.

Using these guidelines, the quality and uniformity of BIAs will improve. More specific instructions on how to perform a budget impact analysis can be found in Mauskopf et al. [12]. These guidelines and instructions, however, do not inform the decision about what is or is not an acceptable budget impact. These issues are briefly discussed in Section 8.3.

8.3   BUDGET IMPACT ANALYSIS AND AFFORDABILITY

An introduction of a new product that is very cost-effective at the individual patient level may result in a large annual budgetary impact at the population level if there is a large eligible population or if the price of the new intervention is very high (e.g., a cure for a chronic condition or genetic disease), and the impact may play a part in policy decisions about treatment guidelines and reimbursement. For example, decisions about the addition of new drugs to the national formulary in Australia are based on expected budget impact as well as the cost-effectiveness of new interventions [13], while the United Kingdom's (UK's) National Institute for Health and Care Excellence (NICE) bases its recommendations for reimbursement only on cost-effectiveness results [14]. However, NICE frequently examines the cost-effectiveness of treatment for different patient subgroups defined by condition severity or treatment history or other patient characteristics to ensure that treatment for all subgroups is cost-effective. NICE can also negotiate price discounts when the budget impact of treatment for their recommended reimbursed population is very high [14]. NICE produces costing templates that present expected budget impacts and that are intended to be used as guidance for budget holders implementing their reimbursement recommendations. These costing templates are typically designed as cost calculators using Microsoft Excel spreadsheet software and have drug- and condition-related costs, provided there are strong clinical trial or observational data to support the estimates of changes in condition-related costs. To address concerns about affordability of new drugs, in April 2017, NICE announced that the National Health Service (NHS) and NICE were introducing a "budget impact test" [15]. The test works in the following way: any new intervention with an expected annual net budget impact in any of the first 3 years of use of more than £20 million will trigger a commercial discussion between NHS England and the company submitting the intervention to NICE. The discussion will explore ways to reduce the budget impact through changes in price or alternative payment mechanisms. If agreement is not reached, NICE recommendations for use will be allowed to be phased in over a longer time period than the current 90 days.

This chapter has focused on how to estimate the budget impact of a single new innovative drug or other healthcare technology. However, payers are also concerned about the aggregate impact of all the new interventions in healthcare that are marketed each year, since this is important for budget planning, premium setting, and/or tax increases. To the extent that information can be provided to budget holders with aggregate estimates of the budget impact of all the new interventions entering the market in upcoming years, this would be very helpful for financial planning.

The independent Institute for Clinical and Economic Review (ICER) in the United States has considered the aggregate impact of new interventions in their value framework; the framework combines a CEA and other intangible factors to determine "care value" and adds a consideration of the budget impact to determine health system value for new interventions [16]. The methods initially used by ICER to estimate budget impact for individual interventions were similar to those described in this chapter, although the rate of uptake of the new drug was not evidence based. Rather, the eligible population was estimated and unmanaged use by this population was assumed over a 5-year time horizon; the costs associated with changes in the treatment mix and in condition-related costs were estimated to determine the likely budget impact. However, using this approach, both ICER and outside groups [6] have determined that the early budget impact estimates made by ICER were higher than those actually observed after the product entered the market. Two of the main causes of higher budget impact estimates were overestimates of the product's uptake and overestimates of the product prices using list prices. To adjust for this overestimation, ICER now produces a range of budget impact estimates based on a range of uptake for the eligible population and a range of US health plan prices reflecting individual plan discounts.

Further, to ensure that the budget impacts of new interventions are affordable, ICER relates the estimated budget impacts to a ceiling level that ICER researchers believe is sustainable for new products coming to market. This ceiling amount is computed each year, starting with estimates of the aggregate amount by which total healthcare budgets can be increased, calculated by multiplying current total healthcare costs by the US expected increase in gross domestic product (GDP) plus 1%. This value was chosen to reflect realistic annual increases for total healthcare costs each year in the United States. In order to translate this figure into a value that would be of concern for an increase in a drug's budget, ICER multiplies the total increase in healthcare spending by the proportion of that spending that is for drugs and then divides this amount by the average number of new molecular entities entering the market each year (using data from drug approvals over the last 2 years). This amount can be compared with the estimated budget impact for each new product for each year, annualized over 5 years. If the estimated budget impact for a new molecular entity at the payer's price and expected uptake is above this amount, ICER provides a warning to payers; this warning from ICER may provide US payers with a negotiating tool for price negotiations or restrictions on product use [17].

There is still a problem for decision makers if the aggregate budget impact of all new products that are cost-effective at current thresholds is higher than GDP plus 1% and price negotiations or restrictions on patient use are not successful. How can these budget restrictions be met?

Cohen et al. stated that the economic and equity rationale for carrying out BIAs is opportunity cost, or benefits forgone, measured in terms of utility or equitable distribution by using resources in one way rather than another [18]. In other words, by choosing to use the budget in one way rather than another, decision makers forego other opportunities to use the same resources. The value of ICER's approach is that it provides a way to estimate what should be considered a large budgetary impact and what is a small one by allowing the healthcare budget to grow by GDP plus 1% (as described previously). Australia and the United Kingdom have also placed what they consider to be a large budgetary-impact limit on their health technology assessment processes. However, this does not solve the problem of how to cope with a situation where the budget impact of all the new interventions together exceeds what is considered affordable within the health system.

REFERENCES

[1] J.A. Mauskopf, S.D. Sullivan, L. Annemans, J. Caro, C.D. Mullins, M. Nuijten, E. Orlewska, J. Watkins, P. Trueman, Principles of Good Practice for Budget Impact Analysis: Report of the ISPOR Task Force on Good Research Practices—Budget Impact Analysis, *Value in Health* 10 (5) (2007) 336–347.

[2] S.D. Sullivan, J.A. Mauskopf, F. Augustovski, J. Jaime Caro, K.M. Lee, M. Minchin, E. Orlewska, P. Penna, J.-M. Rodriguez Barrios, W.-Y. Shau, Budget Impact Analysis—Principles of Good Practice: Report of the ISPOR 2012 Budget Impact Analysis Good Practice II Task Force, *Value in Health* 17 (1) (2014) 5–14.

[3] K. van de Vooren, S. Duranti, A. Curto, L. Garattini, A Critical Systematic Review of Budget Impact Analyses on Drugs in the EU Countries, *Applied Health Economics and Health Policy* 12 (1) (2013) 33–40.

[4] J. Mauskopf, S. Earnshaw, A Methodological Review of US Budget-Impact Models for New Drugs, *Pharmaco Economics* 34 (11) (2016) 1111–1131.

[5] M.S. Broder, J.M. Zambrano, J. Lee, R.S. Marken, Systematic Bias in Predictions of New Drugs' Budget Impact: Analysis of a Sample of Recent US Drug Launches, *Current Medical Research and Opinion* 34 (5) (2017) 765–773.

[6] J.T. Snider, J. Sussell, M.G. Tebeka, A. Gonzalez, J.T. Cohen, P. Neumann, Challenges with Forecasting Budget Impact: A Case Study of Six ICER Reports, *Value in Health* 22 (3) (2019) 332–339.

[7] J.W. Geenen, C. Boersma, O.H. Klungel, A.M. Hövels, Accuracy of Budget Impact Estimations and Impact on Patient Access: A Hepatitis C Case Study, *Eur J Health Econ* 20 (6) (2019) 857–867.

[8] E. Dorman, A.R. Kansal, S. Sarda, The Budget Impact of Introducing Delayed-Release Dimethyl Fumarate for Treatment of Relapse-remitting Multiple Sclerosis in Canada, *Journal of Medical Economics* 18 (12) (2015) 1085–1091.

[9] J.S. Borer, A.R. Kansal, E.D. Dorman, S. Krotneva, Y. Zheng, H.K. Patel, L. Tavazzi, M. Komajda, I. Ford, M. Böhm, A. Kielhorn, Budget Impact of Adding Ivabradine to Standard of Care in Patients with Chronic Systolic Heart Failure in the United States, *Journal of Managed Care & Specialty Pharmacy* 22 (9) (2016) 1064–1071.

[10] J. Mauskopf, Meeting the NICE Requirements: A Markov Model Approach, *Value in Health* 3 (4) (2000) 287–293.

[11] D. Husereau, M. Drummond, S. Petrou, C. Carswell, D. Moher, D. Greenberg, F. Augustovski, A.H. Briggs, J. Mauskopf, E. Loder, Consolidated Health Economic Evaluation Reporting Standards (Cheers)—Explanation and Elaboration: A Report of the ISPOR Health Economic Evaluation Publication Guidelines Good Reporting Practices Task Force, *Value in Health* 16 (2) (2013) 231–250.

[12] J. Mauskopf, S. Earnshaw, A. Brogan, S. Wolowacz, T. Brodtkorb, *Budget-Impact Analysis of Health Care Interventions: A Practical Guide*, Springer International Publishing, Adis, 2017.

[13] J. Mauskopf, C. Chirila, C. Masaquel, K.S. Boye, L. Bowman, J. Birt, D. Grainger, Relationship between Financial Impact and Coverage of Drugs in Australia, *Int J Technol Assess Health Care* 29 (1) (2013) 92–100.

[14] J. Mauskopf, C. Chirila, J. Birt, K.S. Boye, L. Bowman, Drug Reimbursement Recommendations by the National Institute for Health and Clinical Excellence:

Have They Impacted the National Health Service Budget?, *Health Policy* 110 (1) (2013) 49–59.

[15] National Institute for Health and Care Excellence (NICE). Changes to NICE Drug Appraisals: What You Need to Know. 2017. Available at: www.nice.org.uk/news/feature/changes-to-nice-drug-appraisals-what-you-need-to-know. Accessed January 7, 2020.

[16] S.D. Pearson, The ICER Value Framework: Integrating Cost Effectiveness and Affordability in the Assessment of Health Care Value, *Value in Health* 21 (3) (2018) 258–265.

[17] A. Brogan, S. Hogue, R. Vekaria, I. Reynolds, A. Coukel, Understanding Payer Perspectives on Value in the Use of Pharmaceuticals in the United States, *J Manag Care Spec Pharm* 25 (2019) 1319–1327.

[18] J.P. Cohen, E. Stolk, M. Niezen, Role of Budget Impact in Drug Reimbursement Decisions, *Journal of Health Politics, Policy and Law* 33 (2) (2008) 225–247.

9 Multicriteria Decision Analysis for the Healthcare Decision Maker

Sumitra Sri Bhashyam, PhD
Decision Lab UK
London, UK

Kevin Marsh, PhD
Evidera
London, UK

TABLE OF CONTENTS

9.1   INTRODUCTION

> . . . a formalization of common sense for decision problems which are
> too complex for informal use of common sense.
>
> (R. L. Keeney 1982, 806)

Keeney's quote concisely captures the support that multicriteria decision analysis (MCDA) offers decision makers. Decisions can be complex, involving many alternative courses of action, many criteria against which to evaluate these alternatives, uncertainty in the performance against these criteria, and conflicting perspectives. Where this is the case, decision makers risk relying on simplifying heuristics that cannot be guaranteed to reach the "right" decision. MCDA can support decision makers facing such situations to make better, more transparent, and consistent decisions.

We begin by providing a brief introduction to MCDA in the context of healthcare decisions. This is followed by a high-level description of the steps involved in conducting an MCDA. Finally, we illustrate how to implement an MCDA using the example of an individual's choice of contraception.

9.2   MCDA – A BRIEF OVERVIEW

9.2.1   WHAT IS MCDA?

MCDA is a term used to denote a collection of approaches that allow one to formally evaluate alternatives against a set of multiple, often conflicting, objectives, from the perspective of individuals or groups of decision makers and where no dominating course of action is evident [1]. As such, MCDA is a sociotechnical process. It is designed around the social element of the decision, that is, engaging stakeholders within the process, and the technical aspect of how the problem is solved, that is, which method(s) and tool(s) is/are used. Regardless of the method(s) used, the same sequence of steps is broadly used.

MCDA can aid decision making by providing away to structure deliberation, facilitate knowledge transfer, promote better-quality discussions, and to transparently communicate the reasons for decisions [2]. Table 9.1 lists the key benefits of MCDA.

9.2.2   USES OF MCDA

MCDA is a technique that has been widely applied in nonhealth contexts [3, 4]. More recently, there has been an increased interest in the applications of MCDA in health [2, 5]. MCDA can be useful in supporting a wide range of decisions, such as:

TABLE 9.1

The Key Benefits of MCDA

Benefit	Qualification
Completeness	Ensuring that all relevant criteria are considered
Formal incorporation of value judgments	Quantification of stakeholders' value judgments and combination with performance measurement
Understanding	Fostering a shared understanding of a decision problem and identifying areas of important disagreement
Transparency	Forming a transparent link between judgments and decisions

- *Pharmaceutical companies making decisions regarding their pipelines and trial designs.* For example, Allergan conducted an MCDA to support decisions about investment in 59 assets across five therapeutic areas [6].
- *Marketing authorization*: The Innovative Medicines Initiative Pharmacoepidemiological Research on Outcomes of Therapeutics by a European Consortium (IMI PROTECT) applied MCDA to support benefit–risk assessment involved in marketing authorization decisions [7]. For other examples, see Ho et al. [8] and European Medicines Agency [9–11]
- *Reimbursement decisions*: Examples of the use of MCDA to support the evaluation of new medical technologies for reimbursement purposes in Hungary [12], Italy [13], Germany [14], and Thailand [15].
- *Resource allocation decisions*: MCDA was used to support the Isle of Wight Primary Care Trust's allocation of resources across 21 interventions spread across five health priority areas [16].
- *Prescription and shared decision-making decisions*: MCDA was used to support the choice of colorectal cancer screening options [17].

9.3   IMPLEMENTING AN MCDA – AN OVERVIEW OF THE STEPS

Various guidelines for implementing MCDA are available [1, 18–20]; these broadly agree on the sequence of steps as listed in Table 9.2. While the steps are presented in a linear manner, they are often undertaken in an iterative manner, refining the MCDA as learning is gained throughout the process.

9.3.1   STEP 1: PROBLEM STRUCTURING

The first step in implementing an MCDA is to define the decision problem. This involves answering a number of questions, such as: What are the alternatives to be evaluated? Who are the decision makers? What are their objectives? And what type of decision do they have to make? The answer to the last question may be that they need to rank alternatives.

TABLE 9.2

MCDA Steps

Step Description

Step 1. Problem structuring
- Agree on a shared definition of the problem

Step 2: Criteria selection
- Identify criteria important to decision makers

Step 3: Determining the performance of alternatives against criteria
- Gather data to measure performance against each outcome

Step 4: Determining the scores and weights – estimating the values of the outcomes
- Evaluate the scores of outcomes
- Elicit weights (trade-offs) representing the relative importance of the outcomes

Step 5: Evaluation and comparison of alternatives
- Evaluate alternatives
- Interpret and communicate the results
- Conduct a sensitivity analysis

Another important question is whether the decision makers want to apply their own preference in the evaluation or to elicit the preferences of another stakeholder group. For instance, regulators may want to understand patients' preferences, or a reimbursement agency may want to know the preferences of the general population.

A definition of the decision problem can be provided by reviewing documents such as the mission statement of the organization the decision makers represent or the rationale for previous decisions they have made. It is also recommended that the decision makers themselves be consulted. Other expert input can also be useful, such as key opinion leaders and/or patient advocacy groups.

9.3.2 STEP 2: CRITERIA SELECTION

Different decisions will involve different sets of objectives and, thus, evaluation criteria. For instance, a prescription decision may consider clinical outcomes as well as convenience criteria, such as the mode of administration and location of getting a treatment. A resource allocation decision may consider a broader set of criteria, such as equity and budget impact.

Two approaches can be used to generate the list of criteria to include in the MCDA:value-focused thinking (also called top-down approach) and alternative focused thinking (bottom-up approach). The first approach helps identify fundamental objectives and further decomposes them into subobjectives. The second approach is driven by the existing alternatives and their distinguishing characteristics to articulate objectives [21, 22]. While there are strong arguments for using value-focused thinking [22], research also shows that individuals may struggle to think about their fundamental objectives and may need prompts to support articulating what they hope to achieve [23]. This could be done by some preliminary research on existing studies as a starting point to guide the discussions. Franco and Montibeller [21] provide a comprehensive list of tools for generating objectives.

The output from the review can then be validated and refined through discussions with the stakeholders. In contexts where there are numerous stakeholders with differing technical backgrounds, facilitated decision-conferencing workshops can be useful [6].

Once these steps have been conducted, a long list of concepts would have been gathered. In many cases this stage will generate too many criteria to be incorporated into the MCDA. There is no rule as to how many criteria to include although as few criteria should be included as are requisite with the decision. Identifying this number requires making trade-offs between increasing the validity of the decision by using a more complete set of criteria versus the resulting fatigue from the increased length of the decision task [24]. MCDAs in healthcare use between 3 and 19 criteria, with an average of 8.2 [2].

To narrow down the criteria, it is helpful to keep in mind the desirable properties of criteria sets, described in Table 9.3. These will depend on the form of the MCDA aggregation function adopted (see step 5). The most commonly adopted aggregation function in healthcare is an additive model (also referred to as "weighted sum model" or "additive multiattribute value model"). In this model, a numerical score for each alternative on a given criterion is multiplied by the relative weight for the criterion and then summed to get a "total score" for each alternative. While simple to construct and communicate, additive models require adherence to certain criteria set properties, such as preference independence, that is, that the preference for a criterion can be stated without knowing how an intervention performs on another criterion.

TABLE 9.3
Desirable Properties of Criteria [1]

Properties	Description
Unambiguous	A clear relationship exists between consequences and descriptions of consequences using the criteria.
Understandable	Consequences and value trade-offs made using the attribute can readily be understood and clearly communicated.
Direct	The criteria levels directly describe the consequences of interest.
Operational	In practice, information to describe consequences can be obtained and value trade-offs can reasonably be made.
Comprehensive	The criteria levels cover the range of possible consequences for the corresponding objective and value judgments implicit in the criterion are reasonable.
Preferential independence	How much one cares about the performance of an intervention on a criterion should optimally not depend on its performance on other criteria

A common example of preference dependence is a patient's preference for the frequency of administration depending on the mode of administration: preference for the frequency of administration will depend on whether the treatment is administered orally or via injection. Where preference dependence exists, this can be dealt with by restructuring criteria, such as combining the mode and frequency of administration into a single criterion.

To facilitate the application of criteria set properties, the concepts can be organized into groups with the purpose of extracting the essence of what matters to the decision makers. Problem structuring methods, including cognitive maps and strategic options development and analysis (SODA) maps, can be used to achieve this [25, 26] and the resulting criteria can further be organized into a value tree [21, 27]. This exercise is not trivial and will require iterations to arrive at a final list of criteria.

The definition of criteria should consider the types of measurements that are available [28]:

- *Direct or natural measurement* – Whenever possible, this type of measurement is favored as it has a common understanding and directly measures the criterion in question.
- *Proxy measurement or indirect measurement* – Where direct measures are not available, proxies may be required. For example, distance to hospital may be used instead of travel time. An example might be using "commute time" when measuring the distance to receive a treatment.
- *Constructed scale* – In the absence of direct or proxy measures, it may be necessary to construct a scale.

9.3.3   STEP 3: DETERMINING THE PERFORMANCE OF ALTERNATIVES AGAINST CRITERIA

Data to measure the performance of alternatives against criteria can be collected from a range of sources, including trials, observational studies, systematic reviews, and expert opinion. Existing standards for assessing the quality of evidence, such as the Cochrane Risk of Bias tool [29], should be applied.

It is helpful to organize the data in a performance matrix or effects table [10] (as in Table 9.4).

TABLE 9.4

Effects Table

Outcome	Time Point	Unit (Scale)	Intervention 1 (Mean, LCI-UCI)	Intervention 2 (Mean, LCI-UCI)	Min[1]	Max[1]
Outcome 1						
Outcome 2						
Outcome 3						
Outcome 4						

[1]Min and Max denote the range of outcomes between which the interventions perform. LCI = lower confidence interal; UCI = upper confidence interval.

9.3.4   STEP 4: DETERMINING THE SCORES AND WEIGHTS – ESTIMATING THE VALUES OF THE OUTCOMES

Aggregating multiple criteria requires that they be translated onto a single scale. This is undertaken using scores and weights:

- **Scores:** The relative value of changes within a criterion. For example, is a weight loss from 30 to 25 lbs valued the same as a weight loss from 25 to 20 lbs? These are also referred to as partial values, which can be displayed in a value function.
- **Weights:** The relative value of changes on different criteria, or the trade-offs between criteria. For example, how much weight loss would be required to offset an increase in the risk of death?

Eliciting scores and weights from stakeholders can be done using numerous methods, such as the following:

- Stated preference methods, for example, discrete choice experiments [30–32]
- Pairwise comparison, such as the analytical hierarchy process (AHP) [33] or measuring attractiveness by a categorical based evaluation technique (MACBETH) [34]
- Swing weighting method and the bisection method [4]
- Additional methods (see review in Marsh et al. [2, 35])

The selection of the appropriate elicitation methods will depend on the following:

- The sample size achievable
- The number and complexity of the attributes
- The nature of preferences, that is, strength and homogeneity

Further guidance on the selection and implementation of scoring and weighting methods is available [36–40].

9.3.5   STEP 5: EVALUATION AND COMPARISON OF ALTERNATIVES

9.3.6   STEP 5.A: AGGREGATE THE DATA TO OBTAIN THE OVERALL VALUE OF THE ALTERNATIVES

The evaluation of assets using an additive model is done in a relatively simple manner – a weighted average is used to aggregate the weights and the scores. That is, for each criterion, the weight on a criterion is multiplied by the score of an intervention on that criterion. These weighted scores are then summed to give us the overall value of an alternative. This can be done using a calculator, a spreadsheet, or an existing software PROGRAM to support the elicitation of preferences and building a model. Though also valuable, undertaking a probabilistic sensitivity analysis of an additive model will require more sophisticated methods.

Formally, this is done using the following formula to estimate this overall value estimate [1, 41]:

$$U(x) = \sum_{i=1}^{n} w_i \times u_i(x_i) \qquad (1)$$

where

- $U(x)$ is the overall value of an intervention x;
- w_i is the weight attached to criterion i;
- u_i is the score function for criterion $i\sim$;
- x_i is the performance of alternative x against criterion i.

This can be organized as in Table 9.5.

TABLE 9.5

Scores and Overall Values of Interventions

Interventions	Criterion 1	Criterion 2	Criterion 3	Overall Value
Intervention a	$u_1(x_a)$	$u_2(x_a)$	$u_3(x_a)$	$w_1 \times u_1(x_a) + w_2 \times u_2(x_a) + w_3 \times u_3(x_a)$
Intervention b				
Intervention c				
Intervention d				
Weights	w_1	w_2	w_3	

9.3.7 Step 5.b: Testing Assumptions via Sensitivity Analysis

Sensitivity analysis can be used to both validate and test the robustness of an MCDA model.

Quality assurance: Sensitivity analysis can be used to test the behavior of the model by simply changing some of the inputs to see if the results are as expected. A typical test would consist of setting all the weights to 0 and checking that the overall value of alternatives is also 0. Another typical test would consist of setting the scores of a given alternative to 0 and then 100 to test if the overall value is 0 and 100, respectively.

Understanding the robustness of preference ranking: Sensitivity analysis can be used to gain confidence in the ranking of preferred alternatives given that inputs, both value judgments and the performance estimates, are uncertain. Chapters 5 and 6 in Keeney and Raiffa [42] illustrate how to do this.

9.4   USING MCDA TO EVALUATE CONTRACEPTIVE METHODS – AN ILLUSTRATION

This section illustrates the implementation of an MCDA using the example of the decision aid model "My contraception tool" (referred to hereafter as MCT) designed to support an individual's choice of contraception [43]. The illustration is applied from the perspective of a hypothetical individual, Rachael.

9.4.1   STEP 1: PROBLEM STRUCTURING

There are currently 15 available contraceptive methods (listed in Figure 9.1), each with their different benefit–risk profiles, making the choice a complex one.

The MCT asks the stakeholder sociodemographic and medical history questions to determine potential contraindications for certain methods based on the UK Medical Eligibility Criteria (UKMEC). For instance, given she is over 35 years old and a smoker, the combined pill is not an option for which Rachael would be eligible.

9.4.2   STEP 2: CRITERIA SELECTION

To identify the criteria to include in the MCT, the authors conducted an initial literature review, followed by three face-to-face group interviews of 15 women and 5 men. Based on this, 32 concepts were identified, in addition to avoidance of pregnancy and sexually transmitted infections (STIs) outlined in Table 9.6. Longer-term events, such as increased risk of thrombosis and decreased risk of endometrial and ovarian cancers, were excluded from the list due to their probabilities being so low that they would be unlikely to affect the MCT's recommendations.

Within the MCT tool, individuals are asked to choose between 1 and 4 criteria of importance to them within the list of the short-term effects. The attributes that matter most to them in this decision are listed as follows:

- Avoidance of pregnancy
- Avoidance of STI
- Less heavy periods
- Avoiding weight gain
- Avoiding mood changes
- Avoiding remembering to take contraception

9.4.3   STEP 3: DETERMINING THE PERFORMANCE OF ALTERNATIVES AGAINST CRITERIA

The authors of the tool obtained the performance of alternatives from the Faculty of Sexual & Reproductive Healthcare guidelines, relevant Cochrane reviews, or clinical guidance when no performance estimates were available. The evidence used in the MCT was reviewed by a clinical advisor [43].

For illustration, the description of the performances of some of the contraceptives available for Rachael is listed in Table 9.7. In the case of the risk of pregnancy,

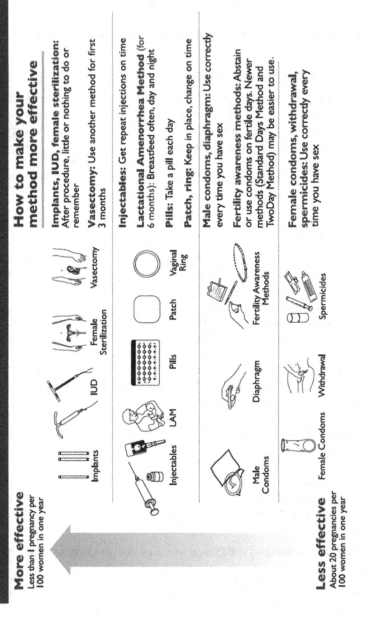

FIGURE 9.1 Contraceptive methods (World Health Organization Department of Reproduction Health and Research (WHO/RHR) and Johns Hopkins Bloomberg School of Public Health/Center for Communication Programs (CCP) [44].

TABLE 9.6

Long List of Attributes

Benefits	Side Effects	Nonclinical Outcomes
	Long-Term Effects	
Avoidance of pregnancy		
Avoidance of STIs		
	Short-Term Effects	
Less heavy periods	Heavier periods	Having to see a doctor or nurse to get
No periods	No periods	contraception
Less painful periods	Painful periods	Having to go to a shop/pharmacy to get
More regular periods	Irregular bleeding or	contraception
Fewer premenstrual	spotting	Having an injection
symptoms	Nausea	Having an implant under the skin in one's arm
Less acne	Weight gain (>2 kg)	Having a vaginal examination at a clinic
	Irritability/depression	Remembering when to take or use contraception
	Breast tenderness	Relying on my partner to remember when to take
	Headaches	or use contraception
	Skin irritation	Genital contact (touching the vagina or penis) to
	Loss of sex drive	use contraception
	Delay in return to fertility	Any interruption during sex to use
		a contraceptive method
		Any loss of sensation/feeling during sex
		Sexual partner knowing of contraceptive use
		Friends or family knowing of contraceptive use

two rows of data are available, that is, with the perfect use of the contraceptive and with its typical use. This is a source of uncertainty which can be tested.

9.4.4 STEP 4: DETERMINING THE SCORES AND WEIGHTS – ESTIMATING THE VALUES OF THE OUTCOMES

9.4.4.1 Determining the Scores

The MCT model assumes that value functions for the clinical criteria are linear, in other words, that Rachael values each incremental added effect equally. To determine the scores for the criteria relating to the inconvenience of the different methods (such as avoiding going to a clinic, relying on a partner, loss of sensation, and remembering to take contraception), Rachael would be asked to provide her own ratings, on a scale from 0 to 1, of how bothersome the criteria level would be. For example, if remembering to take or use a contraceptive method was deemed as "extremely difficult," it is scored as 0.9 or 0.2 if deemed "slightly difficult."

TABLE 9.7

Effects Table for Contraceptive Methods for the Criteria Relevant to Rachael

Outcome	Time Point	Unit (Scale)	Female Sterilization	Male Sterilization	IUS (Mirena)	IUD (Copper T)	Injection	Implant	Male Condom	Female Condom	Worst^	Best^
Pregnancy (perfect use)~	1st year	%	0.5%	0.1%	0.2%	0.6%	0.2%	0.05%	2%	5%	5%	0.05%
Pregnancy (typical use)~	1st year	%	0.5%	0.15%	0.2%	0.8%	6%	0.05%	18%	21%	21%	0.05%
STI	Throughout use	Binary	No protection	No protection	No protection	No protection	No protection	No protection	Protected	Protected	No protection	Protected
Less heavy periods	Throughout use	Ordinal	No change	No change	Reduced/no periods	Heavier periods	Reduced	Reduced/irregular	No change	No change	Heavier periods	Reduced periods
Mood changes	Throughout use	Ordinal	No change	No change	Some evidence of improvement or worsening	No evidence	Some evidence of improvement or worsening	No evidence	No change	No change	Some Evidence	No change/No Evidence
Weight gain	Throughout use	Ordinal	No change	No change	Little evidence	No evidence	Some evidence	No evidence	No change	No change	Some evidence	No change
Remembering use	Throughout use	Ordinal	No	No	No – once every 5–10 years	No – once every 3–5 years	Yes – every 8 or 12 weeks	No – once every 3 years	Yes – each use	Yes – each use	Yes daily	No
Relying on my partner	Throughout use	Ordinal	Not difficult	Not difficult	Not difficult	Not difficult	Slightly difficult	Not difficult	Not difficult	Not difficult	Extremely difficult	Not difficult
Loss of sensation	Throughout use	Binary	No	No	No	No	No	No	Yes	Yes	Yes	No
Avoiding going to a clinic	Throughout use	Binary	No	No	No	No	No	No	Yes	Yes	No	Yes

^ Min and Max denote the range of outcomes between which the interventions perform.

~ Efficacy data from [45].

The darker the shading, the poorer the performance.

9.4.4.1 Determining the Weights

The MCT asks Rachael to indicate how much she is concerned with the different criteria she selected in Step 2 by asking her to move her cursor on a blue bar, which visually represents the relative importance placed on the criteria (see Figure 9.2). Rachael's weights show that avoiding pregnancy is her primary concern, followed by reducing her periods, avoiding weight gain, and, to a lesser extent, not having to remember when to take or use contraception, avoiding feeling irritable or depression, and, finally, avoiding STIs.

9.4.5 STEP 5: EVALUATION AND COMPARISON OF ALTERNATIVES

9.4.6 STEP 5.A: AGGREGATE THE DATA TO OBTAIN THE OVERALL VALUE
OF THE ALTERNATIVES

After normalizing the weights provided by Rachael and using formula (1) in Section 9.3.6, the MCT calculates the overall value of each of the contraceptive

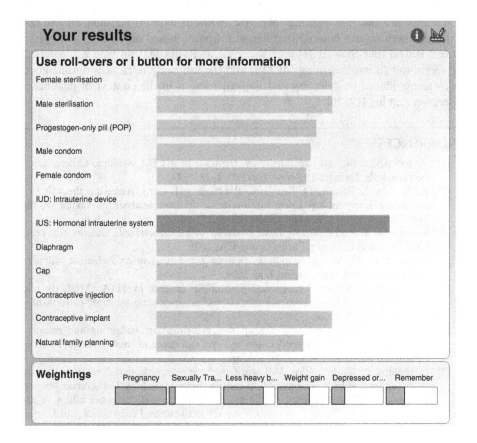

FIGURE 9.2 The MCT results screen with Rachael's selected attributes and weights. (Note: the swing weights displayed on the figure are normalized at the backend to generate the overall value of contraceptive methods) [43, p. 99].

methods available to Rachael, reflecting her priorities (Figure 9.2). Rachel's top two choices are to get a hormonal intrauterine system (IUS), followed by an intrauterine device (IUD) or implant.

9.4.7 STEP 5.B: TESTING ASSUMPTIONS

The MCT allows for Rachel to vary the weights while she analyzes the recommended contraceptive methods. This enables her to see how robust the rankings of contraceptives are to changes in weights.

Another key source of uncertainty lies in the efficacy of the contraceptives, in particular, how well they are used, though this is not explored within the MCT. Conceptually, this would involve evaluating the ranking of contraceptives using different performance estimates such as in the scenario that she was using the contraceptive methods perfectly.

9.5 SUMMARY

This chapter provides an introduction to MCDA and its multiple applications to healthcare decision making. Multiple methods exist to conduct an MCDA and the methods are tailored to different purposes, based on existing good practices. Belton and Stewart [1] and Keeney and Raiffa [42] provide a theoretical background to implementing MCDA, and the following references outline good practice guidance on selecting and implementing it in the context of healthcare decision making [19, 20].

REFERENCES

[1] V. Belton, T.J. Stewart, *An Integrated Approach to MCDA*, Multiple Criteria Decision Analysis, Springer US, New York, 2002, 331–343.

[2] K. Marsh, T. Lanitis, D. Neasham, P. Orfanos, J. Caro, Assessing the value of healthcare interventions using multi-criteria decision analysis: A review of the literature, *PharmacoEconomics* 32(4) (2014) 345–365.

[3] R. Clemen, T. Reilly, *Making Hard Decisions with DecisionTools*, 2nd rev. ed., Duxbury Thomson Learning, Pacific Grove, CA, 2001.

[4] P. Goodwin, G. Wright, *Decision Analysis for Management Judgment*, 4th ed., Wiley, Chichester, West Sussex, UK, 2009.

[5] N. Devlin, J. Sussex, Incorporating multiple criteria in HTA: Methods and Processes, 2011. www.ohe.org/publications/incorporating-multiple-criteria-hta-methods-and-processes.

[6] L. Phillips, C. Bana e Costa, Transparent prioritisation, budgeting and resource allocation with multi-criteria decision analysis and decision conferencing, *Annals of Operations Research* 154(1) (2007) 51–68.

[7] L. Phillips, N. Zafiropoulos, IMI work package 5: supplement 2 to Wave 1. case study report 1: B:Iii:Efalizumab Multi-criteria decision analysis: Decision conference. European Medicines Agency. http://protectbenefitrisk.eu/documents/Phillips_et_al_Supplement_2_to_Wave_1_case_study_report_Efalizumab_Feb2013.pdf., 2013.

[8] M.P. Ho, J.M. Gonzalez, H.P. Lerner, C.Y. Neuland, J.M. Whang, M. McMurry-Heath, A. Brett Hauber, T. Irony, Incorporating patient-preference evidence into regulatory decision making, *Surgical Endoscopy* 29(10) (2015) 2984–2993.

[9] European Medicines Agency, Benefit-risk methodology project. Work package 3 Report: field Tests. EMA/718294/2011. European Medicines Agency. www.ema.europa.eu/docs/en_GB/document_library/Report/2011/09/WC500112088.pdf., 2011.

[10] European Medicines Agency, Benefit-risk methodology project. Work package 4 Report: Benefit-risk tools and processes. EMA/297405/2012 – Revision 1. European Medicines Agency. www.ema.europa.eu/en/documents/report/benefit-risk-method ology-project-work-package-4-report-benefit-risk-tools-processes_en.pdf., 2012.

[11] European Medicines Agency, Benefit-risk methodology project. Update on work package 5: Effects table pilot (Phase I). EMA/74168/2014. European Medicines Agency. www.ema.europa.eu/en/documents/report/benefit-risk-methodology-pro ject-update-work-package-5-effects-table-pilot-phase-i_en.pdf., 2014.

[12] D. Endrei, B. Molics, I. Ágoston, Multicriteria decision analysis in the reimbursement of new medical technologies: Real-world experiences from hungary, *Value in Health* 17(4) (2014) 487–489.

[13] G. Radaelli, E. Lettieri, C. Masella, L. Merlino, A. Strada, M. Tringali, Implementation of EUNETHTA CORE MODEL®in LOMBARDIA: The VTS Framework, *International Journal of Technology Assessment in Health Care* 30(1) (2014) 105–112.

[14] M. Danner, J.M. Hummel, F. Volz, J.G. van Manen, B. Wiegard, C.-M. Dintsios, H. Bastian, A. Gerber, M.J. Ijzerman, Integrating patients' views into health technology assessment: Analytic hierarchy process (AHP) as a method to elicit patient preferences, *International Journal of Technology Assessment in Health Care* 27(4) (2011) 369–375.

[15] S. Youngkong, R. Baltussen, S. Tantivess, A. Mohara, Y. Teerawattananon, Multicriteria decision analysis for including health interventions in the universal health coverage benefit package in Thailand, *Value in Health* 15(6) (2012) 961–970.

[16] M. Airoldi, A. Morton, J.A.E. Smith, G. Bevan, STAR—People-powered prioritization, *Medical Decision Making* 34(8) (2014) 965–975.

[17] J.G. Dolan, E. Boohaker, J. Allison, T.F. Imperiale, Patients' preferences and priorities regarding colorectal cancer screening, *Medical Decision Making* 33(1) (2012) 59–70.

[18] J. Dodgson, M. Spackman, A. Pearman, L. Phillips, *Multi-Criteria Analysis: A Manual*, Eland House, London, 2009.

[19] K. Marsh, M. Ijzerman, P. Thokala, R. Baltussen, M. Boysen, Z. Kaló, T. Lönngren, F. Mussen, S. Peacock, J. Watkins, et al, Multiple criteria decision analysis for health care decision making—Emerging good practices: Report 2 of the ISPOR MCDA Emerging good practices task force, *Value in Health* 19(2) (2016) 125–137.

[20] P. Thokala, N. Devlin, K. Marsh, R. Baltussen, M. Boysen, Z. Kalo, T. Longrenn, F. Mussen, S. Peacock, J. Watkins, et al, Multiple criteria decision analysis for health care decision making—An Introduction: Report 1 of the ISPOR MCDA Emerging good practices task force, *Value in Health* 19(1) (2016) 1–13.

[21] L.A. Franco, G. Montibeller, *Problem Structuring for Multicriteria Decision Analysis Interventions, Wiley Encyclopedia of Operations Research and Management Science*, John Wiley & Sons, Inc., New York, 2011.

[22] R.L. Keeney, *Value-Focused Thinking: A Path to Creative Decision Making*, Harvard University Press, Cambridge, MA, 1996.

[23] S.D. Bond, K.A. Carlson, R.L. Keeney, Generating objectives: Can decision makers articulate what they want? *Management Science* 54(1) (2008) 56–70.

[24] L. Phillips, A theory of requisite decision models, *Acta Psychologica* 56(1–3) (1984) 29–48.

[25] C. Eden, Cognitive mapping, *European Journal of Operational Research* 36(1) (1988) 1–13.

[26] J. Mingers, J. Rosenhead, Problem structuring methods in action, *European Journal of Operational Research* 152(3) (2004) 530–554.

[27] D. von Winterfeldt, B. Fasolo, Structuring decision problems: A case study and reflections for practitioners, *European Journal of Operational Research* 199(3) (2009) 857–866.

[28] R.L. Keeney, R.S. Gregory, Selecting attributes to measure the achievement of objectives, *Operations Research* 53(1) (2005) 1–11.

[29] J.P.T. Higgins, D.G. Altman, P.C. Gotzsche, P. Juni, D. Moher, A.D. Oxman, J. Savovic, K.F. Schulz, L. Weeks, J.A.C. Sterne, The Cochrane Collaboration's tool for assessing risk of bias in randomised trials, *BMJ* 343(oct18 2) (2011) d5928–d5928.

[30] J.F.P. Bridges, A.B. Hauber, D. Marshall, A. Lloyd, L.A. Prosser, D.A. Regier, F. R. Johnson, J. Mauskopf, Conjoint analysis applications in health—A checklist: A report of the ISPOR good research practices for Conjoint Analysis Task Force, *Value in Health* 14(4) (2011) 403–413.

[31] R. Johnson, E. Lancsar, D. Marshall, V. Kilambi, A. Mühlbacher, D. Regier, B. Bresnahan, B. Kanninen, J. Bridges, Constructing experimental designs for discrete-choice experiments: Report of the ISPOR conjoint analysis experimental design good research practices task force, *Value in Health* 16(1) (2013) 3–13.

[32] E. Lancsar, J. Louviere, Conducting discrete choice experiments to inform health-care decision making, *PharmacoEconomics* 26(8) (2008) 661–677.

[33] T.L. Saaty, A scaling method for priorities in hierarchical structures, *Journal of Mathematical Psychology* 15(3) (1977) 234–281.

[34] BANA Consulting, M-MACBETH | A Multiple Criteria Decision Support System, 2017. http://m-macbeth.com/.

[35] K. Marsh, P. Thokala, A. Mühlbacher, T. Lanitis, *Incorporating Preferences and Priorities into MCDA: Selecting an Appropriate Scoring and Weighting Technique*, Multi-Criteria Decision Analysis to Support Healthcare Decisions, Springer International Publishing, New York, 2017, 47–66.

[36] PREFER 2019. Including the patient perspective. Prefer. www.imi-prefer.eu/.

[37] P. Blinman, M. King, R. Norman, R. Viney, M.R. Stockler, Preferences for cancer treatments: An overview of methods and applications in oncology, *Annals of Oncology* 23(5) (2012) 1104–1110.

[38] E.W. de Bekker-grob, C. Berlin, B. Levitan, K. Raza, K. Christoforidi, I. Cleemput, J. Pelouchova, H. Enzmann, N. Cook, M.G. Hansson, Giving Patients' Preferences a voice in medical treatment life cycle: The PREFER Public–Private Project, *The Patient - Patient-Centered Outcomes Research* 10(3) (2017) 263–266.

[39] Food and Drug Administration, Patient Preference Information: Voluntary submission, review in premarket approval applications, humanitarian device exemption applications, and de Novo Requests, and inclusion in device summaries and device labeling. Guidance for industry, Food and Drug Administration Staff, and Other Stakeholders 1500006. www.fda.gov/downloads/medicaldevices/deviceregulatio nandguidance/guidancedocuments/ucm446680.pdf., (2016).

[40] T. Tervonen, H. Gelhorn, S. Sri Bhashyam, J.-L. Poon, K.S. Gries, A. Rentz, K. Marsh, MCDA swing weighting and discrete choice experiments for elicitation

of patient benefit-risk preferences: a critical assessment, *Pharmacoepidemiology and Drug Safety* 26(12) (2017) 1483–1491.

[41] B. Roy, *Multicriteria Methodology for Decision Aiding*, Springer Science & Business Media, New York, 2013.

[42] R.L. Keeney, R. Howard, *Decisions with Multiple Objectives: Preferences and Value Tradeoffs*, Wiley, New York, 1976.

[43] R.S. French, F.M. Cowan, K. Wellings, J. Dowie, The development of a multi-criteria decision analysis aid to help with contraceptive choices: My Contraception Tool, *Journal of Family Planning and Reproductive Health Care* 40(2) (2013) 96–101.

[44] World Health Organization Department of Reproductive Health and Research (WHO/RHR), and Johns Hopkins Bloomberg School of Public Health/Center for Communication Programs (CCP). 2018. Family Planning - A Global Handbook for Providers. Baltimore and Geneva: CCP and WHO. https://apps.who.int/iris/bit stream/handle/10665/260156/9780999203705-engpdf;jsessionid=26F9A8EEF F279EAEDC36F38C60B9911B?sequence=1 ISBN 978-0-9992037-0-5.

[45] J. Trussell, Contraceptive failure in the United States, *Contraception* 83(5) (2011) 397–404.

10 DICE Simulation

A Unifying Modeling Approach for Pharmacoeconomics

J. Jaime Caro, MDCD, FRCPC, FACP
McGill University
Montreal, Canada
Evidera, Boston, USA

Jörgen Möller, MSc
Evidera
London, UK

TABLE OF CONTENTS

10.1 BACKGROUND

Mathematical models have been used to inform decisions in healthcare since at least the 1950s [1] and the underlying theory goes back much further [2]. Economic considerations were also incorporated early on [3]. Initially, these models were mostly based on decision trees, but their lack of explicit consideration of time led to the proposal that state-transition (i.e., "Markov";– see Chapter 4 for more on Markov models) models be used instead [4]. Recognition of the limitations of the state-transition approach brought to the fore the advantages of discrete event simulation [5]. Although other techniques have been used [6], these three comprise the vast majority of the models used in pharmacoeconomics [7], with the cohort Markov approach still the most common one [8]. Until now, these types of models have been viewed as distinct, mutually exclusive approaches [9], with the implication that a modeler must choose among them when designing a solution to a particular problem.

One of the main uses of models in pharmacoeconomics is to inform health technology assessments (HTAs) by agencies that control market access. For this purpose, the model integrates evidence from multiple sources to estimate the expected costs and health consequences of a new technology. As this HTA process may be, by its very nature, adversarial, the manufacturer seeks coverage at a price that is often higher than the agency finds reasonable – the means of estimating the expected consequences are subject to much scrutiny. Thus, the model must be presented to the health authority who needs to be able to evaluate its veracity. Apart from requiring appropriate technical knowhow, this evaluation also depends on the transparency of the submitted model. Given widespread familiarity with spreadsheets, it has become commonplace to request that the model be implemented using this kind of software with the hope that it will be more intelligible than if it is programed in another language.

Unfortunately, spreadsheets were not designed for sequential calculations required in most pharmacoeconomic models. As a workaround, many modelers implement their Markov approach by using sequential spreadsheet rows as a proxy for time, referencing the prior row to apply the changes in state membership each cycle. The resulting linkages can become quite complex and errors are common despite careful verification [10]. An even bigger problem, however, is that constraining the modeling tool to a spreadsheet has perpetuated the restriction to Markov models as implementation of a discrete event simulation in this kind of software is perceived as too onerous [11]. The contortions required to shoehorn the increasingly complex problems into cohort Markov models further complicate the formulas and linkages and increase the propensity for error.

It was against this background that a new modeling approach was sought. It had to free the modeler to properly reflect the necessary aspects of the problem without forcing simplification or unnecessary manipulation, yet it had to remain possible to implement it fully in a spreadsheet without requiring external software or programming. In addition, any new method should not introduce undue complexity and should remain as transparent as possible regardless of the complexity of the model. Flexibility to implement changes or alternative structures was also considered highly desirable. This quest resulted in the development of discretely integrated condition event (DICE) simulation. As it turns out, this approach unifies the common modeling techniques into a single framework.

In this chapter, the fundamental concepts of DICE are explained, the implementation of a DICE model is described, and the handling of the common modeling types is illustrated. The execution of a DICE simulation is detailed and various software variations are considered. Finally, the future directions for DICE are discussed.

10.2 FUNDAMENTALS

There are only two simple concepts in a DICE simulation: conditions and events. A condition is any item of information considered in the model, and an event is a point during execution where at least one condition is modified. The DICE simulation begins by initializing all the conditions to their known values at baseline (the "Start" event) and then proceeds to call each event at its scheduled time; process that event's consequences; and then call the next event, until an event designated "End" is encountered, at which point the simulation stops and the values of those conditions designated as Outputs are reported.

A very simple example is a survival model. In such a model, there are two obvious conditions: *Alive* and *Dead*. If everyone starts alive, then the concern is to record the proportion who die at each point in time of interest. At the **Start**, the simulation enters 100% for *Alive* and 0% for *Dead*. The simulation then advances to the next *TIME* (a condition, of course) where an event, say **Transition**, occurs and applies the *Death* probability (another condition). This results in a change in *Alive* using the simple equation *Alive* × (1−*Death*). Similarly, *Dead* changes to *Dead* + (*Alive* × *Death*). If the interest is in computing survival in life years, then an output condition, *LifeYears*, is defined and it accrues *Alive* × *Interval*, with the latter condition defined as the current *TIME* minus the *Previous Event Time*, a condition that is recorded at each occurrence of **Transition**. (Note that the accrual of life years should happen before the *Death* probability is applied.) This continues until either 100% are *Dead* or another criterion is met, say *TIME* is equal to another condition *Timehorizon*. This calls the **End** event, which stops the simulation and reports the *LifeYears*. What has been described in this simple example is, of course, a cohort Markov model.

It turns out that with these two basic concepts – conditions and events – it is possible to specify just about any pharmacoeconomic model of interest. Conditions can refer to all the characteristics of patients that may be relevant (e.g., age, sex, weight, smoking, biomarker level, EQ5D score, etc.); they can also describe the disease (e.g., subtype, severity, duration, prior treatment, score, etc.); the intervention (e.g., name, class, dose, route, side-effects, formulation, price, etc.); the values to be applied (e.g., utilities, unit costs, etc.); the parameters of equations (e.g., the type of distribution, its shape and scale); the times at which events will occur; model aspects (e.g., structural links, flags and toggles, random numbers, etc.); and, of course, the outputs to be accrued.

The special *output* conditions can be of several types. The simplest are *counters* that record the number of occurrences of a particular item of interest (e.g., deaths, hospitalizations, adverse events, treatment switches, etc.). Another type are *discrete accumulators* that add a quantity every time the corresponding thing happens (e.g., adding the cost of a doctor's visit or of an admission to hospital). Sometimes a quantity *accumulates continuously* over time (e.g., life years, QALYs, daily costs). Finally, there may be a need to *record* how an outcome changes over time (e.g., a Markov trace of a state membership). Regardless of the type, the accrual of outputs must be specified in each event, as appropriate.

The *events* in a DICE model are the points in time where the values of conditions change. These may correspond to an event that happens in the real world (e.g., birth, death, hospitalization, treatment initiation, etc.) or they may be an instance required by the model. The **Start** and **End** events are examples of the latter (mandatory ones), and the **Transition** event in a Markov model is one as well. There is no limitation to the number or nature of events in a DICE model – the modeler may specify as many as required to properly address the problem.

At each event, its consequences must be specified. These generally imply a change in the values of conditions. The simplest action is to **Set** the value of a condition. For example, the next time of occurrence of an event can be set to a very large value to ensure it does not happen again or it can be set equal to *TIME* so that it happens immediately. A related action is to **Update** a value, usually via some sort of calculation. *Age*, for example, is commonly updated by adding *TIME* to the *baseline Age*. Similarly, values are **Accrued** into outputs and more complex formulae can be used to **Calculate** other quantities (e.g., using a Cox proportional hazards equation). Sometimes, it is necessary to **Find** a value in a source table of conditions or to **Select** one according to some index. Finally, a logical expression may be used to **Decide** what happens next.

A DICE model is fully specified by the list of Conditions, including the list of special Output conditions, the list of Events, and the lists of Consequences of each event. These lists constitute the entire model and nothing else is required to detail the structure, inputs, and outputs. The execution of the simulation is carried out by a separate component that is not part of any specific model.

In order to find the next event and actuate its consequences, a *discrete integrator* is needed. This component must be able to read the lists that specify a particular model; it must find the next event and implement its consequences in their specified order and must also detect the **End** event where it stops and reports the outputs. It is convenient if around this core loop the discrete integrator also is able to repeat the simulation for each intervention to be modeled, for each subgroup or individual and for as many replications as the modeler specifies. These "outer loops" are described in more detail later.

10.3   EXECUTING A DICE SIMULATION

Execution of a DICE simulation is carried out by the discrete integrator. An important specification for developing the DICE method was that it must be possible to implement it entirely in a spreadsheet such as MS Excel®; the description here will address the details of this implementation. Needless to say, the same steps can be taken using many other software programs and this is briefly addressed in a subsequent section.

The key to executing a DICE simulation in MS Excel® is to impede the spreadsheet's inherent calculation of all equations at once and replace that by sequential activation of each instruction at the appropriate time. This is done by eliminating the equal signs that signal to Excel that an expression is a formula to be calculated. For example, if a spreadsheet cell contains the formula = *Age* + *Time*, then Excel will look for the cell range named *Age* and add to it the value of the cell named *Time*, placing the result in the cell that contains the formula. If the = is removed, however, Excel interprets *Age* + *Time* as a text phrase and does nothing with it. This successfully blocks execution of the formula until the precise time during the simulation when it needs to be activated.

The next step is to write a macro that reads the text expression and executes the specified formula. This is tantamount to entering the = in front of it. Once the calculation is complete and the result has been stored in some specified cell, the = must be removed again so that the formula reverts to a text expression until the next time it is activated. The macro then places the = in front of the next expression and the execution proceeds. The macro that implements this process is detailed in the following.

For the macro to be able to work, it must also be able to read the lists that fully specify the model. This can be implemented in MS Excel® by taking advantage of the formal Tables object included in the software. An Excel Table is a named set of demarcated columns and rows that has certain properties. By identifying a Table with a unique name, the *discrete integrator* can be directed to the appropriate Table, regardless of how many rows or columns it has or where it is placed in the spreadsheets. Apart from its name, a very useful property of a Table is its number of rows, not including the row holding the column labels. This property can be used to set the limit for the loop that executes the expressions in the table.

The three lists of components (Conditions, Outputs, and Events) are easily placed in named Excel® Tables. Each Table has the name of the component in the first column. The *Conditions* table (Table 10.1 has the current value of each condition in the second column. A third column can be used to store the initial values and the fourth column can hold any clarifying notes. The *Outputs* table can be laid out in a similar manner except there is no initial values column as these always accumulate from zero. The *All Events* table also has the name of each event in the first column (Table 10.2). The second column stores the

TABLE 10.1

Example of a conditions table listing four conditions

Name	Current value	Initial value
ID		1
Sex		Female
Age		64
BioMarker		144

TABLE 10.2

Example of the AllEvents table for a Markov model

Name	CurEventTime	Initial Time To Event	Table	Notes
Start		Now	tblStart	Initializes intervention
Partition		Cycle	tblPartition	Reads the partition curves
End		TimeHorizon	tblEnd	Ends the simulation

TABLE 10.3

Example of a portion of a Consequences table

Type	Name	Expression	Notes
Condition	LOS	Time-TimeAdmitted	Calculate length of stay
Condition	HospCost	LOS*DailyHospCost	Calculate hospital cost
Output	accruedQALY	accruedQALY+(Time-TimePrevEvent)*Utility	Accumulating QALYs
Condition	Utility	utilityStroke	Updating utility
Event	ThisEvent	Never	Do not execute this event again
Condition	NextEventTime	MIN(CurEventTime)	Find next event time
Condition	NextEvent	MATCH(NextEventTime, CurEventTime,0)	Find next event

current time to the next occurrence of that event. This array of event times is called ***CurEventTime***. The third column contains the initial time to that event (if known at the Start). The fourth column is very important as it contains the name of the Table that lists the consequences of that event.

The *Consequences* tables are organized a bit differently (Table 10.3). For convenience, the first column specifies the type of component that a row will act on. Although they are all conceptually conditions, it is useful to distinguish Outputs and Event times from the other Conditions. The second column specifies the name of the Condition, Output, or Event time that will be affected, and the third column contains the text expressions that detail what should happen when the *discrete integrator* activates that row. As already noted, these are devoid of the = that would convert them into Excel formulae, but they must respect Excel syntax so that at the time of activation by the *discrete integrator* they are correctly executed.

10.4   THE DISCRETE INTEGRATOR (DICE MACRO)

The DICE macro consists of a core loop that implements the DICE Consequences tables for one pass between the ***Start*** and the ***End*** events of several outer loops that repeat the execution for each intervention of interest, each subgroup, or individual profile, and for as many replications as the modeler intends

10.4.1   THE CORE LOOP

The core loop executes, for one profile and one intervention, the consequences of each event when it is called. For each selected event, the expressions in the event consequence table are executed one by one starting with the first row. For example, if the consequence table for the event *Hospital Discharge* has the first row in Table 10.3, the macro will subtract the value of the condition TimeAdmitted from the condition Time and store the result in the condition LOS, thus calculating the length of stay. These computations can be done by letting Excel calculate the expression using a normal cell; however, to improve execution speed, it can be done internally in the macro. The Consequence tables may have any number of rows, which the macro activates in the sequential order they are listed. After the first row is calculated and the received value stored in the named item, the next row is executed and so on to the end of that event table.

It can be important to be mindful that the macro calculates the rows in sequence, from top to bottom of the table. For example, if the rows in Table 10.3 were reversed, the calculations would render very different results because LOS needs to be calculated before it is used

Sometimes the reversal is intentional. For example, if the current utility value is for the "healthy" state and the person has a stroke, the QALYs must be accrued before the utility is updated to that poststroke (third and fourth rows in Table 10.3).

When the end of a Consequences table is reached, the macro looks for the next event. The core loop does so by choosing the minimum time from *CurEventTime* list. This is easily ensured by including the last two rows of Table 10.3 at the end of each event consequences table. The first of these rows finds the lowest event time and the second matches that to the corresponding event, yielding its row number in the *All Events* table (Table 10.2). The macro then uses that number to find the name of the Consequences table for that event. Since at the end of each Consequences table the macro checks the *CurentEventTime* list for the minimum time, it will find that the time of the event it is executing remains the lowest time, unless this is explicitly changed. Thus, early on in each event Consequences table the time of that event must be changed to a very high number (conveniently stored in a cell named Never). Or, if it is recurrent, to a time in the future (e.g., TIME + 1). If this is not done, the same event will be repeatedly executed, which leads to an infinite loop. This keeps happening until the *End* event is encountered (which is why an *End* event is mandatory). At that point, the macro executes any expressions in the *End* event and stops the core looping.

10.4.2   THE OUTER LOOPS

Since the core loop handles the events for one profile for one intervention, it needs to be executed multiple times to address any additional interventions and profiles. This is what the outer loops do.

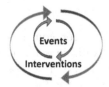

The "closest" loop out from the core events loop is the interventions loop.

This loop adds one to the current Intervention number, reinitializes the Condition values, Event times, and Outputs, and restarts the execution of the core loop. Thus, the values of intervention-specific conditions (e.g., efficacy, dose, cost, etc.) need to be set in the *Start* event. If there are many such conditions, it is convenient to group them in an *Initiate Treatment* event called immediately after *Start*.

Since all interventions are run without changing the profile, nuisance variance is reduced. If it is important that certain random numbers are the same for a given profile across the different interventions, these should be stored as Conditions. The macro will reset them to their initial values (without drawing new random numbers), thus using the same initial values for all interventions when running each profile.

The next loop further out from the core is the Profiles loop. This loop copies the values contained in the next profile into the corresponding Conditions (e.g., Sex, baseline Age, Biomarker level, etc.), and restarts the Interventions and core loops. The macro will loop in this way through all the profiles selected to run in the model.

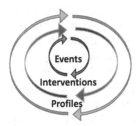

A profile contains the set of Condition values that identify a type of person that will be simulated. In a Markov cohort model, this might be a single profile, or there may be several to represent subgroups (e.g., younger females, younger males, older females, older males). In an "individual patient" model, there will be many profiles. If there are no relevant characteristics to consider, the single profile will consist of the minimum condition required by the DICE macro, which is "ID." There is no upper limit to the number of characteristics that can be stored in the profiles.

The profiles are listed in a profile table (Table 10.4) (side note, for Excel to keep the structure of a table it must have at least two columns, so a placeholder besides the "ID" is required if no other columns are defined), and copied into the condition table in the same order as in the table. Thus, the columns of the profile table should exist as conditions in the condition table in the same order. This Profile will be read into the Conditions table (Table 10.1).

TABLE 10.4

Example of a Profiles table

ID	Sex	Age	BioMarker
1	Female	64	144
2	Male	61	232

Once the values from the Profile table are copied into the Conditions table, any initial values are calculated (e.g., a risk score may depend on characteristics in the Profile) and any random numbers in the Conditions table are sampled. This completes the initial setup for that specific profile; it is stored so it can be used for all interventions (as explained earlier).

If a Profile table consists of multiple profiles, there is a possibility to filter (using the normal, built-in, Excel Autofilter function) the table and DICE will only run the visible profiles. Thus, the desired subgroup can be selected from the entire Profiles table.

Finally, the outermost loop is the Replication loop. This loop restarts all inner loops, reinitializing the profile selection, the intervention number, and the core loop. This will be repeated until the specified number of replications has been executed.

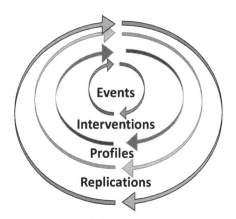

Since this loop will select all new random numbers, it will produce a set of outputs in each replication that differs from previous replications. By running many replications, stochastic uncertainty can be addressed. If no random numbers have been specified (i.e., model is fully deterministic, such as a cohort Markov model), the results would not change unless the inputs change between replications. This is what is done when running a Probabilistic Sensitivity Analysis (PSA), regardless of whether the model itself is deterministic or stochastic.

The number of calculations that is executed is multiplicative, meaning for a simple Markov model with three events (*Start, Transition, End*), a single profile, two interventions, a cycle time of 1 year, and a time horizon of 20 years, there will be 44 events (22 for each of the 2 interventions) to execute (each event having multiple rows to calculate). If a PSA of 1,000 replications is run, the core loop will be run 44,000 times. If there are 100 calculations in the core loop, the macro has to execute 4.4 million computations. If this is converted to an individual simulation with 1,000 profiles, there will be more than 4 billion expressions to calculate. This explains why execution times, especially for PSA, can be extended.

10.5 HOW A DICE SIMULATION INSTANTIATES THE DIFFERENT MODEL "TYPES"

To illustrate how the DICE method unifies the different model "types" under one framework, a simple example will be used. This example is the HSD (Happy–Sad–Dead) model, which starts off all profiles in Happy mood, with a certain probability of becoming Sad that depends on the intervention. Regardless of intervention, a person can become Happy again. Mood affects costs, utility, and the probability of dying.

10.5.1 SURVIVAL PARTITION

In a survival partition model, the cohort is distributed into the three states over time by reading the proportion who are no longer Happy and the proportion who have Died and obtaining the proportion who are Sad by subtraction. In this very simple conceptualization, the return to Happy is not allowed. The transition probabilities out of Happy are converted to a hazard, and since they are specified as constant, an exponential distribution is used to derive the partition curve for proportion still Happy. The transition probabilities to Dead are also converted to a hazard and in the same way used to derive the corresponding survival curve.

The model is implemented in DICE using a *Partition* event plus the mandatory *Start* and *End*. In the *Partition* event, the two curves are read, and the Sad proportion is calculated (Table 10.5). In the *Start* event, the intervention-specific conditions are initialized (Table 10.6). In the *End* event, little is required. The *All Events* table has three rows (Table 10.2). The Conditions table will contain all the conditions specified in these event tables together with their initial values. The Outputs table will list the three outputs specified.

10.5.2 COHORT MARKOV

Converting the survival partition model to a cohort Markov and enabling the transition back from Sad to Happy is fairly simple. In the *All Events* table, the Partition event is renamed Transition and its table specified as tblTransition.

TABLE 10.5
Example of a Partition event table

Type	Name	Expression	Notes
Event	Partition	Time + Cycle	Set next Partition to occur at cycle time
Output	QALY	QALY+Cycle*(Alive*uAlive +Sad*uSad)	Accrue QALYs using average utility
Output	Cost	Cost+Cycle*(Alive*cAlive +Sad*cSad)	Accrue Cost using average costs
Condition	ReadTime	Time + HalfCycle	Allows for half cycle correction
Condition	Alive	Exp(-DeathHazard*ReadTime)	Reads proportion still alive
Condition	Happy	Exp(-HappyHazard*ReadTime)	Reads proportion still happy
Condition	Sad	Alive-Happy	Computes proportion sad
Condition	NextEventTime	MIN(CurEventTime)	Find next event time
Condition	NextEvent	MATCH(NextEventTime, CurEventTime,0)	Find next event

TABLE 10.6
Example of a Start event table

Type	Name	Expression	Notes
Condition	Time	Start	To reset the clock to zero
Event	Start	Never	To avoid infinite loop
Output	Tmt	CHOOSE(IntervNum, "SoC", "UpUpMab")	To label the output according to treatment
Condition	HappyHazard	HappyHazard*CHOOSE(IntervNum, 1,HR)	Set according to treatment hazard ratio
Output	CostTmt	CHOOSE(IntervNum,CostSoc, CostInterv)	Set cost according to intervention
Condition	NextEventTime	MIN(CurEventTime)	Find next event time
Condition	NextEvent	MATCH(NextEventTime, CurEventTime,0)	Find next event

In the *Start* event, the HappyHazard is changed to pHappyToSad (the transition probability) and the adjustment uses a relative risk (RR). The *End* event does not change, but the Partition event is modified to the Transition event by replacing the three state condition rows (Tabke 10.7).

The new conditions replace now unneeded ones in the Conditions table, and that's it.

TABLE 10.7

Rows that replace the three state condition rows in the Partition event table

Condition	HappyDead	pHappyToDead*Happy	Computes happy who are dying
Condition	SadDead	pSadToDead*Sad	Computes sad who are dying
Condition	HappySad	pHappyToSad*Happy	Computes happy who get sad
Condition	SadHappy	pSadToHappy*Sad	Computes sad who get happy
Condition	Dead	Dead+HappyDead+SadDead	Collects proportion in Dead
Condition	Happy	Happy+SadHappy-HappyDead-HappySad	Collects proportion in Happy
Condition	Sad	Sad+HappySad-SadDead-SadHappy	Collects proportion in Sad

10.5.3 INDIVIDUAL MARKOV

In an individual Markov model, the structure is very similar to that of a cohort Markov model, but the transition probabilities are tested using random numbers. Since an individual can only be in one state, the three Cohort model states can be replaced by a single Condition named "status," with 1=Happy, 2=Sad, and 3=Dead. The transition probabilities are then cumulated to a single distribution that reflects the possibilities from each state. For example, if the individual is Sad, then the boundaries of the distribution segments are 0, pSadToHappy, 1-pSadToHappy-pSadToDead, and 1.

To implement this, the seven rows in Transition event that processed the transition probabilities are replaced (Table 10.8):

TABLE 10.8

Rows in the microsimulation Transition event table that replace the seven transition probability rows in the cohort Markov table

Output	QALYs	QALYs+Cycle*Utility	Accrue QALYs
Output	caCost	caCost+Cycle*Cost	Accrue costs
Condition	cumPHappy	CHOOSE(Status, 1-pHappyToSad-pHappyToDead, pSadToHappy,0)	Select cumulative happy probability that applies
Condition	cumPSad	CHOOSE(Status, pHappyToSad, 1-pSadToHappy-pSadToDead,0) + cumPHappy	Select cumulative sad probability that applies
Condition	Status	MATCH(RAND(), cumPArray, 1)	Determine current status
Condition	Utility	CHOOSE(Status,uHappy,uSad,0)	Assign utility according to status
Condition	Cost	CHOOSE(Status,CostHappy,CostSad,0)	Assign cost according to status
Event	End	If(Status=3,Time,End)	If Dead, end simulation

Presumably, the reason to convert to an individual simulation is that pHappy-ToSad depends on some individual characteristics. Suppose that a separate analysis produced a Cox proportional hazards equation:

$$\text{EXP}(0.37 * (\text{Sex} = \text{"Female"}) + (\text{Age} - 70) * 0.027 + 0.00189 * (\text{BioMarker} - 100))$$

If this will not be updated during the simulation, then the baseline Prognostic Index can be computed directly in the Profiles table where Sex, Age, and Bio-Marker are also stored. These conditions are added to the Conditions table and the expression for pHappyToSad is modified in the **Start** event to pHappyTo-Sad*CHOOSE(IntervNum,1,RR)*ProgIndex. The weighted average utility and cost used in the cohort model are no longer appropriate. Instead, the current Utility and Cost are set according to "Status" after this is updated (second to the last two rows in Table 10.8). These are used at the beginning of the Transition event to accrue the QALYs and costs (first two rows in Table 10.8). Finally, since the individual may die at a Transition event, there is no point in continuing to simulate that person, and so a line is inserted after the new Status is determined to end the simulation if it is determined that death will happen (last row of Table 10.8). The Conditions table is then modified accordingly, and the Cohort Markov has been converted to an individual model.

10.5.4 DISCRETE EVENT SIMULATION (UNCONSTRAINED)

The conversion to a discrete event simulation involves a bit more effort since transition probabilities are no longer tested but rather used to determine the time until each event will occur. Thus, the Transition event is deleted and replaced by three events (Table 10.9).

Assuming the individual begins Happy, the time until **GetSad** is selected in the Start event using a random number, and a hazard conditional on treatment and adjusted for the prognostic index (Table 10.10). The time to **Die** is selected in the same way.

TABLE 10.9

Modified AllEvents table for the discrete event simulation

Name	CurEventTime	Initial Time To Event	Table	Notes
Start	Now		tblStart	Initializes intervention
GetSad	Never		tblGetSad	Processes the change of mood to sad
GetHappy	Never		tblGetHappy	Processes the change of mood to happy
Die	Never		tblDie	Processes a death
End	TimeHorizon		tblEnd	Ends the simulation

TABLE 10.10

New rows in the Start event for the discrete event simulation

Event	GetSad	(LN(1-RAND())/-HazardToSad) + Time	Select time to GetSad
Event	Die	(LN(1-RAND())/-HazardToDie) + Time	Select time to Die

TABLE 10.11

Partial Get Sad event table

Type	Name	Expression	Notes
Condition	Interval	Time—TimePrevEvent	Store time from last event
Output	QALYs	QALYs+Interval*Utility	Accrue QALYs
Output	caCost	caCost+Interval*Cost	Accrue costs
Condition	Status	"Sad"	Update the status
Event	Die	Die*(HazardToDie/HazardSadToDie)	Update Time to Die
Event	GetHappy	(LN(1-RAND())/-HazardToHappy)+Time	Update Time to get Happy again
Condition	TimePrevEven	Time	Store time of this event

In the **GetSad** event, the Status needs to change, the time to Die must be recalculated and the time to Get Happy again derived (Table 10.11). The accumulation of Outputs is different now because it happens over a variable period since the fixed cycling no longer takes place. This interval is calculated near the beginning of each event (Table 10.11) and TimePrevEvent is stored near the bottom.

The **GetHappy** event is a mirror image of the **GetSad** one and **Die** is very simple, just calling the **End** event immediately. All new conditions are entered in the table and the conversion is complete.

10.6   ADVANTAGES AND LIMITATIONS

Hopefully, some of the many advantages of DICE simulation have already become evident. They are reiterated here with a few additions and the current limitations of the method are discussed as well.

10.6.1 ADVANTAGES

10.6.1.1 Simplicity

The method relies only on two concepts in a standard basic structure for every model. This means that if you can understand the concept of a condition (piece of information) and an event (point in time where that information changes), then you can assess any DICE model, and with appropriate subject matter knowledge, understand what it is doing [12].

A DICE model is entirely specified in MS Excel®, which is the most common choice for spreadsheet software. This ensures familiarity with the interface and navigation, the commands, and the available functions. All stakeholders have the option to engage early on to work with and review the model since it consists of a standard structure in basic Excel and the files are small and easily shared. Thus, there is no need to acquire or learn new software or find specialized programmers.

The clarity, brevity, and familiarity of a DICE simulation promote the possibility of making models open source, without imposing massive support burdens on the developers. An instruction manual that is generic is easily created and shared. Users can review the model, understand its workings, and if the developers allow it, even modify the structure.

10.6.1.2 Building and Modification

A DICE model is quick to implement, which shifts focus from coding and implementation (as in standard models) to design and development of inputs, especially equations, and ensuring that the model is appropriately reflecting the disease pathways and interventions. Once a modeler has built one DICE and has grasped the simple tables concept, building the next one is very easy and further reduces the emphasis on programming.

Any DICE table can be easily edited, with new elements added by just inserting rows, while no-longer needed ones can be simply deleted. There are no links to rebuild, no live formulas to handle, and the expressions in plain text are easy to check since they are entered only once. By avoiding repetition of formulas, the propensity for errors is minimized. The ease of modification makes changes – even last minute – possible (albeit revalidation should be done).

The flexibility of DICE, as explained in Section 10.5, allows for whatever structure makes sense for the problem. Even multiple types are easy to implement in the same model and Markov elements can be combined with discrete event simulation [13] in hybrid models that fit the problem. Aspects such as nonpersistence, switching treatment, sequential lines, side-effects, clinical decision rules, varying biomarker levels, patient characteristics, and more can be easily included since DICE handles time accurately and simply.

The often-heard lamentation that structural sensitivity analysis is very important but almost impossible to do is relieved. DICE makes it possible to address structural uncertainty in multiple ways, including the simple way of turning on and off events with toggles to incorporate two or more structures in the same framework. A toggle can change the structure from pure cohort Markov model to an individual patient time-to-event model to check if the selected structure has any significant impact on the results.

In the lifetime of a model, new data appear, as well as requests to adapt the model for other jurisdictions. Sometimes this requires changes to the model, if the new data are not directly comparable with the old ones, the new country's treatments paths differ, and so on. Since modifications of the model are easily made, this presents no problem.

10.6.1.3 Transparency

The models being used for HTA assessments are required to be transparent
[14], meaning that it should be possible for someone other than the modeler
to review the model and understand it (sometimes even rebuild it).

With the entire DICE model specified in a set of plain tables, built in Excel
(which is the preferred software of many HTAs [15, 16]), it is easy to accomplish
this. A typical text expression like "QALY+IntervalSincePrevEvent*Utility" is
easy to understand. And with the expression/formula being in one place and not
repeated many times, checking for linking errors is eliminated. Nothing is hidden,
and no part of the actual model is in code.

The macro running the model (looping through the event tables) is general
to all models, is very simple, and is provided open source. An agency reviewing
a model can run it using their own, checked, version of the macro to be certain
that the macro supplied with the model has not been modified.

10.6.1.4 The Method Is Open Source

The DICE method, as well as the macro running the model, is fully open
source and is available to download. The decision to keep it open and available
to anyone has fostered wide acceptance by authorities, clinicians, and other
stakeholders. The DICE consortium that will oversee the official version of the
DICE method and the macro, as well as facilitate updates, is coming together
as a mix of academia, industry, HTA agency, consultancies, and other key
competencies.

10.6.2 LIMITATIONS

10.6.2.1 Execution Speed

The use of Excel® and the transparent and generic way a DICE model is set
up leads to slower execution speeds, particularly if the core macro in VBA is
forced to go back and forth to the worksheets. A bespoke model custom coded
entirely in a fast programming language with all equations and expressions
embedded is certainly much faster but it loses transparency and the reliability
of having everyone depend on the same model engine, regardless of the disease
area or interventions.

There are ongoing efforts to speed up the DICE macro. It is already 20 times
faster than the first open version. It is expected that speed will continue to
improve as ways are found to avoid triggering the worksheets during execution.
In addition, a version of the macro that is written in a fast lower-level language
is in progress. This will increase the execution speed by a thousand times or
more without taking away any of the advantages of DICE.

10.6.2.2 Interaction and Queue Limitations

By design, DICE executes one profile (patient, cohort, subgroup) at a time,
which results in a few limitations. There can be no direct interactions between
profiles. For example, in a model of an infectious disease, it is not possible to

have one person infect another or, based on vaccination coverage, allow herd immunity to develop. Moreover, competition for resources (hospital beds, doctors, etc.) or estimating queuing time in front of constrained resources is not easily possible. For these types of requirements, the solution is to use appropriate sophisticated DES software that includes entities or agents, explicit representation of resources and queues, and other components.

10.6.2.3 Issues with International Excel, Versions, and Operating Systems

Microsoft enables Excel to adjust to local conventions and use either a point or a comma as the decimal separator. Similarly, the list divider (e.g., CHOOSE (InterventionNum, "SoC", "TheNewDrug")) can be a comma or a semicolon. In the normal function of a worksheet, where the expressions have an initial equal sign, and are thus recognized by Excel® as formulas, the components are updated to the local setting of that specific computer, including translations of function names (e.g., "CHOOSE" becomes "ELEGIR" if opened in a computer set to use Spanish as the default). This does not work when the equal sign is removed, turning the expression to pure text. This problem can be overcome either by:

- putting equal signs in all expressions before transferring a DICE workbook from one computer to another with a different language setting;
- opening the model in the recipient computer and verifying that the functions have been translated; or,
- removing the equal signs from all expressions to restore their "text" nature.

A handy utility for doing this is included in the DICE custom ribbon.

Of course, manual translation of the functions, replacement of decimal signs, and list dividers can always be done.

REFERENCES

[1] Ledley RS, Lusted LB. Reasoning Foundations of Medical Diagnosis: Symbolic Logic, Probability, and Value Theory Aid Our Understanding of How Physicians Reason. *Science*. 1959;130(3366):9–21. doi: 10.1126/science.130.3366.9.

[2] von Neumann J. Zur Theorie Der Gesellschaftsspiele. *Mathematische Annalen*. 1928;100:295–320.

[3] Weinstein MC, Stason WB. Foundations of Cost-Effectiveness Analysis for Health and Medical Practices. *New England Journal of Medicine*. 1977;296(13):716–21. doi: 10.1056/nejm197703312961304.

[4] Beck JR, Pauker SG. The Markov Process in Medical Prognosis. *Medical Decision Making*. 1983;3(4):419–58. doi: 10.1177/0272989x8300300403.

[5] Caro JJ. Pharmacoeconomic Analyses Using Discrete Event Simulation. *PharmacoEconomics*. 2005;23(4):323–32. doi: 10.2165/00019053-200523040-00003.

[6] Stahl JE. Modelling Methods for Pharmacoeconomics and Health Technology Assessment. *PharmacoEconomics*. 2008;26(2):131–48. doi: 10.2165/00019053-200826020-00004.

[7]   Caro JJ, Briggs AH, Siebert U, Kuntz KM. Modeling Good Research Practices—
      Overview: A Report of the ISPOR-SMDM Modeling Good Research Practices
      Task Force-1. *Value in Health*. 2012;15(6):796–803. doi: 10.1016/j.jval.2012.06.012.

[8]   Kim H, Goodall S, Liew D. Health Technology Assessment Challenges in Oncology:
      20 Years of Value in Health. *Value in Health*. 2019;22(5):593–600. doi: 10.1016/j.
      jval.2019.01.001.

[9]   Brennan A, Chick SE, Davies R. A Taxonomy of Model Structures for Economic
      Evaluation of Health Technologies. *Health Economics*. 2006;15(12):1295–310. doi:
      10.1002/hec.1148.

[10] Dasbach EJ, Elbasha EH. Verification of Decision-Analytic Models for Health
      Economic Evaluations: An Overview. *PharmacoEconomics*. 2017;35(7):673–83. doi:
      10.1007/s40273-017-0508-2.

[11] Caro JJ, Möller J, Karnon J, Stahl J, Ishak J. *Discrete Event Simulation for Health
      Technology Assessment*. Chapman and Hall/CRC,Boca Raton, Florida.2015.

[12] Caro JJ. Discretely Integrated Condition Event (DICE) Simulation for Pharmacoe-
      conomics. *PharmacoEconomics*. 2016;34(7):665–72. doi: 10.1007/s40273-016-0394-z.

[13] Caro JJ, Moller J. Adding Events to a Markov Model Using DICE Simulation.
      Medical Decision Making. 2018;38(2):235–45. doi: 10.1177/0272989X17715636.
      PubMed PMID: 28675959.

[14] Eddy DM, Hollingworth W, Caro JJ, Tsevat J, McDonald KM, Wong JB. Model
      Transparency and Validation: A Report of the ISPOR-SMDM Modeling Good
      Research Practices Task Force-7. *Value in Health*. 2012;15(6):843–50. doi: 10.1016/
      j.jval.2012.04.012.

[15] Davis S, Stevenson M, Tappenden P, Wailoo A. *NICE DSU Technical Support
      Document 15: Cost-Effectiveness Modelling Using Patient-Level Simulation*. Report
      By the Decision Support Unit, London, 2014.

[16] Merlin T, Tamblyn D, Schubert C. *Guidelines for Preparing a Submission to the
      Pharmaceutical Benefits Advisory Committee, Version 5.0*. Australian Government,
      Department of Health,Canberra, Australia.2016.

11 Some Problems/ Assumptions in Pharmacoeconomic Analysis

Stuart Birks, PhD
Massey University
Palmerston North, NZ

Alan Haycox, MD
University of Liverpool
Liverpool, UK

TABLE OF CONTENTS

11.1   INTRODUCTION

Previous chapters have outlined four commonly used evaluation techniques, cost–benefit analysis (CBA), cost-effectiveness analysis (CEA), cost–utility analysis (CUA) and cost-minimisation analysis (CMA), which are all used to assist in decision-making. It might be thought that this only involves undertaking the calculations and then applying a decision rule. For example, the simplest rule in CBA is to proceed in all cases in which CBA gives a positive net present value where benefits exceed costs, so a net gain to society is achieved. However, it may not be desirable to rely solely on such a decision rule. The rule can result in poor decisions when there are mutually exclusive alternatives. Mutually exclusive alternatives occur when there is a specific resource which, if used on one project, is no longer available for others (hence, there is an opportunity cost in terms of alternative options foregone). For example, a piece of land could be used for a hospital or a rest home but not both. Even if both give positive net present value, only one of them can be undertaken. In this situation, it is suggested that the one with the highest net present value be chosen to achieve the greatest benefit for society. In addition, there may be reservations about the distributional effects of this approach. These arise because gains and losses are simply added up to get a net present value, meaning that some people may gain substantially while others may lose. The decision maker may be concerned about the resulting distribution of costs and benefits, rather than just their totals. This is just one of several criticisms that can be raised about the approach. For a broadly based critical perspective on the application of neoclassical microeconomics to policy decisions, see Chapter 14 of Hunt [1].

A more fundamental concern is the allocation of decision-making responsibility. At one extreme, decisions could be made entirely according to a mechanical decision rule whereas, at the other extreme, decision makers could have full discretion in their choices. In a democracy elected representatives are entrusted to make decisions on people's behalf, and they may be able to add societal insights that cannot be incorporated into mechanistic approaches. They may be able to incorporate preferences, as with distributional aspects, or there may be specific local considerations not covered in general evaluations. In practice, small, routine decisions are likely to be made according to established rules, whereas larger, one-off decisions are more commonly made by appointed/elected decision makers.

Briefly, then, a purely mechanical approach may not always be satisfactory as the technique and the decision rule may not always give the optimal answer and it might be considered important that the final decision be left to elected representatives. In other words, the actual **process** of policy making/decision-making may be important. Tyler [2] describes the importance of **procedural justice**, suggesting that people are more willing to accept decisions, even those that are against their interests, if they believe that the processes followed were fair. In recent decades, an emphasis on 'evidence-based policymaking' would suggest a mix of technical analysis and political input, with the former serving to inform the latter.

11.2   STEPS IN THE TECHNICAL ANALYSIS

In making any resource allocation decision there will undoubtedly be a multitude of factors to consider. However, a decision rule approach requires that the mass of relevant information be somehow condensed into a single number. Three steps are involved. First, the components in relation to the specific problem must be identified and measured. This can be difficult and will involve expertise beyond that commonly possessed by an economist. In other words, a cross-disciplinary approach is required. A health specialist may be aware of the relevant clinical dimensions associated with a treatment and an economist should understand the economic dimensions. However, perhaps neither is well informed on the psychological and social factors that may affect preferences and perceived costs and benefits. The current move by some academic economists into the growing area of "happiness research" indicates both recognition of our lack of understanding of this issue and acknowledgement of its possible importance [3]. The need for a mix of health and economic information is clearly described from the introduction to Dasbach, Elbasha and Insinga [4] and Goldie et al. [5] beginning with a reference to health, economic and national policy perspectives.

Second, some or all of the selected components of costs and benefits will have to be valued. To the extent that the analysis is based on dollar values, market or other prices ("shadow prices") must be determined. Shadow prices are needed if there is no market for the item or if it is considered that the market prices are misleading. Moreover, as some costs and benefits occur in the future, estimates will have to be made as to future prices, along with a mechanism for comparing values over time. Goldie et al. refer to the quality adjustment of life expectancy as a form of valuation [5]. For this to be the case, the basic unit of "currency" utilised is a healthy year of life.

Third, some form of analysis will have to be undertaken to convert the information into the measures to which the decision rule can be applied. These might be net benefits, benefit:cost ratios or cost per quality-adjusted life year (QALY), for example.

11.3   POTENTIAL PROBLEM AREAS

Analytical techniques are applied at each step in the analysis, and it is important to assess the value and appropriateness of such techniques. To what extent do they address the issues in such a way as to give the "right" answers or are they simply commonly accepted methods? In other words, are they based on logic and proof or rhetoric and persuasion? Ideas change over time, and methods applied and accepted in the past may be considered unsatisfactory now just as present approaches will almost certainly be interpreted as being suboptimal in the future. To some degree, we are simply faced with a problem of having to make difficult decisions, so we rely on approaches that will hopefully give reasonable results in the majority of situations. Such techniques remove some of the responsibility from the decision makers on the basis that they followed "best practice," rather than acting subjectively or according to personal prejudice. In this section, two broad aspects of analysis are considered. First, we look at discounting, then we consider the identification of preferences as a basis for measuring or valuing costs and benefits.

11.3.1 DISCOUNTING

Aggregation is the process of grouping together items and treating them as if they are the same. We aggregate diverse expenditures by using dollar values as a common measure. We give figures for the number of patients treated, even though individual treatments may vary. There is an assumption that all patients are the same. Similarly, in Goldie's model, it is assumed that "all persons residing in a particular health state are indistinguishable from one another" [5]. Aggregation is central to the process of reaching one number on which to apply a decision rule.

Frequently we must aggregate over time. When dollar values are used, it is commonly accepted that a dollar today is not equivalent to a dollar next year. At the very least, a dollar today could be set aside to earn interest, thereby having a value greater than one dollar by next year. For this and other reasons, it is widely accepted that, when aggregating monetary values over time, we should adjust for timing. Hence, we could compound the values to give some value in the future, taking into account the interest that could be earned. More commonly, we would follow this process in reverse, by discounting future values to give a measure of "present value" (PV).

At its simplest interpretation, given a sequence of payments over time, the PV of the sequence is the sum of money that, if held today, could be invested at the specified interest rate so as to allow the holder to just recreate the payments. There are other interpretations that can apply when other discount rates are used. These are based on other reasons for having positive "time preference," whereby the present is valued more highly than the future. For example, if I could earn 10% annual interest, then $100 today could turn into $110 in one year and $121 in two years. If I wanted to spend $100 this year, $110 next year and $121 the year after, then it would not matter if I were paid those sums at those times, or if I received $300 now. With $300 now, I could spend $100 now, while investing $100 for one year and $100 for two years. Alternatively, if I could also borrow at 10% interest and I wanted to spend $300 now, then it would not matter whether I received all $300 now, or three yearly payments of $100, $110 and $121. The nature of the required calculations is described in the Appendix to this chapter.

In summary, *if it is possible to borrow or lend at the same rate of interest,* then it is possible to convert any pattern of payments and receipts over time into any other pattern so long as they both have the same PV (calculated by discounting at that rate of interest). The PV figure gives us all the information we need. Aggregation over time is acceptable because timing is not important.

11.3.1.1 What Discount Rate?

It is well recognised that streams of monetary values over time can be combined through discounting. The discussion above indicates one possible justification for this approach, subject to the assumption that borrowing and lending are possible at a rate of interest equal to the discount rate. It is an approximation for several reasons.

a) Borrowing and lending rates commonly differ.

b) There may be further distortions due to differing tax treatments of interest earned and paid. Interest income may be taxed, but it may be possible to set it off against losses elsewhere. Interest payments may be made from after-tax income (as with home mortgages), or be considered as a deductible expense, as with mortgage interest on investment properties, thereby coming out of before-tax income.

c) Interest payments and receipts will be measured differently if considered from the point of view of individuals (concerned about the effect on them, and hence looking at the net-of-tax sums), or the government or society, concerned about the overall effect from their perspectives.

d) Interest rates are also sensitive to inflation. Lenders commonly want higher interest when inflation is high. The extra interest is really a response to the falling purchasing power of the money they have lent. There is therefore a capital repayment component in the interest payment. Economists talk of nominal and real interest rates. Nominal rates are those actually charged or paid. Real rates are the percentages paid after adjusting for the distorting effects of inflation. As a simple example, if the nominal interest rate is 10% and inflation is 10%, then $100 lent for a year would give the lender $110 at the end of the year. This is just enough to buy what could have been bought with $100 at the start of the year, so the lender is no better off. The $10 interest is nothing more than a part of the repayment of capital, and the real interest rate is zero. Moreover, if tax on interest must be considered, this means that inflation is causing a portion of the real capital to be taxed on repayment.

Prevailing interest rates are set through financial markets and are influenced by market demand and supply. It could be considered that this process fails to reflect society's preferences. For example, it is sometimes suggested that individuals, thinking of themselves, may have a shorter time horizon than society as a whole which may be considering future generations. Placing a lower value on the future equates to discounting at a higher rate. It is therefore widely thought that the individual/private discount rate is too high, and that the social discount rate should be lower.

Goldie et al. adopt a societal perspective, discounting future costs and life years at an annual rate of 3% [5]. If we use a discount rate other than that at which we can borrow or lend, then our interpretation of discounting breaks down. It would not be possible to switch between any two payment streams of the same PV. Some other justification for ignoring timing would then be required.

An alternative interpretation might be that we are indifferent between the two streams, so timing is not important. This does cause a problem, however. If we are indifferent at the chosen discount rate, and we can borrow and lend at another rate, then we have an incentive to actively borrow or lend. Consider a social discount rate of 5% and a prevailing interest rate of 10%. Society would be indifferent between $100 now and $105 next year, but $100 now could earn interest and become $110 in a year's time. Society (or the government on society's behalf) has an incentive to defer $100 of spending now, so as to be able to spend $110 next year. If the rates are constant, it has an incentive to defer every $100 of spending now, and it could also defer every $110 of spending next year so as to be able to spend $121 the following year, and so on. In fact, if the social rate is lower than the market rate, it would make sense to defer all spending indefinitely!

More probably, the more current spending is curtailed, the greater the value that would be placed on an additional dollar of current spending, and the more future potential spending is increased, the lower the value seen in an additional dollar spent in the future. This is an example of marginal analysis, which is widespread in economics. Additional costs and benefits are unlikely to be constant as quantities increase. This indicates a limitation of cost-effectiveness measures or cost:benefit ratios which, being ratios, conceal the scale of activity at which they were calculated. There is no reason to assume the same cost-effectiveness for a screening program reaching 70% of a target population and the same program reaching 90% of the population. As Goldie states, "screening is not equally accessible to all groups of women" [5], and Dasbach describes Taira's finding of cost-effectiveness varying with coverage [4].The social and private rates would therefore move closer together. As we do not see major spending deferral, perhaps the difference in rates is very small. Alternatively, if the decision is political, then public decisions (including the choice of discount rate) may be shaped by the expression of individual preferences through the political process, or through politicians placing emphasis on short-term, political considerations.

11.3.1.2   First-best and Second-best Solutions

Economic analysis frequently aims to describe a "best" solution based on structures assumed in economic theory under conditions of perfect competition. These solutions have been referred to as "first-best" solutions. Perfect competition is seldom if ever observed in real-world markets and hence first-best solutions may therefore not be the best in real-world practice. The optimal decision for the real world, recognising the inevitable distortions from perfect competition, is called the second best. Lipsey and Lancaster's article is a classic treatise on the Theory of Second Best [6]. The points they raise are relevant here. The argument that future benefits would be undervalued in evaluations using standard discount rates should be considered in the context of the operation of the economy as a whole. Note that a common approach in economic theory is to make an implicit assumption that other parts of the economy are functioning properly. The undervaluing of future benefits is then the only distortion to consider. In other words, we could aim for a "first-best" solution. However, if there are distortions elsewhere that cannot be removed, then a first-best solution is not attainable. The problem then becomes far more complex.

In making the case for lower or zero discount rates for health benefits, it has been suggested that there would be underinvestment in health care if standard discount rates are used. However, a case could also be made that there is underinvestment in numerous private sector areas. The argument goes as follows. Private sector investors are aware that outcomes are uncertain. If an investment turns out badly, the costs to them can be severe. They are therefore likely to want a higher expected return to compensate them for the risks they face. This is called risk aversion. The outcome of numerous private investments from the perspective of society as a whole is far less uncertain. Some projects succeed, others fail, and there is some averaging out overall. From a social perspective, therefore, it is desirable for many individual risks to be ignored. Therefore, there are potential private sector investments that are socially desirable but are not undertaken due to risk aversion. The private sector is under-investing. Healthcare investments and private sector non-healthcare investments are competing against each other for limited funds. If lower requirements are set for health investments, more of them will be approved, further reducing (or "crowding out") other investment.

This is a major problem as the world assumed by the theory is a simplification which ignores a range of real-world distortions and suboptimalities which limit the practical value of the theory. At the same time, decisions must be made on some basis. The term used to describe simplified approaches to decision-making is "heuristics." Perhaps, then, theory could be considered as giving an analytic basis for some heuristic approaches that we can and do use as a loose guide to our decision-making. They may be helpful, but they are approximations which will not always give us the most appropriate answers.

11.3.2 Discounting Non-monetary Units

A clear distinction separating CMA, CEA and CUA from CBA is that the latter requires dollar values to be placed on all the costs and benefits that are considered. In contrast, CMA, CEA and CUA include non-monetary measures. As mentioned previously, one popular non-monetary measure in health economics is the QALY. Hence, CEA is often applied in terms of cost per QALY gained from treatments. For the purposes of illustration of non-monetary measures, the following discussion will consider just life years. For a novel (and fictional) approach to placing a monetary value on life, see Johnson [7].

The problem of discounting non-monetary units can be considered in two steps. First, is it meaningful to add up quantities and then undertake analyses in relation to the totals? Second, if the answer to the first question is "yes," should we then adjust for the timing of the quantities by discounting (i.e. discounting at a non-zero rate)? The first question is important because it asks what meaning can be given to the units used. Discussion on discounting such units commonly focuses only on the second question, as if the question were solely one of deciding whether to discount at a non-zero rate, and, if so, what rate should be chosen.

11.3.2.1   Is It Meaningful to Simply Add up Quantities?

Consider the outcome of a treatment being measured in terms of increased life expectancy, or life years gained. Is it meaningful to talk of total life years? It might be helpful to think of some other item, such as motor vehicles. Would we find it helpful to consider the number of motor vehicles produced in a year or in a decade? Motor vehicles include motorcycles, cars, buses, trucks and even motor boats. Even taking cars alone, there are numerous makes and models. The differences may be unimportant, but an annual data series showing motor vehicles by volume could look very different from a series by value, which can be affected by the types of vehicles produced. Nevertheless, volume figures are sometimes presented as an indication of output. What about volume figures for a decade? It would be rare for economists to refer to numbers such as these. They may be used for descriptive purposes but are unlikely to be used for analysis, especially in relation to costs. Timing of production might be considered important, and costs over a decade would almost certainly be discounted. If we find it misleading with cars, would it not be equally misleading with life years?

There is a fundamental process involved when we are adding up in this way. Whenever we group items, whether quantities or values, we are **aggregating**, and are therefore at risk of encountering aggregation problems. These arise because aggregation can involve the loss of information or misleading simplifications. The key requirement for aggregation is homogeneity of the components of the aggregate. When an aggregate variable (such as total output) is used in a specific analysis, a context is defined. This includes the variable's relationships with other variables (such as total cost). There is no loss of information if the relationships are identical for each component of the aggregate (such as each motor vehicle). Conversely, if the relationships differ, we are approximating (as with using an estimate of average cost). Birch [8] gives an example of the Simpson paradox, where one treatment appears better than another when considering a sample from a population as a whole, but the results are reversed when considering the population divided into two subgroups, rich and poor, for which the effects differ. Similarly, if we are using aggregate output when our real concern is with benefits, there is an implicit assumption that all units provide equal benefit. Aggregation of health state values is discussed in Brazier et al. [9]. They assume that some form of aggregation is acceptable. Their focus is on the method of aggregation, questioning whether the mean or median response should be used. This indicates a further set of options to consider when constructing an aggregate.

Hence, we are making implicit homogeneity assumptions as soon as we group life years in the context of a cost-effectiveness analysis.

11.3.2.2 What Do Discounted Quantities Actually Mean?

Consider now the concept of discounting motor vehicle production as we might discount dollar values. With annual value of production figures, we could calculate their PV through discounting at an appropriate rate. So, instead of simply adding up motor vehicles, a volume measure, can we make some equivalent adjustment for the actual year in which the vehicles are produced? The result would not be in the same units as the undiscounted total. Just as we talk of PV, which is different from the sum of annual dollar values, we would have to talk of some unit such as "present motor vehicles." The production of 100,000 motor vehicles a year for ten years would not give us one million motor vehicles. At a 10% discount rate it would equate to the production of 675,904 "present motor vehicles". Can we be comfortable with this concept? We do not use it when considering motor vehicles. Should we use it when considering life years? Instead of referring to a life expectancy at birth of 75 years, should we discount at 10% per annum and talk of a life expectancy of eleven "present years"?

There is a way that this approach can be explained. It is not that we are avoiding valuing life years. Rather, without open acknowledgement, we are implicitly valuing them, but in another currency. The prices of all life years at the same time are assumed equal. This, in relation to quality-adjusted life years, has been encapsulated in the expression that a QALY is a QALY is a QALY (see, for example [10],). If we think of it, this may not be something we are willing to accept. The position runs counter to that expressed in the "fair innings" viewpoint, which is based on the idea that people who have already lived a certain amount of time have had a fair innings, whereas younger people deserve more [11]. Considering fair innings, it may be paradoxical that people's preferences are used to estimate specific QALYs, but they are ignored when aggregating QALYs.

If life years are then discounted to calculate present life years, it is assumed that the implicit values of a life year change in a systematic way according to the timing. All that is missing from this approach for us to be able to go from present life years to dollars is an exchange rate.

The length of life issue raises another possible complication. What if the effects of a treatment for an individual can be felt over several years? The effects may well differ according to the age, and hence the life expectancy, of the patient. Consider, for example, a treatment with the simple effect that it prevents instant death, after which the individual can live as normal. This might give 10 years of life to a 75-year-old but closer to 60 years of life to a 25-year-old. In other words, the effects of a treatment could depend not only on the treatment itself but also on the types (or age groups) of individuals treated. Should treatments then be assessed in relation to each type separately? Even when assessed for one group, results may vary. For the analysis to produce a single figure, this uncertainty will have to be ignored.

11.3.2.3   What Discount Rate Should Be Used?

This issue is discussed in detail in Neumann's update of Gold et al.'s classic book [12].The question of choice of discount rate is generally posed in terms of a search for some constant rate to apply. Hence there is an implicit assumption that the rate does not vary over time. However, there is much controversy about the choice of discount rates and whether costs and benefits should be discounted at the same or different rates. In recognition of this, Drummond and Jefferson [13] suggest that sensitivity analyses should be undertaken using alternative discount rates, including zero. One reason why zero discount rates have been suggested in both the health and the environmental area is that the benefits are likely to be felt some time in the future, whereas many costs are incurred now. It has been argued that discounting at a positive rate counts against activities with more distant benefits. Discounting at a zero rate results in these benefits being more prominent and is, therefore, thought by some to be more desirable. The argument is flawed. It is claiming that the approach should be taken not because of some inherent validity in the reasoning, but because the results more closely reflect the advocates' wishes. However, a discount rate should not be chosen simply because it gives the result we want. There should be some stronger rationale. If the results are considered unacceptable when using an economically justified discount rate, then perhaps the problem lies elsewhere in the analysis. For example, perhaps we should consider the (explicit or implicit) values placed on the future benefits.

Those who want a lower or zero discount rate are really saying that the analysis is based on prices of future life years that are too low. A zero-discount rate means that we should be prepared to set aside as much now to gain a future life year as we are willing to spend for an extra life year this year. That same sum would grow over time, so more is effectively being allocated per life year in the future. When applied to the environment, the argument could be that future consequences of environmental damage are greater than currently commonly believed, and the costs of repairing the damage will rise if the problem is not addressed soon. However, logic aside, it may be politically easier and more persuasive to use the argument that discounting shows a lack of concern for the future, hence the call for a zero-discount rate for environmental issues.

If we treat discounting (including at a zero rate) as a means of condensing a series of life years over time into one number, we could apply the same test as for PV. If two series equate to the same total number of present life years, is it possible to convert from either series into the other? If so, then we could consider them equivalent, and the actual timing unimportant. Can we forego current life years in exchange for future life years or vice versa? For individuals, this may be difficult, although there could be some scope for shifting quality of life from one year to another. For society as a whole, there is more flexibility. Nevertheless, the ability to shift may not match the discount rate being used for financial transactions.

Failing the ability to shift, would we be comfortable with an assumption that we (or society) are indifferent between the two series? One interpretation of discounting is based on "time preference", with the view that people value the present more highly than the future. For a person to be indifferent between two sums of money, one now and the other at some time in the future, it would generally be expected that the future sum would be larger (and, if discounted to the present, the discounted value would equal the sum available now). It is not clear that we would view years of life in the same way. First, mainstream economics assumes that people get utility from the consumption of goods and services. The more they consume, overall, the greater their utility. Were it possible to simply suspend a year of life, so as to live it sometime in the future, then it would also be possible to leave wealth to accumulate, enjoying the much larger sum at the later date. Given that possibility, a year of life in the future would be far preferable to a year of life now. Put more simply, if life will be so much better in the future, it is preferable to increase future life rather than life in the present (for individuals or for society as a whole). This raises a fundamental issue. While there are attempts to limit world population growth, large sums are being spent on health care, including health care of the elderly. Analyses such as CMA, CBA and CEA are concerned with efficient use of resources, given specified objectives, focusing on costs and benefits for people who are alive. Future generations only have an indirect say in these decisions to the extent that they are a factor influencing the preferences of the current population. Besides efficiency, we are also concerned about equity issues and perhaps broader aspects of an implicit social contract. For these, the distribution of costs and benefits is important. People's perceptions of the decision-making processes may also be important, as can be seen in literature on procedural justice. This is the reverse of the monetary evaluation, one argument of which states that people will be better off in the future, so an additional dollar then would be valued less than an additional dollar now. This is based on the concept of diminishing marginal utility. Note that the link between utility and wellbeing is more complex than assumed in current mainstream microeconomics. Earlier thinking on utility was not restricted to it being a function of goods and services (see [14]), and developments in the area of happiness research are also based on a broader view [15]. As a curiosity, Jeremy Bentham, the most prominent name associated with utilitarianism, is reported to have said that he would rather live the rest of his life one year per century[16].

In summary, there is no clear and generally accepted answer as to what discount rate should be chosen, or even if the aggregation and discounting process has any validity. At best, it could perhaps be argued by analogy that if an approach is valid for monetary measures, then a similar method may suit non-monetary measures. A deeper investigation of the assumptions required for this raises serious concerns. An alternative approach could be to forego the attempt to find a single number, presenting instead a broader range of information to assist decision makers. This point has been made in Bos, Postma and Annemans [17].

11.3.3 MEASURING PREFERENCES

Mainstream economic theory includes the assumption that people's preferences are exogenous and therefore taken as given and determined outside the
theory. This is understandable, given the emphasis on static analysis and
ceteris paribus assumptions in this body of theory. Static analysis does not
consider adjustments over time, and at any one time, preferences are fixed. In
addition, under the economic "ideal" of perfect competition, people are
assumed to be perfectly informed. Even where imperfect information is
assumed, it is interpreted as the information being incomplete, rather than
actually false, or misleading. This does not reflect the real world. In practice,
issues are highlighted, opinions are shaped, people are persuaded to see things
from particular perspectives, and understanding is influenced by experience,
the media and the attitudes of others.

11.3.3.1 Whose Preferences?

QALYs or other measures, including monetary valuations, are required for
assessing outcomes or benefits, and sometimes costs, associated with interventions. Goldie et al. considered costs and clinical benefits, but recognised the
need for data on patient and parent preferences [5]. There are not well-
functioning markets for all the aspects that should be considered. Preferences
must be deduced by other means. One approach is by asking people, as with
stated-preference techniques. For a brief overview of stated preference techniques in healthcare evaluations, including discussion of problems and limitations, see Bridges [18]. However, this begs the question of who should be
asked, and how?

When considering the effects of a healthcare intervention, some studies ask
healthcare professionals, others ask patients and yet others ask the general
public. These may give different answers. They have differing levels of understanding, their emotional commitments to the issues may differ, and they are
taking different perspectives. Moreover, people's preferences may change
according to their circumstances. A specific problem has been identified with
patients' preferences, namely "peak" effects and "end" effects [19]. People's
remembered perceptions are heavily influenced by the extremes (peaks) and by
the situation at the end, as with pain that suddenly stops, compared to an
equivalent pain that then gradually eases, with the former being considered
worse. An additional dimension is the extent to which findings from a study
can be applied. Do they relate to that study sample alone, or are they more
useful than that? In other words, there are issues of transferability and gener-
alisability ([20], Chapter 10).

When obtaining survey results, information is passed on to the participants.
The results can depend on people's prior knowledge and the information
given. In addition, views can change when people are responding in
a communal situation where there has been some general discussion. It is not
clear whether these changes are due to people refining their views or adapting
so as to appear to conform to the general view. This has been discussed in

a health context [21], also raising the point that individuals' valuations may differ depending on whether they are considering a personal or societal perspective. A similar point has been made in Richardson and Smith [22] on willingness to pay for a QALY. Group influence on expressed views has also been discussed in the broader context of deliberative democracy [23].

Whereas markets provide a price (hopefully the equilibrium price), surveys give individual preferences. These must then be combined to get an overall figure. Utility theory and welfare economics stress that a person may be able to indicate a preference ordering, stating if A is preferred over B, but this is an ordinal measure. As such, it does not say by how much A is preferred, nor is it possible to compare the degree of one person's preference to that of someone else. For that, cardinal measures are required. Nevertheless, some method of aggregation is required so as to combine individual preferences to obtain a measure for the evaluation. Wiseman [24] uses two alternative methods to show that the choice of method can affect the result. It is therefore not enough to know that preferences have been elicited.

These issues have been widely discussed in the health economics literature but more subtle problems with preferences that have been largely ignored by economists involve sociolinguistics and discourse analysis. It is to these that we now turn.

11.3.3.2   The Role of Process and Persuasion

While the comments below are raised in the context of pharmacoeconomics, they have a wider relevance in terms of economic approaches more generally, and in relation to public deliberation on policy issues.

Techniques are applied, and their results may have an impact on decisions that are made. Are the techniques legitimate? How much weight should be placed on the results? If they are accepted, is this because of the inherent merit of the studies, or is there just some tacit agreement to be persuaded by these analyses?

Adam Smith, sometimes referred to as the "father" of modern economics, gave a series of lectures on rhetoric in 1762 and 1763 [25]. This was not remarkable at the time. Smith reflected a long tradition (dating back to classical Greece) where both logic and rhetoric were considered central to a good education. Briefly, we could consider logic to be concerned with proof, whereas rhetoric is concerned with persuasion. When describing the rhetoric of political debate, whereby policy decisions are made, Smith used the term "deliberative eloquence". People are not necessarily swayed by detailed, technical, logical arguments. It is more likely that they would be persuaded by simple points and rhetorical techniques such as humour, the use of analogy, or appeals to authority or to emotion.

While this perspective could be used to consider political debate, it has also been suggested that the same techniques may influence our understanding of economics. This point is discussed at length in a book called *The Rhetoric of Economics* [26]. McCloskey considers the extent to which accepted economic findings do not have a firm basis in logic. There are numerous examples.

Economic theory might conclude, within a narrowly defined theoretical framework, that competition is desirable. We cannot logically claim that this result applies in the real world without showing that the theory reflects the real world. Failing that, an acceptance of the view requires a leap of faith. We are persuaded, but not on the basis of logic.

Literature on the processes of policy making can also be seen to draw on the scholarship of rhetoric. Dunn [27], for example, lists eleven "modes of argumentation." These are ways in which positions can be presented so as to persuade people to a particular viewpoint. Logic is not mentioned, and the presentation of logical arguments may not be very effective in comparison to other approaches – advertising and celebrity endorsement immediately come to mind. The results of studies may be convincing, although this is not necessarily related to the quality of the studies themselves. McCloskey [26] devotes much attention, in her book and elsewhere, to the distinction between statistical significance and economic or policy significance. She stresses that many refereed studies fail to note the difference, resulting in questionable policy conclusions. See also Chapter 6 by Donaldson et al. [28]. Persuasive methods include "authority," the use of a source or personality that people trust, and "analogy", applying an approach in one context that people already accept in another (even though it may not, in fact, be suitable). Some of the techniques that analysts apply may have achieved acceptance on such grounds as well.

Literature on critical discourse analysis focuses on the use of selected words to emphasise a particular perspective and on broader approaches to "frame" issues in desirable ways. Fairclough [29] refers to "ideological-discursive formations" which groups may use to define debate in a way that favours their perspective. Attitudes to health conditions may differ according to whether they are seen as resulting from individual behaviour or as a consequence of social circumstances, for example.

Such analyses could be considered as "macro" approaches to rhetoric, as compared to traditional rhetoric, which is "micro" in focus, looking at individuals in debate. This is drawing on the economic distinction between microeconomics, looking at individual units or markets, and macroeconomics, which considers a broad-brush approach to the economy as a whole. Public perceptions and media presentation of issues will be heavily influenced by dominant terminology and frames. Considine [30] describes policy as the result of competition between groups, each trying to create the dominant perspective. In a similar vein, other literature emphasises the setting of agendas [31–33].

Public perceptions are shaped by the information that is transmitted in these processes. It might be hoped that debate in the media would result in an informed public. Bourdieu doubts this. He suggests that television favours people he terms "fast thinkers."[34] He does not mean that they actually think quickly. Rather, they can give quick answers that will be accepted. Far from thinking, they are simply tapping in to currently held beliefs, thereby getting instant audience acceptance and giving the appearance of being knowledgeable. His point could apply to much of the mass media. Consequently, dominant frames are emphasised, prior beliefs reinforced and false perceptions perpetuated. This can have a significant impact on people's understanding of issues and priorities, at least those for which they have little or no direct personal experience.

11.4　CONCLUSION

The title of this book indicates that the aim is to go from theory to practice. Terms used in several texts on economic evaluation in health are best practice or the current convention. This is no mistake. Theory is not conclusive on the methods to be used. In fact, it could be argued that any approach taken is subject to valid criticisms. There is often a conflict between theory and practice. Analysts are charged with undertaking assessments and making policy recommendations. They cannot avoid the issues by saying that the data do not exist or the theories are deficient. In many cases, *ad hoc* or pragmatic approaches may be used, while theories are being developed in parallel or subsequently. In some areas of economics, theories have been developed in an attempt to find a rationale for existing analytical practices. Indicative planning is one example (see [35]).

Where theories are used, they could be questioned in terms of their own validity (given their assumptions), and in terms of their applicability in a particular situation. In relation to the latter, assumptions may be made as a basis for an approach, after which the conclusions could be treated as if they apply regardless of the assumption. This is a problem when assumptions are not explicitly stated, as with exogenous preferences. Debates on approaches also indicate that methods are sometimes chosen not based on their legitimacy, but because they give the desired results. More generally, approaches may be chosen less on the basis of logic and more based on rhetoric or persuasion. They are plausible, or appealing.

This does not mean that pharmacoeconomic analyses are necessarily giving wrong results but, rather, we cannot be necessarily certain that they in all cases will derive better answers than alternative analytical approaches. In such circumstances, it is important that health economists exhibit a certain degree of humility by at least acknowledging the limitations of our understanding.

APPENDIX ON DISCOUNTING

Mathematically, discounting can be considered as follows:

Imagine investing $X at a rate of interest, r, for one year, with the interest to be paid at the end of the year. You would get back your $X, plus $rX in interest, or $(1+r)X in total. It has grown by a factor (1+r). In other words, on this basis, $1 now is equivalent to $(1+r) next year and $(1+r)^n$ in n years' time. Consider this process in reverse. $1 next year can be obtained by investing \$1/(1+r) now. We would say that the PV of \$1 next year, discounted at a rate, r, is \$1/(1+r).

If you were to invest \$X for additional years, the sum would increase by a factor of (1+r) each year. After two years, you would have $\$(1+r)^2 X$, and after n years you would have $\$(1+r)^n X$. Considering this in reverse, \$1 in n years' time is equivalent to $\$1/(1+r)^n$ now.

We can apply this to a stream of dollar sums, X0 to Xn, for years 0 (the present) to n. This would give us the PV of the sums of money. The formula would be:

$$PV = X_0 + (1/(1+r))X_1 + \left(1/(1+r)^2\right)X_2 + \left(1/(1+r)^3\right)X_3 + \dots$$
$$+ (1/(1+r)^n)X_n$$

REFERENCES

[1]   Hunt EK: *History of Economic Thought: A Critical Perspective*, 2nd edn. New York, NY: HarperCollinsPublishers; 1992.

[2]   Tyler T: **Social Justice: Outcome and Procedure**. *International Journal of Psychology* 2000, **35**(2): 117–125.

[3]   Veenhoven R: *World Database of Happiness, Erasmus University Rotterdam*. Rotterdam, 2009 Erasmus University Rotterdam.

[4]   Dasbach EJ, Elbasha EH, Insinga RP: **Mathematical Models for Predicting the Epidemiologic and Economic Impact of Vaccination against Human Papillomavirus Infection and Disease**. *Epidemiol Rev* 2006, **28**(1): 88–100.

[5]   Goldie SJ, Kohli M, Grima D, Weinstein MC, Wright TC, Bosch FX, Franco E: **Projected Clinical Benefits and Cost-effectiveness of a Human Papillomavirus 16/18 Vaccine**. *J Natl Cancer Inst* 2004, **96**(8): 604–615.

[6]   Lipsey RG, Lancaster K: **The General Theory of Second Best**. *The Review of Economic Studies* 1956, **24**(1): 11–32.

[7]   Johnson BS: *Christie Malry's Own Double-entry*. London: Picador; 2001.

[8]   Birch S: **Making the Problem Fit the Solution: Evidence-based Decision Making and "Dolly" Economics**. In: *Evidence-based Health Economics: From Effectiveness to Efficiency in Systematic Review*. Edited by Donaldson C, Mugford M, Vale L. London: BMJ; 2002: 133–147.

[9]   Brazier J, Ratcliffe J, Salomon J: *TsuchiyaA: Measuring and Valuing Health Benefits for Economic Evaluation*. Oxford: Oxford University Press; 2007.

[10] **Scientific and Social Value Judgements** [www.nice.org.uk/niceMedia/Pdf/boardmeeting/brdmay04item6.pdf]

[11] Nord E: **Severity of Illness and Priority Setting: Worrisome Lack of Discussion of Surprising Finding**. *Journal of Health Economics* 2006, **25**(1): 170–172.

[12] Neumann, PJ Sanders, GD Russell, LB Siegel, JE Ganiats. TG*Cost-effectiveness in Health and Medicine*, 2nd edn. New York: Oxford University Press; 2016.

[13] Drummond MF, Jefferson TO: **Guidelines for Authors and Peer Reviewers of Economic Submissions to the BMJ**. *British Medical Journal* 1996, **313**(7052): 275–283.

[14] Bentham J: *An Introduction to the Principles of Morals and Legislation*. New York: Hafner; 1973.

[15] Layard PRG: *Happiness: Lessons from a New Science*. New York: Penguin Press; 2005.

[16] Hazlitt W: *The Spirit of the Age, Or, Contemporary Portraits*. London: Oxford University Press; 1904.

[17] Bos JM, Postma MJ, Annemans L: **Discounting Health Effects in Pharmacoeconomic Evaluations: Current Controversies.** *PharmacoEconomics* 2005, **23**(7): 639–649.

[18] Bridges JFP: **Stated Preference Methods in Health Care Evaluation: An Emerging Methodological Paradigm in Health Economics.** *Applied Health Economics and Health Policy* 2003, **2**(4): 213–224.

[19] Oliver A: **Should We Maximise QALYs?: A Debate with respect to Peak-End Evaluation.** *Applied Health Economics and Health Policy* 2004, **3**: :61–66.

[20] Glick H, Doshi J, Sonnad S, Polsky D: *Economic Evaluation in Clinical Trials.* Oxford: Oxford University Press; 2007.

[21] Akunne A, Bridges J, Sanon M, Sauerborn R: **Comparison of Individual and Group Valuation of Health State Scenarios across Communities in West Africa.** *Applied Health Economics and Health Policy* 2006, **5**: :261–268.

[22] Richardson J, Smith RD: **Calculating Society's Willingness to Pay for a QALY: Key Questions for Discussion.** *Applied Health Economics and Health Policy* 2004, **3**: :125–126.

[23] Ryfe DM: **Does Deliberative Democracy Work?** *Annual Review of Political Science* 2005, **8**(1): 49–71.

[24] Wiseman V: **Aggregating Public Preferences for Healthcare: Putting Theory into Practice.** *Applied Health Economics and Health Policy* 2004, **3**: :171–179.

[25] Smith A: *Lectures on Rhetoric and Belles Lettres: Delivered in the University of Glasgow by Adam Smith, Reported by a Student in 1762-63.* London: Nelson; 1963.

[26] McCloskey DN: *The Rhetoric of Economics,* 2nd edn. Madison, Wis.: University of Wisconsin Press; 1998.

[27] Dunn WN: *Public Policy Analysis: An Introduction,* 3rd edn. Upper Saddle River, NJ: Pearson Prentice Hall; 2004.

[28] Donaldson C, Mugford M, Vale L eds.: *Evidence-based Health Economics: From Effectiveness to Efficiency in Systematic Review.* London: BMJ; 2002.

[29] Fairclough N: *Critical Discourse Analysis: The Critical Study of Language.* London: Longman; 1995.

[30] Considine M: *Making Public Policy: Institutions, Actors, Strategies.* Cambridge: Polity Press; 2005.

[31] Cobb R, Ross M eds.: *Cultural Strategies of Agenda Denial: Avoidance, Attack, and Redefinition.* Lawrence: University Press of Kansas; 1997.

[32] Hilgartner S, Bosk CL: **The Rise and Fall of Social Problems: A Public Arenas Model.** *The American Journal of Sociology* 1988, **94**(1): 53–78.

[33] Rochefort R, Cobb R eds.: *The Politics of Problem Definition: Shaping the Policy Agenda.* Lawrence, Kan.: University Press of Kansas; 1994.

[34] Bourdieu P: *On Television.* New York: New Press; 1998.

[35] Masse P: **French Methods of Planning.** *The Journal of Industrial Economics* 1962, **11**(1): 1–17.

12 Patient-Reported Outcome Measures

Dianne Bryant, MSc, PhD
Western University
London, Ontario, Canada

Andrew Firth, MSc
Western University
London, Ontario, Canada

Gordon Guyatt, MD, MSc
McMaster University
Hamilton, Ontario, Canada

Renée J.G. Arnold, PharmD, RPh
Icahn School of Medicine at Mount Sinai
Arnold Consultancy & Technology, LLC
New York, NY, USA

TABLE OF CONTENTS

12.1   PATIENT-REPORTED OUTCOME MEASURES

A patient-reported outcome (PRO) is a direct subjective assessment by patients about aspects of their health, including symptoms, function, emotional well-being, quality of life, utility, and satisfaction with treatment. PROs ask patients to evaluate the impact and functional implications of the disease or treatment to reflect their interpretation of the experience, which is influenced by their internal standards, intrinsic values, and expectations. As such, PROs provide unique information that is unavailable from other sources [1].

Direct measurement of health from the patient's perspective is an increasingly used outcome measure in clinical trial research. In such a case, use of PRO instruments (i.e., a *questionnaire* plus the information and documentation that support its use) is a means to capture PRO data used to measure *treatment benefit* or risks [2]. This phenomenon reflects a shift away from an exclusive emphasis on safety and efficacy, and from research that in the past focused narrowly on laboratory and clinical indicators of morbidity. Measuring patients' experience and the extent to which they can function in their daily activities is crucial when the primary objective of treatment is to improve how the patient is feeling. In fact, even when the goal of treatment is to reduce the incidence of seemingly straightforward outcomes like stroke or myocardial infarction, capturing the variability in patients' function and feelings will provide important complementary information if variability in the adverse morbid outcome varies in severity (e.g., a mild versus severe stroke). In fact, many regulatory bodies allow use of PRO data collection to support claims in approved medical product labeling. The evaluation of a PRO instrument to support claims in medical product labeling includes the following considerations:

- The population enrolled in the clinical trial
- The clinical trial objectives and design
- The PRO instrument's conceptual framework
- The PRO instrument's *measurement properties (see 12.4)*

Endpoint models (e.g., if treatments of a disease or its symptoms are the primary/secondary endpoints) are critical to the success of appropriate PRO selection and usage. Several analyses of the success of PROs in support of labeling claims, both in the United States and European Union (EU), demonstrated that the EU was more than twice as likely as the United States to grant PRO claims (19% vs. 47% for United States and EU, respectively) [3]. Only 16.5% of the 182 New Drug Applications (NDAs) had PRO labeling during the period 2011 to 2015, a decline from 24% of NDAs being granted at least one PRO label from 2006 to 2010, probably due to the publication of the FDA guidance [4]. However, similar percentages of PRO-dependent NDAs (e.g., for approvals in diseases, such as asthma or major depressive disorder, that traditionally rely on PROs for evaluating treatment benefit) had PRO labeling in the United States during the period of 2006 to 2010 (46.9%) as those in the period of 2011 to 2015 (46.0%) [4]. More than ¾ of the claims were for primary, disease-based (vs. symptom-based) endpoints [4].

12.2 HEALTH AND HEALTH MEASUREMENT

12.2.1 THE WORLD HEALTH ORGANIZATION

The World Health Organization (WHO) defines health as a state of complete physical, mental, and social well-being [5]. The WHO's International Classification of Functioning, Disability, and Health (ICF) [6] was developed to provide a standard language and framework to describe and measure health and health-related states. Within the ICF system, health outcomes are classified according to the effect upon body function, body structure, limitations in activities, and limitations in participation. Health outcomes that measure body function include measures of physiological functions of body systems (e.g., ejection fraction, glucose level, depression, pain, etc.). Outcomes that measure body structures include measures of anatomical parts and their components (e.g., x-ray to measure fracture healing, computed tomography to measure tumor size, etc.). Activity is defined as the performance of an action, whereas participation, more broadly, is defined as involvement in meaningful activities and fulfillment of roles that are socially or culturally expected of that person. Impairments are problems with body functions or structures. Having an impairment of a body structure (e.g., disc hernia) or function (e.g., reduced range of motion) may contribute to limitations in activities, including activities of daily living, walking, or driving a car, that might also contribute to restrictions in participation. Comprehensive assessment of an individual's health will include measures of body systems and function, as well as limitations in activities and participation.

12.2.2 HEALTH-RELATED QUALITY OF LIFE

Health-related quality of life (HRQoL) instruments measure the broad concept of health (physical, mental, and social well-being) by inquiring into the extent of difficulty with activities of daily living (including work, recreation, and household management) and how difficulties affect relationships with family, friends, and social groups, capturing not only the ability to function within these roles but also the degree of satisfaction derived from doing them. HRQoL instruments often contain items that measure body function (e.g., pain, depression, anxiety) and limitations with activities and participation.

Within the construct of HRQoL, it is common to come across the terms *disease-specific* and *generic*. A disease-specific measure is tailored to inquire about specific aspects of health that are affected by the disease of interest (e.g., specific to acne). In contrast, a generic instrument measures general health status, including physical symptoms, function, and emotional dimensions of health relevant to all health states, including healthy individuals [7].

Disease-specific instruments are more responsive to small but important changes in health than are generic measures [8]. Because the items on a disease-specific HRQoL instrument are so focused on a particular disease, however, they cannot be used to compare the impact of one disease with another. In fact, in some cases, disease-specific measures are so specific that comparisons between different populations within the same disease are not possible (e.g., pediatric versus adult populations). On the other hand, generic HRQoL instruments are useful when measuring the impact of a specific illness or injury across different diseases, severities, and interventions [7].

A number of previously widely used health profiles such as the Sickness Impact Profile (SIP) [9–14] and the Nottingham Health Profile [15–19] are now of largely historical interest; health profiles developed from the Medical Outcomes Study, including the 36-Item Short-Form Health Survey (SF-36) [20–22] and 12-Item Short-Form Health Survey (SF-12) [23] have come to dominate the field of generic health status measurement.

12.2.3   ECONOMIC EVALUATION OF HEALTH

When making decisions on behalf of patient groups, decision makers must weigh the benefits and risks of treatment but must also consider whether the benefits are sufficient to merit the health care resources that must be spent to provide them. Limited societal resources necessitate that in order to add a program, society must forgo some other benefit—if the envelope for health spending is fixed, then another health program must be reduced. An economic analysis can inform these decisions. The primary distinction between this paradigm and HRQoL is the inclusion of explicit valuation of both resource consumption and patient-important benefit and harm.

Economic analyses include methods to evaluate different effects (death, effects of stroke on HRQoL, effect of reduction in acne on HRQoL) in the same metric. One way to create the same units is through the concept of preferences. Utilities and values are different types of preferences. Whether you are dealing with utilities or values depends on how questions on measurement instruments are framed; are participants being asked to consider outcomes that are certain (values) or uncertain (utilities)?

The Standard Gamble is the classical method of measuring utility, based directly on the axioms first presented by von Neumann and Morgenstern (utility theory) that describes how a rational individual "ought" to make decisions when faced with uncertainty [24]. During administration of the Standard Gamble, the participant suffering from a health problem, such as severe hip osteoarthritis (in reality or hypothetically), imagines that there is an intervention that will result in a return to perfect health but that there is a risk of death associated with the intervention. Participants are asked to specify the largest probability of death they would be willing to accept before declining the intervention and choosing to remain in their current (suboptimal) health state. The larger the probability of death that the subject is willing to accept, the lower value they place on their current health state. The utility of the present health state—as in all utility measures—is placed on a continuum between death (typically given a value of 0) and full health (typically given a value of 1.0).

For instance, let us assume an individual suffering from severe hip osteoarthritis would be indifferent between his or her current health state and the gamble when the probability of dying is 50%. This would mean that the utility the individual places on a year in this health state is 0.5, in contrast to a year in perfect health, which would be worth 1.0—hence the concept of the QALY (quality-adjusted life year).

The Time Trade-Off [25] is a measure of values. It asks participants to imagine living their lives in their current health states and to contrast this with the alternative of perfect health in exchange for a shorter lifespan (preference-based measure). The administrator provides alternatives of years of life in the present health state versus years of life in perfect health. The more years a subject is willing to sacrifice in exchange for a return to perfect health, the worse the subjects perceive their current health state (see Figure 12.1 for an example with human immunodeficiency virus [HIV]). Utility is calculated by subtracting the number of years sacrificed from the number of years of life remaining divided by the number of years remaining. The number of years remaining is estimated using actuarial tables. So, for instance, if an individual with 30 years of life remaining with severe hip osteoarthritis was ready to trade off 15 of those years to achieve 15 years in full health, the QALYs allocated to 1 year with arthritis would be 0.5.

Another common value-based measure is the feeling thermometer (FT). When completing the FT, participants rate their health status using a visual analog scale

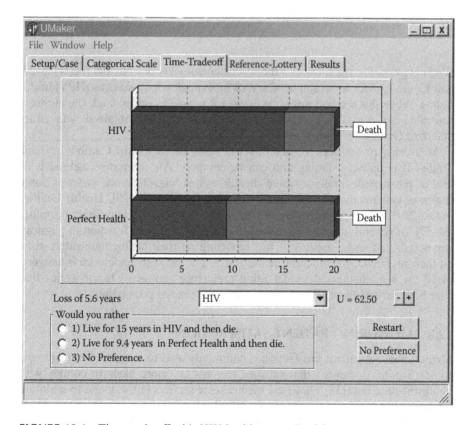

FIGURE 12.1 Time trade-off with HIV health states. Participants are asked to express their preference for living with HIV for 15 years and then dying or living in perfect health for an increasing number of years (less than 15 years) and then dying, until the point of indifference (no preference). Reproduced with permission from U–Maker (Sonnenberg).

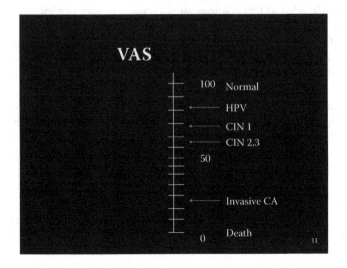

FIGURE 12.2   Visual analog scale.
HPV = human papillomavirus, CIN = cervical intraepithelial neoplasia, CA = cancer.

(VAS) presented in the form of a thermometer from 0 (worst) to 100 (best) [25–27] (see Figure 12.2 for an example of a VAS for human papillomavirus [HPV] health states). While this method might be easier for people to understand, the numbers generated are often quite skewed and higher than those obtained with either Standard Gamble or Time Trade-Off.

Measuring preferences for health states using the Standard Gamble or Time Trade-Off is time-consuming and can be complex. An alternative method is to use a pre-scored, multi-attribute health status classification system. Some common systems include the Quality of Well-Being Scale [28], Health Utilities Index [29–32], European Quality of Life Scale (EQ-5D) [33], and Short Form 6D [34–37]. In general, patients are asked to rate their ability to function in physical, emotional, and social aspects of life, reporting on their health state rather than on their preference for different health states. The patient's preference is assigned based on a mathematical model using preference ratings of health states that have been derived from a random sample of the general population.

12.3   MEASURING PATIENT SATISFACTION

Measurement of patient satisfaction is commonly used to evaluate treatment outcomes. Studies document that satisfied patients are more likely to comply with treatment protocols [38, 39], to use medical care services [40, 41], and to maintain a relationship with a specific provider [42]. Lack of clarity concerning the meaning of satisfaction has, however, been identified as a major weakness [43–49]. Patient ratings of satisfaction are generally directed at either the process of care or treatment outcome [50], the latter of which is of most interest to clinicians.

Satisfaction may be best thought of as a construct, like health, that cannot be measured directly. Those who have investigated items that are important to patients in determining satisfaction have recommended going beyond inquiry about physical symptoms and function of the diseased body part to include items that probe satisfaction with resolution of social effects of the disease [51, 52]. Some have suggested that patient expectations and experiences play a role in defining satisfaction, though the evidence is inconsistent [53, 54].

Experts in the field of measurement of patient satisfaction with treatment outcomes suggest that researchers should develop satisfaction instruments in much the same way they would approach the development of a new measure of quality of life, including the use of qualitative methods for item generation [50, 55]. In consulting with the patients, the main objective should be to identify contexts in which the affected body part has different meanings and tailor questions about satisfaction accordingly.

As with HRQoL, the challenge in developing an instrument to measure satisfaction is capturing the necessary content to appropriately measure the construct. In fact, several authors who have compared satisfaction ratings between measures on the same patients have found substantial differences [56, 57]. To date, most existing instruments were developed from the perspective of the provider or institution and not the patient.

Like HRQoL, several types of satisfaction measures exist. For example, there are global ratings that contain one or two general questions about overall satisfaction, or multidimensional indexes that probe different aspects of satisfaction, including such things as emotions, desires, perceptions, and expectations.

One disadvantage of global ratings is that they do not capture what patients are considering when reporting their satisfaction. Because of this, global instruments are generally found to be unreliable and tend to be highly skewed [46, 57–59]. As with HRQoL, there are also generic and disease-specific instruments to measure satisfaction. Generic instruments can be used to assess satisfaction in any population, whereas disease-specific scales are designed for use in specific patient populations. The pros and cons of generic versus disease-specific instruments are like those outlined in Section 12.2.2.

12.4   WHAT ARE THE PROPERTIES OF A GOOD MEASUREMENT INSTRUMENT?

The choice of instrument should align itself with the objectives of the clinician, researcher, or policy maker. If the instrument is to be developed de novo, the iterative nature of this process must be considered (see Figure 12.3 [2]). The intent may be to (1) discriminate between patients with different disease severity at a point in time (e.g., whose asthma is impairing function to a greater degree and who to a lesser degree), (2) predict patient outcome (e.g., functional status may predict mortality in heart failure patients), or (3) evaluate change following an intervention (e.g., which stroke patients have improved and which have not). To be useful for application in a research and clinical setting for the first two

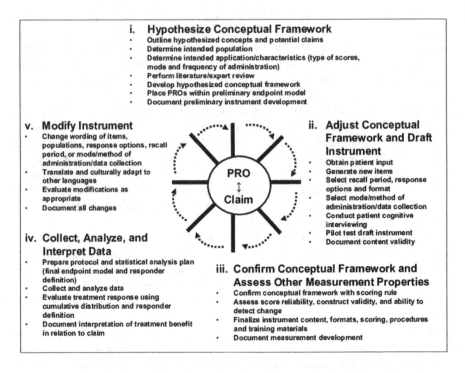

i. **Hypothesize Conceptual Framework**
- Outline hypothesized concepts and potential claims
- Determine intended population
- Determine intended application/characteristics (type of scores, mode and frequency of administration)
- Perform literature/expert review
- Develop hypothesized conceptual framework
- Place PROs within preliminary endpoint model
- Document preliminary instrument development

v. **Modify Instrument**
- Change wording of items, populations, response options, recall period, or mode/method of administration/data collection
- Translate and culturally adapt to other languages
- Evaluate modifications as appropriate
- Document all changes

PRO ↕ Claim

ii. **Adjust Conceptual Framework and Draft Instrument**
- Obtain patient input
- Generate new items
- Select recall period, response options and format
- Select mode/method of administration/data collection
- Conduct patient cognitive interviewing
- Pilot test draft instrument
- Document content validity

iv. **Collect, Analyze, and Interpret Data**
- Prepare protocol and statistical analysis plan (final endpoint model and responder definition)
- Collect and analyze data
- Evaluate treatment response using cumulative distribution and responder definition
- Document interpretation of treatment benefit in relation to claim

iii. **Confirm Conceptual Framework and Assess Other Measurement Properties**
- Confirm conceptual framework with scoring rule
- Assess score reliability, construct validity, and ability to detect change
- Finalize instrument content, formats, scoring, procedures and training materials
- Document measurement development

FIGURE 12.3 Conceptual framework for a patient-reported outcome (PRO).

intentions, instruments must be valid (measure what they are supposed to measure—discriminative validity) and reliable (provide consistent ratings between repeated measures in a stable population). If the intention is to evaluate change following treatment, the instrument must be valid (longitudinal validity) and responsive (able to detect important change, even if the magnitude of the change is small).

12.4.1 VALIDITY

An assessment of the validity of a new instrument is an evaluation of whether the instrument measures what was intended. Researchers developing instruments with the greatest potential for validity will have, in choosing items, consulted with patients, and perhaps clinician experts or patients' family members, who have experience with the disease to ask how the disease affects their lives.

One of the first steps in selecting an instrument is to review the items that make up the questionnaire. In some cases, the authors of an instrument will describe its content or include the instrument in an appendix (more common in online publications than in hard copy) so that clinicians can use their own experiences to decide whether what is being measured reflects what is important to patients (*face validity*) in a comprehensive way (*content validity*).

Readers or researchers can use several strategies to provide empirical evidence of the validity of the outcome measure. For example, they can investigate the *criterion validity* of the instrument, which is an assessment of whether the instrument behaves the way it should when compared with a gold standard measurement of the construct (e.g., the gold standard for virtual colonoscopy using imaging approaches is standard colonoscopy). Although measures of body function and structure are likely to have a gold standard reference, there is no gold standard for quality of life.

Construct validity assesses the extent to which the instrument relates to other measures of theoretical concepts (constructs) in the way that it should. Types of construct validity include convergent and discriminant validity. *Convergent validity* examines the degree to which interpretations of scores on the instrument being tested are like the interpretation of scores on other instruments that theoretically measure similar constructs. For example, we would expect that patients with poorer performance on a 6-minute walk test will have more dyspnea in daily life than those with better walk test scores, and we would expect to see substantial correlations between a new measure of emotional function and existing emotional function questionnaires.

Discriminant validity predicts weaker correlations with less closely-related measures. For instance, one might expect a lower correlation between spirometry and daily dyspnea than between the walk test and daily function. To improve the strength of the inference, investigators pre-specify the magnitude of the correlation that is expected (e.g., no correlation $r<0.20$; weak r 0.20–0.35; moderate $r>0.35$–0.50; strong $r>0.50$). They would then administer multiple instruments (spirometry, walk test, other dyspnea questionnaires, global ratings of function) to a group of patients suffering from chronic obstructive pulmonary disease (COPD) to determine the agreement between predicted and observed correlations. The better the agreement between predicted and observed correlations, the stronger is the evidence for construct validity.

The appropriate way to design a study to investigate these types of validity for a discriminative instrument is by looking at the correlations between measures at a single point in time. Such correlations reflect an instrument's *cross-sectional construct validity.*

Conversely, the appropriate way to measure validity for evaluative instruments is by looking at the correlations in change over time between measures. For example, COPD patients who deteriorate in their 6-minute walk test score should, in general, show increases in dyspnea, whereas those whose exercise capacity improves should experience less dyspnea; a new emotional function measure should show improvement in patients who improve on existing measures of emotional function. Such correlations reflect an instrument's *longitudinal construct validity.*

12.4.2 RELIABILITY

Reliability is defined as the extent to which an instrument is free from measurement (random) error. In practice, reliability refers to the extent to which an instrument discriminates between individuals in a population in a consistent manner when respondents are in stable health.

The mathematical relationship that defines reliability can be explained by the ratio of the variability in scores between patients to the total variability (i.e., between and within patient variability). Scores obtained on a reliable instrument will demonstrate relatively small differences between scores upon repeated administrations in patients who are stable in their condition (i.e., small within-person variability). Reliability will always appear to be greater when measured in a heterogeneous population, with greater variability in scores between patients (e.g., includes patients with no limitations to those with severe limitations) than in a homogeneous population.

An instrument free of random error will have a reliability of 1.0 if there is some between-patient variability. As the amount of random error increases in relation to the between-patient variability, the measure of reliability will approach 0. Common expressions of the magnitude of reliability are *Kappa*, when the scale is categorical, and *intraclass correlation coefficient* (ICC) when the scale is continuous. Several potential influences may affect the reliability of an instrument, including learning effects, regression to the mean, alterations in mood, circumstance and conditions of administration, and the length of time between assessments. It is also possible that real changes have occurred between consecutive assessments. The most important frequently neglected determinant of reliability is the variability in patient status on the underlying attribute.

Different techniques to measure the reliability of an instrument include test–retest and inter-rater. *Test–retest reliability* is a measure of the magnitude of the agreement between ratings in repeated administrations of the instrument in a population with a stable health condition. There is no gold standard time frame between subsequent administrations of the instrument; repeated administrations too close together face criticisms that high levels of agreement reflect patients' ability to remember previous responses, whereas administrations at large intervals run the risk of real changes having occurred within the sample of patients. In general, convention would suggest that any time from 1 to 4 weeks is appropriate, but this will be largely determined by the length of time that patients are expected to remain stable in their condition.

Inter-rater reliability is a measure of the magnitude of the agreement between ratings given by different raters administering the same instrument in a population with a stable health condition. The literature contains some discussion around study design for inter- and intra-rater reliability, which suggests that the timing of ratings (e.g., time of day), by different raters, location, and patient position, may influence agreement between raters [60]. Depending on the instrument, raters may be able to assess the same patient at fairly tight intervals, whereas other outcomes may need to be measured on different days (e.g., measuring maximum strength that requires recovery time).

Internal consistency reliability is quite different from test–retest and inter-rater reliability, and measures the extent to which items in an instrument yield similar scores in the same patients on a single administration. The internal consistency reliability coefficient (R) is used to calculate the standard error of measurement (SEM), which provides an easily defined estimate of the reproducibility of individual measurements (SEM = $\sigma(1-R)^{1/2}$) and can be used to determine whether true change has occurred within an individual ($\sqrt{2} \times$ SEM) [61]. Internal consistency is very limited as a measure of reliability because it relates only to the correlation between items on a single administration and makes no attempt to assess the degree of variability on repeated administration of a measure.

12.4.3   Sensitivity to Change, Responsiveness, and Minimally Important Difference

Many people use the terms "sensitivity to change" and "responsiveness" interchangeably, but by some definitions, there are important differences. Sensitivity to change has been defined as the ability of an instrument to measure true change in the state being measured regardless of whether it is relevant or meaningful to the patient or clinician [62]. In contrast, responsiveness has been defined as the ability of the instrument to detect change that is important to the patient in the state being measured even if that difference is small [62, 63]. It follows that the minimally important difference (MID) is defined as the smallest difference in score in the outcome of interest that informed patients or informed proxies perceive as important, either beneficial or harmful, and that would lead the patient or clinician to consider a change in management [64, 65].

The magnitude of change that constitutes an MID for many objective outcomes may be intuitive to the clinician (changes in platelet count or serum creatinine). For most PRO measures, however, the magnitude of change that constitutes an MID is not self-evident, creating difficulties with interpreting the results of studies that report changes in PROs. In studies that show no difference in HRQoL when patients receive a treatment versus a control intervention, clinicians should look for evidence that the instrument has been shown to be responsive to small- or moderate-sized effects in a similar population in previous investigations. In the absence of this evidence, it is unknown whether the intervention was ineffective or whether the instrument was not responsive.

12.5   INTERPRETING THE RESULTS OF A STUDY THAT DESCRIBES PATIENT-REPORTED OUTCOMES

Physicians often have limited familiarity with methods of measuring how patients feel or their ability to do the things they need or want to do. At the same time, published articles recommend administering or withholding treatment based on its impact on patients' well-being.

In clinical research, physicians are limited to recruiting a sample of patients from the overall population of interest. The aim is to recruit a sample that is representative of the population of interest, test the sample, then use the results to make conclusions about the population [66]. Unfortunately, the sample does not always accurately reflect the population patients were recruited from, and even well-planned studies with *a priori* sample size calculations and pragmatic inclusion/exclusion criteria (that account for variability in the population) can fall victim to random sampling error. Random sampling error is particularly problematic in studies with small numbers, purely due to a greater chance of recruiting a non-representative sample. Studies with strict eligibility criteria that intentionally recruit non-representative samples are also biased and, in this situation, recruiting more patients will not negate these issues. Relying on a single point estimate of statistical significance (e.g., the mean difference in Knee Injury and Osteoarthritis Outcome Scores between groups and the resulting p-value) to determine the success of treatment is problematic, as it may lead to imprecise conclusions about the overlying study population. Statistical significance is an especially poor way to interpret results, as it also lacks context when it comes to the size and importance of the effect and the reproducibility of the findings [67]. Researchers have advocated that studies instead present and interpret confidence intervals (CIs), a range of values estimating the precision of the study statistic and what is likely to be true in the population [68–70].

One of the strengths of precision estimates is that they can be presented around any parameter estimate regardless of the study statistic being used. The most commonly used interval is a 95% CI, which relates to the 5% significance level in that it represents a range of values where the population parameter is expected to fall that are extreme enough to not be rejected at that level [66]. If we were to repeat a study many times using a representative sample of patients and constructed a 95% CI each time, then 95% of those intervals will include the true value of the parameter in the population. Individuals can then interpret the results of a study using the upper and lower boundaries of the 95% CI, which indicate the magnitude and direction of the effect. If both ends of the CI represent the same conclusion, such as improved PRO scores, then clinicians can say the results are definitive and that treatment improves PROs [71]. If the upper boundary shows improvement and the lower boundary shows declining scores, then the clinician can interpret the results as indeterminate, meaning the study lacks the precision to conclude whether treatment is harmful or beneficial. Clinicians should also observe the width of the CI as a measure of precision, as a wide, definitive CI may have boundaries that represent drastically different effects, while a narrow CI provides a more certain estimate of the effect.

Evaluating the upper and lower CI boundaries for a PRO is more difficult than interpreting precision estimates for a more objective outcome. For instance, consider an adequately powered randomized controlled trial comparing experimental medication versus the gold standard to prevent subsequent heart attack in patients with coronary artery disease (CAD). The reported 95% CI for the relative risk of subsequent heart attack ranges from 0.62 to 0.81 (p<0.05), indicating that experimental medication reduces the risk of an event by 19% to 38%. The outcome here is easily interpretable, with both boundaries of the 95% CI, demonstrating a sizeable reduction in the number of events and indicating that the experimental medication is effective. In the same study, patients also completed the Seattle Angina Questionnaire (SAQ) [72], a valid and reliable PRO for patients with CAD. The reported 95% CI for mean difference in SAQ scores is 7.2 to 11.8 points (p<0.05) in favor of the experimental group. The CI demonstrates improvement in patient-reported health for both the lower and upper boundaries, but how should a clinician interpret this score? Is this considered to be significant improvement; did the experimental medication lead to greatly improved quality of life?

Physicians require more information if they are going to make clinical decisions based on the results from studies presenting PROs. The 95% CI nicely summarizes the precision of the study and how much to trust the result, but it lacks context when considering the importance of PROs and the meaningfulness of the observed effect. Thus, if a measure is to be clinically useful, its scores must also be interpretable. Interpretability is greatly enhanced if we know the magnitude of the change in score that is important—the MID.

Strategies to define important change have included distribution-based approaches and anchor-based approaches. In general, distribution-based approaches relate the magnitude of the effect to some measure of variability. For example, in a simple before–after comparison, one could calculate the difference between scores before and after treatment divided by the standard deviation of scores at baseline; the resultant statistic is coined the "effect size." In a parallel group design, the effect size is generated by calculating the difference in scores between the treatment and control group divided by the standard deviation of the change that patients experienced during the study.

A rough rule of thumb for interpreting effect sizes is that changes of a magnitude of 0.2 represent small changes, 0.5 moderate changes, and 0.8 large changes [73]. Interpretation using effect sizes remains problematic because it is sensitive to the homogeneity of the distribution of the sample of patients who participated in the study (i.e., estimates of variability will vary from study to study). In other words, the same difference between treatment and control will appear as a large effect size if the sample is homogenous (patients are similar and thus there is a small between-patient variability, which defines the standard deviation) and as a small effect size if the sample is heterogeneous (patients are dissimilar and thus there is large between-patient variability).

On the other hand, anchor-based approaches involve comparing the magnitude of the change observed on a PRO to an anchor or independent standard that is itself interpretable. The anchor may be defined by achieving change on some external criteria, for example, changing category increasing on a well-known classification system for disease or functional severity (e.g., moving from New York Heart Association Functional Classification III to II) or moving in or out of a diagnostic category (e.g., from depressed to non-depressed, or the reverse).

Another common anchor-based approach, the global rating of change, follows patients longitudinally and asks them to report whether they got better, stayed the same, or got worse. If better or worse, patients rate how much change has occurred—for example, they may rate the degree of change from 1 (minimal change) to 7 (a very large change), where 1 to 3 indicates a small but important change. In the most common way of using this approach, the investigators estimate the MID as the average of the change scores on the PRO that corresponds to a small but important change (that is, the average change in patients who have rated themselves as 1 to 3 on the degree of change rating).

It should be noted that most MIDs available in the literature represent within-patient change, or the number of points on a scale by which an individual must change to be considered important. In most clinical research studies, we are comparing two groups that both receive treatment and are each expected to improve, meaning differences as large as the within-patient MID will rarely be observed. The between-groups MID is considered to be roughly 20%–40% of the reported within-patient MID [74].

12.6 EXAMPLES OF USE OF PROS

12.6.1 HRQoL IN HPV DECISION-ANALYTIC MODELING

Goldie and colleagues [75] used age-specific quality weights for non-cancer states (range was 0.92 in women aged 25–34 years to 0.74 in women older than 85 years) based on data from the Health Utilities Index (Mark II Scoring System) and quality weights for the time spent in cancer health states (range was 0.65 for Stage I to 0.48 for Stage IV invasive cervical cancer) from utility estimates by the Institute of Medicine's Committee to Study Priorities for Vaccine Development. These weights were then multiplied by the time spent in the health state and then summed to calculate the number of QALYs in the cost-effectiveness model.

12.6.2 PROs IN ATOPIC DERMATITIS

In a recent cross-sectional study using data from 6 academic medical centers in the United States collected by a self-administered internet-based questionnaire, 1519 adult patients with atopic dermatitis (AD) were stratified by AD severity as mild or moderate/severe using the Patient-Oriented Scoring Atopic Dermatitis (PO-SCORAD) [76]. The study objective was to characterize the patient-reported burden of AD, a complex, immune-mediated, chronic inflammatory skin disease characterized by pruritus [77, 78], with regard to impact of disease severity and inadequate control in adults from clinical settings using multiple PRO measures. Outcomes included validated measures and standalone questions assessing itch (pruritus numerical rating scale; PO-SCORAD itch VAS), pain (numerical rating scale), sleep (PO-SCORAD sleep VAS; sleep interference with function), anxiety and depression (Hospital Anxiety and Depression Scale), and HRQoL (Dermatology Life Quality Index). Among the 1519 adult patients with AD, patients with moderate/severe AD (n = 830) reported more severe itching and pain, greater adverse effects on sleep, higher prevalence of anxiety and depression (417 [50.2%] vs 188 [27.3%]), and greater HRQoL impairment in comparison to those with mild AD (n = 689). The 103 patients with moderate/severe AD with inadequate disease control[1] despite treatment with systemic immunomodulators or phototherapy (55.7%) reported higher burdens of itch and sleeping symptoms vs. patients with controlled disease, including more days per week with itchy skin (5.7 vs 2.7) and higher proportions with itch duration greater than half a day (190 [22.8%] vs 20 [2.9%]). Sleep symptoms included trouble sleeping (3.9 vs 1.1 on the PO-SCORAD VAS), longer sleep latency (38.8 vs 21.6 minutes), more frequent sleep disturbances (2.6 vs 0.4 nights in past week), and greater need for over-the-counter sleep medications (324 [39%] vs 145 [21%]), thus confirming the high disease burden on adult patients, as well as equating it with disease severity.

12.7   INCORPORATING PROS INTO CLINICAL PRACTICE: BEYOND RESEARCH

Shared decision-making between patients and clinicians has been discussed for at least the past 18 years as potentially helpful in enhancing patient engagement, improving patient satisfaction and general amelioration of patient outcomes during clinical encounters; yet, it has been difficult to implement their use in routine clinical practice [79]. The US National Institutes of Health (NIH) even funded development of the Patient Reported Outcomes Measurement Information System, which created a bank of PRO measures for use across health conditions and was meant to extend from research into practice [80]. The US Medicare Merit-Based Incentive Payment System was also purporting to establish payment structures for collection and reporting of PROs in 2016, but an admittedly small survey (100 hospitals) [81] showed that fewer than 20% had implemented such measures to guide clinical care. Indeed, many have cited cost and time, interruption of workflow and other logistical concerns (such as increased burden on staff and patient time), incompatible technologies (e.g., not allowing quick integration of generated reports into EMRs), concerns about the reliability of results (e.g., from fitness trackers), and need to accommodate the end user. Some of these can be addressed with the use of patient portals, allowing administration of these questionnaires at home and having results at the ready during the office visit; tablet computers in the waiting room; and greater user-centered design and usability testing with different constituencies (e.g., the elderly or disabled with larger font sizes, better tactile experiences), among other tactics [79, 81]. Patients are also becoming more involved, an example being development of the FasterCures Patient Perspective Value Framework (PPVF), which enables understanding value from a patient perspective along 5 domains: patient preferences, patient-centered outcomes, patient and family costs, quality and applicability of evidence, and usability and transparency [82, 83]. In fact, FasterCures and Avalere codeveloped a prototype shared decision making tool for patients with advanced breast cancer [82].

---

1 Inadequately controlled AD was defined as patients who somewhat or completely disagreed with the statement "I feel my current treatments are effective in controlling my atopic dermatitis"; all other responses were considered controlled AD.

12.8   NEWER CONCEPTS: EQUITY, AUGMENTED COST-EFFECTIVENESS ANALYSIS AND MULTICRITERIA DECISION ANALYSIS

Multiple authors have written and spoken about the inadequacy of the QALY to incorporate all measures of value, such as equity, into the decision about value and cost-effectiveness [84–87]. Cookson introduced the concept of the equity impact plane, which allows consideration of trade-offs between improving total health and equity objectives for severely ill patients [84–86, 88]. Extended cost-effectiveness analysis (ECEA) broadens the concept of utility beyond just incremental cost and incremental effectiveness to include measures of financial risk protection and income distribution consequences. Augmented CEA (Figure 12.4), a further option to expand this approach, introduces additional value measures, such as insurance value and equity [85, 87]. A further and possibly more comprehensive measure of value is by using a technique called multicriteria decision analysis (MCDA), which is the weighted sum of partial utility scores (see Chapter 9 for more information on MCDA and the QALY) [84, 85, 88]. Another way of extending the QALY beyond "average" utility values is an effort to replace the EQ-5D with a new measure of quality of life,—the E-QALY,—which will capture domains such as cognition; coping, autonomy, and control; feelings and emotions; self-identity; physical sensations; activity; and relationships and social connections [89]. The EuroQOL group,

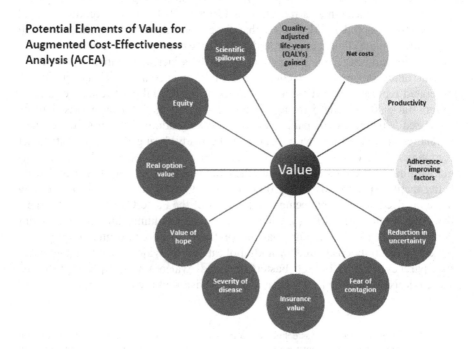

FIGURE 12.4   Permission granted from AMCP to republish this figure.

which is developing the new instrument in conjunction with NICE, is now at the stage of psychometric survey and valuation, proceeding through to implementation.

Several US government-backed measures have been initiated to promote patient-focused drug development, including release of a guidance on voluntary collection of patient preference information (PPI)[2] during US Food and Drug Administration (FDA) premarket review of medical devices (premarket approval, humanitarian device exemption application or de novo request) and passage of the 21st Century Cures Act, which directs the FDA to "incorporate patients' experiences, perspective, needs and priorities in drug development and evaluation" [90]. In the former, quantitative PPI is meant to provide information on the trade-offs patients are/are not willing to make for specified outcomes, such as means of implantation, duration of effect, duration and frequency of use, and utility of the device. While not strictly a PRO, which is meant to measure a patient's perceptions of health status before, during, and after therapy, patient preference studies are related in that they are designed to measure "what specified type of therapy or attributes of a given therapeutic or diagnostic strategy a patient might prefer," such as those measures used in discrete choice experiments.

12.9 SUMMARY

PRO measures provide information gathered directly from the patients about their experiences with the disease and its treatment. Because of the unique perspective offered by patient-reported instruments, direct measurement of health from the patient's perspective is popular and has replaced more objective measures as the primary outcome of interest for a broad spectrum of clinical conditions. For the purpose of evaluating studies that include PROs, it is important to understand the fundamentals of reliability, validity, and responsiveness of the outcome measure being used in addition to appraising the validity of the study. To make wise management decisions, patients and clinicians need to know the magnitude of the effect of treatments on a variety of outcomes, including PROs. Investigators must choose an informative method to present their findings to enhance the interpretability and applicability of their results in a clinical setting.

REFERENCES

[1] M.L. Rothman, P. Beltran, J.C. Cappelleri, J. Lipscomb, B. Teschendorf, Patient-reported outcomes: conceptual issues, *Value in Health* 10 (Suppl 2) (2007) S66–S75.
[2] U.S. Department of Health and Human Services, Food and Drug Administration, Center for Drug Evaluation and Research (CDER), Center for Biologics Evaluation and Research (CBER), Center for Devices and Radiological Health. (CDRH), *Guidance for Industry Patient-reported Outcome Measures: Use in Medical Product*

2 Defined as "qualitative or quantitative assessments of the relative desirability or acceptability to patients of specified alternatives or choices among outcomes or other attributes that differ among alternative health interventions."

Development to Support Labeling Claims, Office of Communications, Division of Drug Information Center for Drug Evaluation and Research Food and Drug Administration, Rockville, MD, 2009.

[3] C. DeMuro, M. Clark, L. Doward, E. Evans, M. Mordin, A. Gnanasakthy, Assessment of PRO label claims granted by the FDA as compared to the EMA (2006–2010), *Value in Health* 16 (8) (2013) 1150–1155.

[4] A. Gnanasakthy, M. Mordin, E. Evans, L. Doward, C. DeMuro, a review of patient-reported outcome labeling in the United States (2011–2015), *Value in Health* 20 (3) (2017) 420–429.

[5] Preamble to the Constitution of the World Health Organization as adopted by the International Health Conference. Official Records of the World Health Organization, no. 2, p. 100 and entered into force on 7 April 1948 19–22 June, 1946. signed on 22 July 1946 by the representatives of 61 States. New York.

[6] World Health Organization, *Towards a Common Language for Functioning, Disability, and Health: ICF the International Classification of Impairment, Disability, and Health*, Report No: WHO/EIP/GPE/CAS/01.3, World Health Organization, Geneva, 2002.

[7] D. Jackowski, G. Guyatt, A guide to health measurement, *Clinical Orthopaedics and Related Research* 413 (2003) 80–89.

[8] S. Wiebe, G. Guyatt, B. Weaver, S. Matijevic, C. Sidwell, Comparative responsiveness of generic and specific quality-of-life instruments, *Journal of Clinical Epidemiology* 56 (1) (2003) 52–60.

[9] M. Bergner, R.A. Bobbitt, W.B. Carter, B.S. Gilson, The sickness impact profile: development and final revision of a health status measure, *Medical Care* 19 (8) (1981) 787–805.

[10] M. Bergner, R.A. Bobbitt, S. Kressel, W.E. Pollard, B.S. Gilson, J.R. Morris, The sickness impact profile: conceptual formulation and methodology for the development of a health status measure, *International Journal of Health Services* 6 (3) (1976) 393–415.

[11] M. Bergner, R.A. Bobbitt, W.E. Pollard, D.P. Martin, B.S. Gilson, The sickness impact profile: validation of a health status measure, *Medical Care* 14 (1) (1976) 57–67.

[12] A.F. de Bruin, M. Buys, L.P. de Witte, J.P.M. Diederiks, The sickness impact profile: SIP68, a short generic version. First evaluation of the reliability and reproducibility, *Journal of Clinical Epidemiology* 47 (8) (1994) 863–871.

[13] A.F. de Bruin, J.P.M. Diederiks, L.P. De Witte, F.C.J. Stevens, H. Philipsen, The development of a short generic version of the sickness impact profile, *Journal of Clinical Epidemiology* 47 (4) (1994) 407–418.

[14] A.F. de Bruin, J.P.M. Diederiks, L.P. de Witte, F.C.J. Stevens, H. Philipsen, Assessing the responsiveness of a functional status measure: the sickness impact profile versus the SIP68, *Journal of Clinical Epidemiology* 50 (5) (1997) 529–540.

[15] S.M. Hunt, J. McEwen, The development of a subjective health indicator, *Sociology of Health and Illness* 2 (3) (1980) 231–246.

[16] S.M. Hunt, J. McEwen, S.P. McKenna, Measuring health status: a new tool for clinicians and epidemiologists, The *Journal of the Royal College of General Practitioners* 35 (273) (1985) 185–188.

[17] S.M. Hunt, S.P. McKenna, J. McEwen, E.M. Backett, J. Williams, E. Papp, A quantitative approach to perceived health status: a validation study, *Journal of Epidemiology & Community Health* 34 (4) (1980) 281–286.

[18] S.M. Hunt, S.P. McKenna, J. McEwen, J. Williams, E. Papp, The Nottingham health profile: subjective health status and medical consultations, *Social Science & Medicine. Part A: Medical Psychology & Medical Sociology* 15 (3 Pt 1) (1981) 221–229.

[19] S.M. Hunt, S.P. McKenna, J. Williams, Reliability of a population survey tool for measuring perceived health problems: a study of patients with osteoarthrosis, *Journal of Epidemiology & Community Health* 35 (4) (1981) 297–300.

[20] C.A. McHorney, W. Johne, R. Anastasiae, The MOS 36-Item Short-Form Health Survey (SF-36): II. Psychometric and clinical tests of validity in measuring physical and mental health constructs, *Medical Care* 31 (3) (1993) 247–263.

[21] C.A. McHorney, J.E. Ware, J.F. Rachel Lu, C.D. Sherbourne, , The MOS 36-Item Short-Form Health Survey (SF-36): III. Tests of data quality, scaling assumptions, and reliability across diverse patient groups, *Medical Care* 32 (1) (1994) 40–66.

[22] J.E. Ware, C.D. Sherbourne, The MOS 36-Item Short-Form Health Survey (SF-36): I. Conceptual framework and item selection, *Medical Care* 30 (6) (1992) 473–483.

[23] J.E. Ware, M. Kosinski, S.D. Keller, A 12-Item Short-Form Health Survey: construction of scales and preliminary tests of reliability and validity, *Medical Care* 34 (3) (1996) 220–233.

[24] J. Von Neumann, O. Morgenstern, *Theory of Games and Economic Behaviour*, Princeton University Press, Princeton, NJ, 1944.

[25] H. Schünemann, Evaluation of the minimal important difference for the feeling thermometer and the St. George's Respiratory Questionnaire in patients with chronic airflow obstruction, *Journal of Clinical Epidemiology* 56 (12) (2003) 1170–1176.

[26] M.A. Puhan, G.H. Guyatt, V.M. Montori, M. Bhandari, P.J. Devereaux, L. Griffith, R. Goldstein, H.J. Schünemann, The standard gamble demonstrated lower reliability than the feeling thermometer, *Journal of Clinical Epidemiology* 58 (5) (2005) 458–465.

[27] H.J. Schünemann, L. Griffith, D. Stubbing, R. Goldstein, G.H. Guyatt, A clinical trial to evaluate the measurement properties of 2 direct preference instruments administered with and without hypothetical marker states, *Medical Decision Making* 23 (2) (2003) 140–149.

[28] R.M. Kaplan, J.P. Anderson, T.G. Ganiats, The quality of well-being scale: rationale for a single quality of life index, in: S.M. Walter, R.M. Rosser (Eds.), *Quality of Life Assessment: Key Issues in the 1990s*, Springer, Dordrecht, Netherlands, 1993, pp. 65–94.

[29] M.H. Boyle, W. Furlong, D. Feeny, G.W. Torrance, J. Hatcher, Reliability of the Health Utilities Index—Mark III used in the 1991 cycle 6 Canadian General Social Survey Health Questionnaire, *Quality of Life Research* 4 (3) (1995) 249–257.

[30] D. Feeny, W. Furlong, M. Boyle, G.W. Torrance, Multi-attribute health status classification systems. Health utillities index, *PharmacoEconomics* 7 (6) (1995) 490–502.

[31] G.W. Torrance, D.H. Feeny, W.J. Furlong, R.D. Barr, Y. Zhang, Q. Wang, Multiattribute utility function for a comprehensive health status classification system. Health utilities index mark 2, *Medical Care* 34 (7) (1996) 702–722.

[32] G.W. Torrance, W. Furlong, D. Feeny, M. Boyle, Multi-attribute preference functions, *PharmacoEconomics* 7 (6) (1995) 503–520.

[33] G. EuroQol, EuroQol–a new facility for the measurement of health-related quality of life, *Health Policy* 16 (3) (1990) 199–208.

[34] J. Brazier, J. Roberts, M. Deverill, The estimation of a preference-based measure of health from the SF-36, *Journal of Health Economics* 21 (2) (2002) 271–292.

[35] J. Brazier, J. Roberts, A. Tsuchiya, J. Busschbach, A comparison of the EQ-5D and SF-6D across seven patient groups, *Health Economics* 13 (9) (2004) 873–884.

[36] S.A. Kharroubi, J.E. Brazier, J. Roberts, A. O'Hagan, Modelling SF-6D health state preference data using a nonparametric Bayesian method, *Journal of Health Economics* 26 (3) (2007) 597–612.

[37] A. Tsuchiya, J. Brazier, J. Roberts, Comparison of valuation methods used to generate the EQ-5D and the SF-6D value sets, *Journal of Health Economics* 25 (2) (2006) 334–346.

[38] J. Raper, B.A. Davis, L. Scott, Patient satisfaction with emergency department triage nursing care: A multicenter study, *Journal of Nursing Care Quality* 13 (6) (1999) 11–24.

[39] J.W. Thomas, R. Penchansky, Relating satisfaction with access to utilization of services, *Medical Care* 22 (6) (1984) 553–568.

[40] Y. Lee, J.D. Kasper, Assessment of medical care by elderly people: general satisfaction and physician quality, *Health Serv Res* 32 (6) (1998) 741–758.

[41] M.S. Marquis, A.R. Davies, J.E. Ware, Patient satisfaction and change in medical care provider: A longitudinal study, *Medical Care* 21 (8) (1983) 821–829.

[42] S.A. Wartman, L.L. Morlock, F.E. Malitz, E.A. Palm, Patient understanding and satisfaction as predictors of compliance, *Medical Care* 21 (9) (1983) 886–891.

[43] S. Abramowitz, A.A. Coté, E. Berry, Analyzing patient satisfaction: A multianalytic approach, *QRB—Quality Review Bulletin* 13 (4) (1987) 122–130.

[44] R. Fitzpatrick, A. Hopkins, Problems in the conceptual framework of patient satisfaction research: an empirical exploration, *Sociology of Health and Illness* 5 (3) (1983) 297–311.

[45] P.L. Hudak, P.D. McKeever, J.G. Wright, Understanding the meaning of satisfaction with treatment outcome, *Medical Care* 42 (8) (2004) 718–725.

[46] D. Locker, D. Dunt, Theoretical and methodological issues in sociological studies of consumer satisfaction with medical care, *Social Science & Medicine. Medical Psychology and Medical Sociology* 12 (4A) (1978) 283–292.

[47] J. Sitzia, N. Wood, Patient satisfaction: A review of issues and concepts, *Social Science & Medicine* 45 (12) (1997) 1829–1843.

[48] B. Williams, Patient satisfaction: A valid concept?, *Social Science & Medicine* 38 (4) (1994) 509–516.

[49] B. Williams, J. Coyle, D. Healy, The meaning of patient satisfaction: an explanation of high reported levels, *Social Science & Medicine* 47 (9) (1998) 1351–1359.

[50] P.L. Hudak, J.G. Wright, The characteristics of patient satisfaction measures, *Spine* 25 (24) (2000) 3167–3177.

[51] P.L. Hudak, S. Hogg-Johnson, C. Bombardier, P.D. McKeever, J.G. Wright, Testing a new theory of patient satisfaction with treatment outcome, *Medical Care* 42 (8) (2004) 726–739.

[52] P.L. Hudak, P. McKeever, J.G. Wright, Unstable embodiments: A phenomenological interpretation of patient satisfaction with treatment outcome, *Journal of Medical Humanities* 28 (1) (2007) 31–44.

[53] R.L. Kane, M. Maciejewski, M. Finch, The relationship of patient satisfaction with care and clinical outcomes, *Medical Care* 35 (7) (1997) 714–730.

[54] S. Linder-Pelz, Social psychological determinants of patient satisfaction: A test of five hypotheses, *Social Science & Medicine* 16 (5) (1982) 583–589.

[55] M.R. Lynn, B.J. McMillen, The scale product technique as a means of enhancing the measurement of patient satisfaction, *Canadian Journal of Nursing Research* 36 (3) (2004) 66–81.

[56] C.K. Ross, C.A. Steward, J.M. Sinacore, A comparative study of seven measures of patient satisfaction, *Medical Care* 33 (4) (1995) 392–406.

[57] J.E. Ware, Effects of acquiescent response set on patient satisfaction ratings, *Medical Care* 16 (4) (1978) 327–336.

[58] Health Services Research Group, A guide to direct measures of patient satisfaction in clinical practice, *CMAJ* 146 (10) (1992) 1727–1731.

[59] R. Blais, Assessing patient satisfaction with health care: did you drop something?, *Canadian Journal of Program Evaluation* 5 (1990) 1–13.

[60] R. Hays, R. Anderson, D. Revicki, Assessing the reliability and validity of measurement in clinical trials, in: M.J. Staquet, R.D. Hays, P.M. Fayers (Eds.), *Quality of*

Life Assessment in Clinical Trials: Methods and Practice, Oxford University Press, Oxford, 1998, p. 169.

[61] P.W. Stratford, C.H. Goldsmith, Use of the standard error as a reliability index of interest: an applied example using elbow flexor strength data, *Physical Therapy* 77 (7) (1997) 745–750.

[62] M.H. Liang, Longitudinal construct validity: establishment of clinical meaning in patient evaluative instruments, *Medical Care* 38 (2000) II-84–II-90.

[63] B. Kirshner, G. Guyatt, A methodological framework for assessing health indices, *Journal of Chronic Diseases* 38 (1) (1985) 27–36.

[64] H.J. Schünemann, G.H. Guyatt, Commentary-Goodbye M(C)ID! Hello MID, where do you come from?, *Health Services Research* 40 (2) (2005) 593–597.

[65] H.J. Schünemann, M. Puhan, R. Goldstein, R. Jaeschke, G.H. Guyatt, Measurement properties and interpretability of the Chronic Respiratory Disease Questionnaire (CRQ), *COPD: Journal of Chronic Obstructive Pulmonary Disease* 2 (1) (2005) 81–89.

[66] L. Portney, M. Watkins, *Foundations of Clinical Research: Applications to Practice*, 3rd ed., Pearson Education Inc, Upper Saddle River, NJ, 2009.

[67] R. Wasserstein, N. Lazar, The ASA's statement on p-values: context, process and purpose, *The American Statistician* 70 (2) (2016) 129–133.

[68] A.S. Rigby, Getting past the statistical referee: moving away from P-values and towards interval estimation, *Health Education Research* 14 (6) (1999) 713–715.

[69] M.J. Gardner, D.G. Altman, Confidence intervals rather than P values: estimation rather than hypothesis testing, *British Medical Journal (Clinical Research Ed.)* 292 (6522) (1986) 746–750.

[70] J. Ranstam, Why the P-value culture is bad and confidence intervals a better alternative, *Osteoarthritis Cartilage* 20 (8) (2012) 805–808.

[71] G. Guyatt, R. Jaeschke, N. Heddle, D. Cook, H. Shannon, S. Walter, Basic statistics for clinicians: 2. Interpreting study results: confidence intervals, *Canadian Medical Association Journal* 152 (2) (1995) 169–173.

[72] J.A. Spertus, J.A. Winder, T.A. Dewhurst, R.A. Deyo, J. Prodzinski, M. McDonell, S.D. Fihn, Development and evaluation of the Seattle Angina Questionnaire: a new functional status measure for coronary artery disease, *Journal of the American College of Cardiology* 25 (2) (1995) 333–341.

[73] J. Cohen, *Statistical Power Analysis for the Behavioral Sciences*, 2nd ed., Lawrence Erlbaum Associates, Hillsdale, NJ, 1988.

[74] C.H. Goldsmith, M. Boers, C. Bombardier, P. Tugwell, Criteria for clinically important changes in outcomes: development, scoring and evaluation of rheumatoid arthritis patient and trial profiles. OMERACT Committee, *The Journal of Rheumatology* 20 (3) (1993) 561–565.

[75] S.J. Goldie, M. Kohli, D. Grima, M.C. Weinstein, T.C. Wright, F.X. Bosch, E. Franco, Projected clinical benefits and cost-effectiveness of a human papillomavirus 16/18 vaccine, *Journal of the National Cancer Institute* 96 (8) (2004) 604–615.

[76] E.L. Simpson, E. Guttman-Yassky, D.J. Margolis, S.R. Feldman, A. Qureshi, T. Hata, V. Mastey, W. Wei, L. Eckert, J. Chao, R.J.G. Arnold, T. Yu, F. Vekeman, M. Suarez-Farinas, A. Gadkari, Association of inadequately controlled disease and disease severity with patient-reported disease burden in adults with atopic dermatitis, *JAMA Dermatology* 154 (8) (2018) 903–912.

[77] M. Boguniewicz, D.Y. Leung, Atopic dermatitis: a disease of altered skin barrier and immune dysregulation, *Immunological Reviews* 242 (1) (2011) 233–246.

[78] J.P. Kim, L.X. Chao, E.L. Simpson, J.I. Silverberg, Persistence of atopic dermatitis (AD): A systematic review and meta-analysis, *Journal of the American Academy of Dermatology* 75 (4) (2016) 681–687 e11.

[79] D.C. Lavallee, K.E. Chenok, R.M. Love, C. Petersen, E. Holve, C.D. Segal, P. D. Franklin, Incorporating patient-reported outcomes into health care to engage patients and enhance care, *Health Affairs (Millwood)* 35 (4) (2016) 575–582.

[80] Northwestern University, Health Measures: Overview, 2019. www.healthmeasures. net/explore-measurement-systems/overview. (Accessed January 17 2019).

[81] Health Catalyst, Survey: fewer than 2 in 10 hospitals regularly use patient-reported outcomes despite Medicare's impending plans for the measures, 2016. www.health catalyst.com/news/survey-fewer-than-2-in-10-hospitals-regularly-use-patient- reported-outcomes/. (Accessed January 19 2019).

[82] J. Seidman, Current value frameworks: what's new?, in: *ISPOR Summit: New Approaches to Value Assessment: Towards More Informed Pricing in Healthcare,* ISPOR, Washington, DC, 2018.

[83] M.I.A. Avalere, Integrating the Patient Perspective into the Development of Value Frameworks, in: FasterCures (Ed.) 2016.

[84] C. Phelps, Novel approaches to value assessment, beyond the cost-effectiveness framework, in: *ISPOR Summit: New Approaches to Value Assessment: Towards More Informed Pricing in Healthcare*, ISPOR, Washington, DC, 2018.

[85] C.E. Phelps, G. Madhavan, Using multicriteria approaches to assess the value of health care, *Value in Health* 20 (2) (2017) 251–255.

[86] R. Cookson, A.J. Mirelman, S. Griffin, M. Asaria, B. Dawkins, O.F. Norheim, S. Verguet, A. J Culyer, Using cost-effectiveness analysis to address health equity concerns, *Value in Health* 20 (2) (2017) 206–212.

[87] L.P. Garrison, Jr., P.J. Neumann, R.J. Willke, A. Basu, P.M. Danzon, J.A. Doshi, M.F. Drummond, D.N. Lakdawalla, M.V. Pauly, C.E. Phelps, S.D. Ramsey, A. Towse, M.C. Weinstein, A health economics approach to us value assessment frameworks; summary and recommendations of the ISPOR special task force report [7], *Value in Health* 21 (2) (2018) 161–165.

[88] S. Griffin, Distribution cost-effectiveness analysis, in: *ISPOR Summit: New Approaches to Value Assessment: Towards More Informed Pricing in Healthcare,* ISPOR, Washington, DC, 2018.

[89] N. Devlin, Extending the cope of PROs and QALYs, in: *ISPOR Summit: New Approaches to Value Assessment: Towards More Informed Pricing in Healthcare,* ISPOR, Washington, DC, 2018.

[90] A. Ambegaonkar, Recent initiatives in US drug policy to promote innovation, value, access and affordability, *Value & Outcomes Spotlight* November/December (2018) 28–30.

13 Sensitivity Analysis

Prof Maarten J. Postma
University of Groningen
Groningen, Netherlands

TABLE OF CONTENTS

13.1 INTRODUCTION

With the widespread use of modeling in pharmacoeconomics (PE), sensitivity analysis has become an important tool for investigating the models being developed and used. In this respect, modeling is conceived as the simulation of complex systems in reality. In particular, a model may be defined as a simplification of such complex relationships, as simple as possible, yet reflecting all relevant aspects of reality. We know that such a model has to be both internally and externally valid, but in addition, it is important to know its properties regarding the changes in the outcomes in relation to changes in the inputs or parameters. The set of parameters reflects those characteristics of reality, which were deemed relevant for simulating the specific realities of interest. The latter may be the costs, savings, and health gains of a specific therapeutic treatment. The parameters may be concerning epidemiology, progression of disease, and unit costs. The generic investigation of these changes in the outcomes in relation to changes in the input parameters is generally labeled sensitivity analysis (SA).

This chapter deals with SA of models in all of its dimensions. The role envisaged for SA will be discussed by considering the PE guidelines throughout the world. Most country-specific guidelines do specify a particular role of SA for judging the appropriateness of models and for selecting those analyses that reflect state-of-the-art PE analysis. Relevance of such PE guidelines is high as, often, reimbursement filings for new drugs must adhere to these and might be denied if this is not the case. Indeed, in the Netherlands, Gardasil® (4-valent *Human Papillomavirus* (HPV) vaccine) has been denied reimbursement within the reference pricing system for individual use due to an inadequate PE reimbursement file (www.cvz.nl). In particular, absence of full and adequate SA on all parameters considered relevant was the primary critique.

After discussing the PE guidelines around the world, this chapter will focus on the terminology surrounding SA. All types will be formally defined and illustrated, often using work on the HPV vaccine. Next to the different types of SA, scenario analysis will be discussed as yet another technique that is sometimes seen as part of SA, however, does exhibit its own specific features, warranting separate consideration and explicit distinguishing from SA.

13.2   PE GUIDELINES AROUND THE WORLD

Various countries around the world have now specified PE guidelines on how to perform a state-of-the-art and good-practice PE analysis. Often, these PE guidelines are formally required for drug reimbursement files submitted by manufacturers to local and national authorities, for example, to have a new drug admitted to reference pricing systems. The International Society for Pharmacoeconomics & Outcomes Research (ISPOR) has summarized the PE guidelines for those countries that have them available. Table 13.1 shows country-specific guidelines referring to SA, both regarding ranges and values for parameters to be investigated and regarding exact methods to be used (Table 13.1 is directly taken from the website www.ispor.org, by selecting countries and individual guidelines). Notably, some countries that do have PE guidelines lack specific ones for SA. In particular, this was the case for Australia, Denmark, Israel, Russia, Taiwan, and South Korea. All other countries included in ISPOR's overview do specify formal requirements for SA.

Table 13.1 shows that PE guidelines often require that SA be undertaken "for key (uncertain) variables over plausible ranges or 95% confidence intervals for parameter values if available." Regarding the techniques, all types are generally advised:

- One-way or univariate SA, in which one (key/uncertain) parameter is varied at a time;
- Two-way or bivariate SA, if two parameters are both varied at the same time;
- Multivariate SA, if multiple parameters (notably more than two) are varied at the same time;
- Best-case analysis, reflecting a specific type of multivariate SA in which all parameters are set at those values in the pre-specified ranges to render the most favorable cost-effectiveness ratio;
- Worst-case analysis, reflecting a specific type of multivariate SA in which all parameters are set at those values in the pre-specified ranges to render the most unfavorable cost-effectiveness ratio; and
- Probabilistic SA, also referred to as Monte Carlo analysis, reflecting the most comprehensive type of analysis in which, for all key and

TABLE 13.1

Country-Specific Pharmacoeconomic Guidelines on Sensitivity Analysis: Parameters and Value Ranges to be Investigated and Methods to be Used (Univariate or One-Way, Bivariate or Two-Way, and Multivariate and Probabilistic Sensitivity Analysis)

	Austria	Baltic (Latvia, Lithuania, Estonia)	Belgium	Brazil & Cuba	Canada	China Mainland	Finland	France	Germany	Hungary	Ireland	Italy
Sensitivity analysis-parameters and range	All key uncertain parameters, within a defined area, or probabilistic	Main assumption variables, confidence interval	Interval estimates should be presented for each parameter in the economic evaluation. All different aspects of uncertainty should be addressed. Confidence interval around the ICER; Cost-effectiveness plane; cost-effectiveness acceptability curve; Tornado diagrams.	For all uncertain parameters, a plausible range must be defined for each parameter	Capture the full range of variability or uncertainty that is relevant for each model input.	All key uncertain parameters, within a defined area, or best/worst case scenario	On uncertain parameters at credible range	Maintain uncertain variables.	The individual input parameters are varied within a range, which may be based on realistic considerations or a schematic variation. Details are given in the guideline.	On uncertain parameters.	Justify the choice of variables and ranges used.	Those parameters which have the most influence on the final results. Effectiveness use CI, range of cost decided by author.
Sensitivity analysis-methods	One-way, multi-way, may be probabilistic analysis	Details of the statistical tests performed	Probabilistic sensitivity analyses should be performed on all uncertain parameters in a model.	One-way, multi-way, probabilistic analysis when adequate	One-way, two-way, multi-way, scenario analysis, Monte Carlo simulation	One-way, multi-way, may be probabilistic analysis Details should be given of the statistical tests performed	Not specific	A distinction is made between univariate and multivariate analysis, and also between first order and second order analysis.	A probabilistic analysis or a different multivariate approach. Details are given in the guideline.	One-way, two-way.	Details should be given of the statistical tests performed	Better showing simultaneous effect of the variations for the more important parameters

TABLE 13.1
(Continued)

	New Zealand	Norway	Poland	Portugal	Scotland	Spain	Sweden	Switzerland	The Netherlands	UK (England & Wales)	United States of America
Sensitivity analysis-parameters and range	All assumptions should be subject to SA.	All key uncertain parameters, within a defined area, or best/worst case scenario	On uncertain parameters at credible range.	Key uncertain parameters. For population data, use CI; others, justified intervals used in detail on the basis of empirical evidence.	Present the associated 95%CI.	Uncertain parameters, using ± 2 SD, or favorable and unfavorable extreme values	At central assumptions and parameters	The variation range accepted for key parameters should be plausible	All key uncertain parameters, within a defined area and best/ worst case scenario	All inputs used in the analysis will be estimated with a degree of impression. The most appropriate ways of presenting uncertainty are confidence ellipses and scatter plots on the cost-effectiveness plane and cost-effectiveness acceptability curves.	All uncertain parameters, high/low value, best/worst scenario, 95% CI, variable distribution.
Sensitivity analysis-methods	Univariate, Multivariate (best and worst case estimate)	One-way, multi-way, probabilistic SA.	One-way, multi-way, may be probabilistic analysis	Not specific	Prefer probabilistic SA (Monte Carlo simulation or Bayesian approach)	Not specific	Not specific	The sensitivity of study conclusions should be examined in detail.	One-way, multi-way and probabilistic analysis	Probabilistic SA.	At a minimum, univariate SA should be undertaken and for important parameters, multivariate SA. Where parameter uncertainty is a major concern, simulation should be undertaken.

Source: directly extracted from a selection on PE-guidelines at www.ispor.org.

uncertain parameters, probability distributions are specified and multiple simulations are performed. Now that we have noted its importance, illustrated by the inclusion of specific requirements for SA in PE guidelines, the different types of SA will be discussed in the next sections, in many cases illustrated by work on the HPV vaccine published in a supplement of the journal *Vaccine* [1].

13.3 SENSITIVITY ANALYSIS

SA is often explicitly differentiated from the so-called "base-case analysis [2]." In the base case, parameter values are all set at their most likely values. Base-case parameter values result in the base-case estimate for the cost-effectiveness ratio, typically representing a point estimate. For example, in their analysis on multi-regional health-economic outcomes of HPV vaccination, Rogoza et al. estimated base-case cost-effectiveness of HPV vaccination at 12 years of age at €22,672 per life-year gained (€18,472 per QALY) and £21,962 per life-year gained (£18,037 per QALY) for the Netherlands and the UK, respectively (Table 13.2) [3].

Also, it is often argued that parameter values should be set conservatively in the base case if uncertainty is high and specification of most-likely values is difficult. For example, for the HPV vaccine, exact full duration of protection is obviously not yet known given the current maximum length of clinical trials at around 6 years. It could, thus, be argued that base-case analyses on the cost-effectiveness of the HPV vaccine should not use durations of protection beyond 6 years, let alone lifelong protection, despite the knowledge that protection is still high after 6 years and is not likely to wane within the next few years. Alternatively, a most likely and probably still conservative period of 10 years could be used.

Taking another look at Table 13.2, it classically presents point estimates for cost-effectiveness. Obviously, this is not the only information that we want; base-case numbers alone do not provide us with all of the information required for full insight into decision-making regarding, for example, reimbursement of the HPV vaccine. SA typically adds crucial information to the base-case analysis: (i) it shows how a plausible range for uncertain key parameters translates into ranges for cost-effectiveness rather than point estimates only and (ii) it shows how changes in the input parameters affect the cost-effectiveness outcomes.

13.3.1 DETERMINISTIC SA

All SAs, except for probabilistic SA, are sometimes labeled as deterministic. In uni-, bi-, and multivariate SA, generally, probabilities, rather than full density functions (often represented as histograms of probability distributions of continuous random variables), are applied. In fact, pre-defined inputs for parameter values are entered into the PE model and outcomes for these inputs are listed. If all key parameters are varied, one-by-one, using such predefined ranges (e.g., plus and minus 20% of base-case values), the SA is univariate or one-

TABLE 13.2

Per Woman Discounted Total Lifetime Costs, QALYs, and Life Years (LYs), with Discounted and Non-Discounted[a] Cost-Effectiveness Ratios for Current Screening and Vaccination Compared with Current Screening in Five Regions[b]

	Canada	Netherlands	Taiwan	United Kingdom	United States
Costs					
No vaccine	CA$906	€123	NT$4112	£216	US$2144
Vaccine	CA$1163	€403	NT$14,911	£409	US$2232
Incremental	CA$258	€280	NT$10,879	£193	US$87
QALYs					
No vaccine	28.689	42.344	27.759	25.518	28.359
Vaccine	28.700	42.359	27.776	25.529	28.370
Incremental	0.011	0.015	0.017	0.011	0.011
LYs					
No vaccine	28.696	42.348	27.763	25.521	28.365
Vaccine	28.704	42.360	27.777	25.530	28.372
Incremental	0.008	0.012	0.015	0.009	0.008
Incremental cost-effectiveness					
Discounted, per QALY	CA$22,532	€18,472	NT$632,559	£18,037	US$7828
Discounted, per LY	CA$31,817	€ 22,672	NT$738,972	£21,962	Dominates[c]
Undiscounted, per QALY	CA$1249	€ 5679	NT$93,508	£1449	US$11,156
Undiscounted, per LY	CA$1554	€ 6785	NT$105,267	£1627	Dominates

Source: Rogoza et al. [3], Only Slightly Adapted Lay-Out, Reproduced with Permission.

[a] Costs, LYs, and QALYs are discounted according to region-specific guidelines (www.ispor.org).

[b] Results are expressed in country- or region-specific currencies.

[c] Vaccination and screening are cost saving and more effective compared to screening alone.

way. One-way SA is often represented using Tornado diagrams. Figure 13.1 shows an example of a Tornado diagram for an analysis of HPV vaccination – again of young teenage girls – in this case for Ireland. The Figure is extracted from Suárez et al. in a specific multi-regional analysis on HPV vaccine cost-effectiveness, with specific focus on vaccine characteristics and alternative vaccination assumptions and scenarios [4]. As such, the paper uses SA as an instrument to investigate impacts of alternative characteristics and assumptions. It clearly shows that the price of the vaccine is an important and influential parameter; however, cost-effectiveness in this analysis is most sensitive to the discount rate.

Figure 13.2 shows an example of a bivariate, or two-way, SA, also extracted from Suárez et al. [4]. In this particular case, the percentage of cross-protection

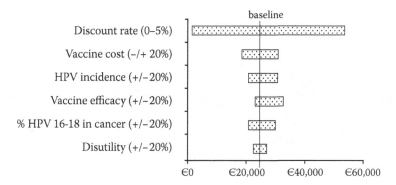

FIGURE 13.1 Tornado diagram of multiple one-way sensitivity analyses on the incremental cost-effectiveness (€/QALY) for vaccinating young teenage girls against HPV in Ireland: sensitivity analysis on parameter uncertainty and variability by varying each parameter ±20% and the discount rate between 0% and 5% (Source: Suárez et al. [4], figure legend slightly adapted to suit this paper, reproduced with permission).

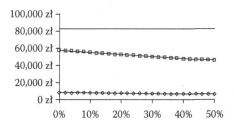

FIGURE 13.2 Two-way sensitivity analysis on the incremental cost-effectiveness (Zloty/QALY) for vaccinating young teenage girls against HPV in Poland: discounting (squares) or non-discounting (diamonds) versus percentage cross-protection against some non-vaccine serotypes at efficacies from 0 to 50%, line represents the potential threshold for favorable cost-effectiveness at 3 times GDP per capita (Source: Suárez et al. [4], figure legend slightly adapted to suit this paper, reproduced with permission).

for some non-vaccine serotypes was investigated in conjunction with discounting outcomes against Polish PE guideline values versus undiscounted outcomes. It can be seen from the lines that the undiscounted results are quite insensitive to inclusion of assumed cross-protection, whereas the discounted results do show some relevant sensitivity. Two-way SA is typically represented by different lines, as in Figure 13.2. Alternatively, a 3-dimensional graph can be constructed, as was done, for example, by Hubben et al. to depict the dependencies on discount rates for health and costs separately for infant pneumococcal vaccination in the Netherlands (Figure 13.3) [5, 6].

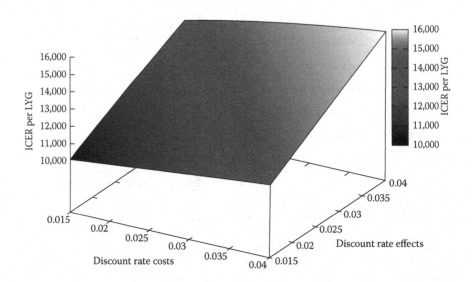

FIGURE 13.3 Two-way sensitivity analysis on the incremental cost-effectiveness in € per life-year gained (LYG) for vaccinating infants with the 7-valent pneumococcal conjugate vaccine in the Netherlands: discounting of costs (on x-axis) versus discounting of health (effects) (Sources: Hubben et al. & Postma [5] [6], figure legend slightly adapted to suit this paper, reproduced with permission).

Rozenbaum et al. typically present a best-case and a worst-case cost-effectiveness for their analysis on antenatal HIV testing in the Netherlands [7]. Taxonomy in best- and worst-case analyses can sometimes be a bit counter-intuitive as, for example, in this specific publication, a higher prevalence of HIV among pregnant women contributes to an improved cost-effectiveness. Yet, a higher prevalence is difficult to be envisaged as "best" in many other respects. In particular, the authors estimated that antenatal HIV testing would cost €6495 per life-year gained in the best case (maximum cost-effectiveness ratio), whereas antenatal testing would be cost saving in the worst case.

13.4 PROBABILISTIC SA

Probabilistic SA concerns the assignment of formal probability distributions or density functions to specific parameters in the model. Probabilistic SA is sometimes referred to as stochastic SA. This type of analysis was first suggested by Doubilet et al. [8]. Generally, these probability distributions are designed for the mean values of the selected parameters (second-order SA), rather than for the sample data from which the estimated mean is derived (first order). Using these distributions, typically 1000 or more simulations are done using random draws from the defined distributions in each simulation. Each individual one (often referred to as "replicate") from these multiple simulations translates into an estimate of the incremental cost-effectiveness ratio. Again from the study by Suárez et al. [4], Figure 13.4 shows a scatter plot of 10,000 replicates around the base-case estimate of cost-effectiveness for vaccinating young teenage girls against HPV in Ireland. Both non-discounted as well as discounted outcomes using a 3.5% discount rate (according to the UK PE guideline) are shown.

Probabilistic SA is often further represented in a cost-effectiveness acceptability curve (CEAC). The CEAC shows, for a range of acceptability or willingness-to-pay (often denoted with λ), the proportions in the scatter plot, which are below each individual λ. Figure 13.5 shows the corresponding CEAC to the scatter plot in Figure 13.4. Additionally, a CEAC with 2% discounting is included in the Figure, possibly better reflecting the Irish underlying time preference (*see* Chapter 11 on discounting). For example, it can be read that with a discount rate of 3.5%, approximately 80% of replicates correspond to a cost-effectiveness ratio below €50,000 per QALY. Also, 95% of replicates, or more, provides an acceptable cost-effectiveness if λ is chosen at €40,000 or over using a discount rate of 2%.

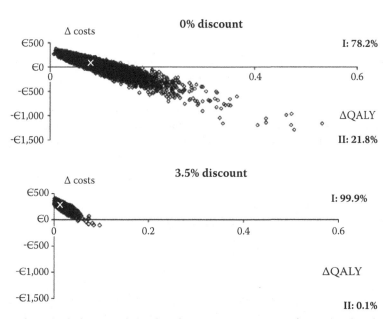

Replicates in the bottom right hand quadrant indicate QALYs gained at a reduced cost; replicates in the top right hand quadrant indicate QALYs gained at an increased cost.

FIGURE 13.4 Scatter plot from the probabilistic sensitivity analysis on the incremental cost-effectiveness (€/QALY) for vaccinating young teenage girls against HPV in Ireland: non-discounted (0%) and discounted (3.5%) results are shown for the base case (x) and for 10,000 replicates (diamonds), I and II represent the first two quadrants from the cost-effectiveness plane, no replicates in the other two quadrants (Source: Suárez et al. [4], figure legend slightly adapted to suit this paper, reproduced with permission).

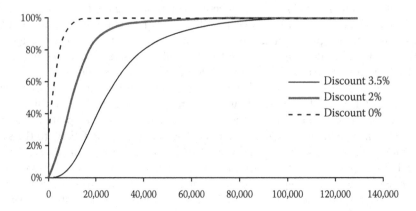

FIGURE 13.5 Cost-effectiveness acceptability curve on the incremental cost-effectiveness (€/QALY) for vaccinating young teenage girls against HPV in Ireland for three levels of discounting with willingness-to-pay (λ) on the x-axis, represented by €/QALY, and the proportion of replicates below the λ threshold on the y-axis; corresponding to the scatter plot in Figure 13.4 (Source: Suárez et al. [4], figure legend slightly adapted to suit this paper, reproduced with permission).

Of course, the major issue in probabilistic SA concerns the exact choice and specification of the probability distributions for the mean parameter values. In the absence of adequate information, often uniform or triangle distributions are taken over plausible ranges with the base-case parameter values as midpoints or expected values. In particular, for both of these types of distributions, a minimum and maximum are defined, with equal probabilities for each value in between for the uniform distribution and increasing probabilities from the minimum or maximum if moving to the pre-defined top of the triangle. Also, referring to the central limit theorem, normal distributions are often considered. Indeed, Suárez et al. [4] used uniform distributions for parameters such as unit costs and screening coverage, and normal distributions for vaccine effectiveness and sensitivity of screening. De Vries et al. [9] used normal and triangle distributions for transition probabilities in the decision tree reflecting progression to aspergillosis and candidosis underlying their analysis of cost-effectiveness of itraconazole prophylaxis against invasive infections for neutropenic cancer patients. Also, Postma et al. [10] used normal and uniform distributions for average length of stay, antibiotic prescriptions, and indirect costs of production losses in their analysis of the cost-effectiveness of treatment with oseltamivir for influenza patients. Additionally, in line with theories underlying the formal estimation of relative risks (RR), they used lognormal distributions for RRs regarding advantages of oseltamivir treatment on antibiotic prescriptions, hospitalizations, deaths, and production losses.

Briggs advocates the use of beta distributions for specific parameters [11]. Beta distributions model events that take place within minimum and maximum values. Given their natural limitation between 0 and 1, these distributions are particularly suitable for risks (e.g., of dying or hospitalization). In particular, in an analysis on beta-blocker therapy for chronic heart failure, beta distributions were used for risks of initial, 2nd, 3rd, and 4th or more hospitalizations and for risks of dying at home or in hospital, next to lognormal distributions for RRs and normal distributions for unit costs [11].

With the majority of PE models being defined in MS Excel™ and TreeAge Pro (TreeAge Software Inc.), it is relevant to briefly consider how both packages facilitate PSA. In particular, PSA is a built-in feature of TreeAge Pro, with a function of Monte Carlo analysis as an explicit analytic option. For Excel, several add-ons that allow PSA exist. For example, @Risk (Palisade) has been explicitly developed and often used for this purpose [10].

13.5 SCENARIO ANALYSIS

Not always formally distinguished as such, it does make sense to briefly consider scenario analysis as a specific type of SA. Scenario analysis is sometimes defined as exploring possible future paths given specific decisions and actions taken in the present. PE modeling, in a sense, also involves present decisions – for example, on which social time preference to choose, which price to set for a new drug – with impacts on cost-effectiveness in (near) future years. Some of the parameters in the model merely reflect decisions by policy makers (which discount rate to choose), manufacturers (pricing), and other stakeholders. These parameters can thus be seen as reflecting instrumental variables, i.e., instruments with which cost-effectiveness can be guided, rather than chance variables impacting probabilistically on the cost-effectiveness outcome. Varying these instrumental variables/parameters, therefore, also reflects the results of choices more so than the results of uncertainty.

For those parameters reflecting instrumental variables in the PE model, it wouldn't make sense to include them in PSA. The effects on the outcomes of varying this set of parameters could be labeled scenario analysis and would typically closely resemble a univariate SA on these parameters. The discount rate and prices of the new product investigated (e.g., of the HPV vaccine) are typical examples of parameters not to be included in PSA but in scenario analysis. As scenario analysis obviously closely resembles univariate SA, it is indeed often done as part of univariate SA and not formally distinguished as such.

13.6 SUMMARIZING

This chapter reviewed methods currently used in SA for PE models. In particular, we considered deterministic versus probabilistic SA, univariate versus multi-variate analysis and scenario analysis as a specific form of SA.

REFERENCES

[1] Franco EL, Drummond MF Eds.. Health economics of HPV Vaccination for cervical cancer prevention: historical developments and practical applications. *Vaccine* 2008;26(Supplement 5).

[2] Gold MR, Siegel JE, Russel LB, Weinstein MC (Eds.). *Cost-effectiveness in Health and Medicine*. New York: Oxford University Press, 1996.

[3] Rogoza RM, Ferko N, Bentley J, Meijer CJLM, Berkhof J, Wang K-L, Downs L, Smith JS, Franco EL. Optimization of primary and secondary cervical cancer prevention strategies in an era of cervical cancer vaccination: a multi-regional health economic analysis. *Vaccine* 2008;26S:F46–F58.

[4] Suárez E, Smith JS, Bosch FX, Nieminen P, Chen C-J, Torvinen S, Demarteau N, Standaert B. Cost-effectiveness of vaccination against Cervical Cancer: a multi-regional analysis assessing the impact of vaccine characteristics and alternative vaccination scenarios. *Vaccine* 2008;26S:F29–F45.

[5] Hubben GAAE, Bos JM, Glynn DM, Van der Ende A, Van Alphen L, Postma MJ. Enhanced decision support for policy makers using a web interface to health-economic models - Illustrated with a cost-effectiveness analysis of nation-wide infant vaccination with the 7-valent pneumococcal conjugate vaccine in the Netherlands. *Vaccine* 2007;25:3669.

[6] Postma MJ. Public health economics of vaccines in the Netherlands: methodological issues and applications. *J Public Health* 2008;16:267–73.

[7] Rozenbaum MH, Verweel G, Folkerts DKF, Dronkers F. Van den Hoek JAR, hartwig NG, De Groot R, Postma MJ. Cost-effectiveness estimates for antenatal HIV testing in the Netherlands. *Int J STD & AIDS* 2008;19:668–75.

[8] Doubilet P, Begg CB, Weinstein MC, Braun P, McNeil BJ. Probabilistic sensitivity analysis using Monte Carlo simulation. A practical approach. *Medical Decision Making* 1985;5:157–77.

[9] De Vries R, Daenen S, Tolley K, Glasmacher A, Prentice A, Howells S, Christopherson H, de Jong – van den Berg LT, Postma MJ. Cost effectiveness of Itraconazole in the prophylaxis of invasive fungal Infections. *PharmacoEconomics* 2008;26:75–90.

[10] Postma MJ, Novak A, Scheijbeler HWKFH, Gyldmark M, Van Genugten MLL, Wilschut JC. Cost effectiveness of Oseltamivir treatment for patients with Influenza-like Illness who are at increased risk for serious complications of influenza. *PharmacoEconomics* 2007;25:497–509.

[11] Briggs AH. Handling uncertainty in economic evaluation and presenting the results. In: Drummond M, McGuire A (Eds.) *Economic Evaluation in Health Care*. New York: Oxford University Press, 2001; pp. 172–214.

14 Use of Pharmacoeconomics in Drug Reimbursement[1]

What Can We Learn from International Experience?

Chris Sampson, MSc, PhD
Office of Health Economics
London, UK

Margherita Neri, MSc
Office of Health Economics
London, UK

Kyann Zhang, MSc
Office of Health Economics
London, UK

TABLE OF CONTENTS

1 Including revised content from the first edition of this book.

14.1   INTRODUCTION

Recent years have seen a proliferation of health technology assessment (HTA) policies and practices being implemented around the world. HTA agencies have been created to provide formal structures and processes for decision-making about the pricing and reimbursement of pharmaceuticals. In many countries, pharmacoeconomic studies are a requisite component of reimbursement consideration. Countries with diverse institutional and cultural profiles have adopted HTA policies and have, in light of this diversity, pursued different tactics [1]. This variation extends to the ways in which pharmacoeconomic analyses are conducted and considered.

The proliferation of HTA around the globe provides a wealth of insight and experience on the use of pharmacoeconomics. As countries without formal HTA processes become the exception, rather than the rule, there is an interest from such jurisdictions in the adoption of HTA more fully. Perhaps the most notable absence of publicly funded centralised HTA is in the United States, where many policymakers have remained sceptical or even belligerent, and the influence of pharmacoeconomic analyses has been limited (see more on this later in the chapter). Likewise, the growing international experience provides lessons for established HTA bodies in addressing current and future challenges.

HTA is arguably lacking in a standard definition [2]. However, we can assert that it is fundamentally about determining the value of health technologies. HTA is an evidence-based multidisciplinary endeavour that should support transparent and unbiased decision-making [3]. Decision makers are often tasked with allocating fixed budgets, meaning that it is necessary to consider costs as well as consequences for health outcomes – and other societal objectives – in order to achieve an efficient health system. In this regard, pharmacoeconomics has become a cornerstone for the assessment of health technologies, informing appraisal decisions.

In this chapter, we provide a broad overview of HTA experience around the globe, considering some of the lessons that might be learned by existing and future HTA bodies alike, with a focus on the ways in which HTA bodies have used pharmacoeconomic analyses to support decision-making.

14.2   THE GLOBAL DEVELOPMENT OF HTA

14.2.1   EUROPE

The first HTA initiatives in Europe began in the 1970s as a response to increasing concerns about the cost and quality of health care, equity in access and ethical questions around the use of health technologies [4]. In this period, health economists and health systems' stakeholders took part in cross-national meetings and conferences, which aimed to establish consensus on the need for a comprehensive and systematic assessment of the way in which investments in health care are made [5].

These initiatives led to the establishment of the first national HTA agency, the Swedish Council on Health Technology Assessment (SBU). Created in 1987, the SBU was mandated to inform the Swedish government about the value of health technologies. In the decade that followed, other European countries, such as Denmark, Finland, Norway, Spain and the United Kingdom, formally set up their own agencies and began to refine the concepts and various possible designs of HTA [6, 7]. By the mid-2000s, HTA had gained mainstream popularity as a policy tool to inform the allocation of healthcare resources. Many more countries in Europe started to build national HTA capacity, often in the form of institutions financed by public resources but with independent status and adopting an advisory role [6].

The National Institute for Health and Care Excellence (NICE) in the United Kingdom has become one of the most influential HTA bodies in the world. NICE was established in 1999 to issue guidance on the use of health technologies to the National Health Service (NHS) in England and Wales. As part of NICE's technology appraisal processes, manufacturers prepare submissions in accordance with the institute's methodological guidelines. In general, submissions include decision-analytic cost-effectiveness models (see Chapters 1, 2, 4 and 7 for more on this topic) that estimate the cost per quality-adjusted life year (QALY) gained.

In most Western European countries, HTA is a well-established and advanced decision-making tool in healthcare policymaking. However, in Central and Eastern Europe (CEE), HTA is in an earlier stage of development. In some countries, including Hungary and Poland, the role of HTA is recognised and investments to build a national capacity have been undertaken. Yet, most CEE countries have not implemented comprehensive and transparent decision-making frameworks [8, 9]. Weak HTA structures and a lack of clear roadmaps have left health decision-making in CEE susceptible to political influences. Additionally, where local evidence is scarce and international HTA findings are used without the necessary adaptations, the assessments may result in biased decisions [8].

Since the early days of HTA, the European Union (EU) has played an important role in the development and expansion of HTA. In the 1990s and early 2000s, the EU funded four key cross-national initiatives that explored opportunities for joint assessment, improvement and harmonisation of HTA methods, effective dissemination and increased impact of findings among European countries [5]. These were the EUR-ASSESS (1994–1997), the HTA Europe (1997–1998), the ECHTA/ECAHI (1997–1999) and the European network for HTA (EUnetHTA) Projects (2006–2008). The original EUnetHTA Project took place under the auspices of a network of public HTA agencies and academic institutions, as well as ministries of health and international organizations. The network that forms the basis of EUnetHTA is still active today and counts over 80 member institutions throughout 28 European member states [10]. A notable achievement of the EUnetHTA Project has been the HTA Core Model, an assessment framework formed by nine domains covering clinical, organizational, economic and patient aspects of health technologies [11]. The framework was developed to improve collaboration among HTA agencies by encouraging non-duplication of evidence and to improve the transparency of procedures and usability of the available evidence across European countries.

Over time, EUnetHTA has grown and continued to receive funding for activities targeting the global development of HTA and cross-border HTA collaboration, such as the EUnetHTA Collaboration (2009) and three consecutive EUnetHTA Joint Action (JA) programmes (2010–2012; 2012–2015; 2016–2020). These programmes have made contributions towards the practical uptake and improvement of the HTA Core Model. For example, the HTA Core Model has been used in several joint assessments, where a chosen number of new pharmaceuticals is appraised collectively by EUnetHTA partners of different European countries and the results can be adapted for use in national contexts [11].

14.2.2 ASIA

During the past few decades, there has been growing recognition of a role for HTA in the pricing and reimbursement of new health technologies in Asia. In the 1990s, South Korea was the first country to introduce economic evaluations as part of its decision-making process, based on the practices of countries with established HTA processes such as Australia, Canada and the United Kingdom [12]. South Korea's healthcare infrastructure is relatively well developed compared to many other countries in Asia [13], with a universal national health system in place since 1989. HTA assessments are currently carried out by the National Evidence-based Healthcare Collaborating Agency established in 2009.

As a lower middle-income country, Thailand was an early adopter of HTA, with several initiatives from the 1990s onwards [14]. Thailand's Health Intervention and Technology Assessment Program was established in 2007, both generating and reviewing cost-effectiveness evidence, and the country recently published formal HTA guidelines [15].

Asia's largest economies – China, India and Japan – have recently begun to formalise economic considerations into healthcare decision-making. Universal health coverage has been available in Japan since 1961, with the entire population covered by either public or association-managed health insurance. Evidence from economic evaluations has in principle been included in the process for the reimbursement of new medicines in Japan since 1992, with relevant data submitted to the Ministry of Health, Labour and Welfare (MHLW). However, a lack of clear rules regarding how this information would be used in the pricing of new drugs meant that assessments were rarely actually submitted, and for the most part were used to compare prices, as opposed to assessing cost-effectiveness [16]. A new formalised system was introduced in 2019 [17]. The Central Social Insurance Medical Council (Chuikyo), a separate body within the MHLW, provides recommendations for pricing of medical products. The drug pricing system in Japan remains complex and includes criteria under which a premium (up to 90%) may be applied for drugs that are considered innovative [18].

For both South Korea and Japan, the availability of health outcomes data is a strength in facilitating further development and implementation of HTA. However, challenges remain with respect to the consistency in the way that cost-effectiveness outcomes are assessed, as well as the ways in which HTA outcomes are incorporated into pricing and reimbursement decisions. One possible barrier to the consistent use of cost-effectiveness evidence in Asian countries is the lack of a universal health system, such as in the cases of China and India.

While the majority of China's population (around 97%) are covered under three public health insurance schemes, these schemes are funded and managed separately, with funding pooled at various government levels, resulting in different reimbursement rates [19]. Recently, there has been more political coordination at the national level, with responsibility designated to the National Health Commission in 2018. The China National Health Development Research Centre, established in 1991, has more recently launched an evidence network to support HTA through providing a framework for pooling and integrating HTA resources at the national level. The network also seeks to engage internationally to share experience and skills [19].

In India, the health system is complex and fragmented, with only a small proportion of people covered by government schemes, and decision-making for health technologies has not historically been employed at the national level. The recent establishment of a dedicated HTA body (HTAIn) has formed part of the effort by the Ministry of Health and Family Welfare to incorporate HTA into health sector decision-making [20].

In general, there has been a shift in Asia towards increased incorporation of HTA processes in decision-making for new health technologies. Countries in Asia conducting HTA have largely followed the processes developed by countries with established HTA bodies. For instance, Singapore established the Agency for Care Effectiveness in 2015, relying on the expertise of HTA specialists from Australia, Canada and the United Kingdom through the appointment of an International Advisory Panel; however, it is recognised that there is currently a gap in local capabilities to perform such assessments [21].

14.2.3 THE REST OF THE WORLD

Australia was a forerunner in HTA and has influenced many other countries. Pharmacoeconomic studies have been part of manufacturers' submissions to the Pharmaceutical Benefits Advisory Committee (PBAC) since 1993. The PBAC's recommendations are used as the basis for listing drugs on the Pharmaceutical Benefits Schedule, which receive public subsidy. Manufacturers' submissions are prepared in accordance with guidelines provided by PBAC and assessed by an independent review group. A decision is made to recommend the listing of the drug – or to reject or defer the application – with the final price agreed upon by a separate committee.

Canada also has a strong commitment to HTA, with organisations originally developing at the provincial level. The Canadian Agency for Drugs and Technologies in Health (CADTH) was established in 1989 and has evolved to become the central agency for the coordination of HTA in Canada, providing guidance on methodological standards for manufacturer submissions. CADTH was established with the goal of standardising access to new drugs across the country, though provincial decision-making remains strong, with some provinces occasionally adopting a view that diverges from the CADTH recommendation.

The United States has historically had a decentralised and fragmented set of HTA processes and policies. The Effective Health Care programme at the Agency for Healthcare Research and Quality reviews evidence and generates analytic tools. The Centers for Medicare and Medicaid Services hosts the Medicare Coverage Advisory Committee, with each state Medicaid programme employing some form of HTA and some participating in the Drug Effectiveness Review Project. In the private sector, pharmacy benefit managers and other companies undertake HTA operations. More recently, both private and public sector stakeholders have begun to make use of recommendations by the Institute for Clinical and Economic Review (ICER), which was founded in 2006 as an independent organization. It has grown to prominence in recent years as pharmaceutical pricing has developed into a mainstream political issue. ICER review evidence and conduct de novo pharmacoeconomic analyses to support their recommendations about the value of health technologies (see Chapter 15 on value-based pricing).

There are now very few parts of the world without any form of HTA used to guide reimbursement decision-making. Even in resource-constrained settings, low-income countries are using HTA methods at the national level, including the consideration of cost-effectiveness evidence [7].

14.3   THE ROLE OF PHARMACOECONOMICS IN HTA

Many HTA agencies have evolved following a similar set of core objectives, but the underlying structures and operational protocols vary substantially [4]. For example, European HTA agencies differ with respect to the target audience (e.g. national, regional or hospital-based), the scope of the assessments (e.g. pharmaceuticals, models of care, medical devices), their mandates and their linkage with the decision-making process [22]. In practice, this diversity reflects the variety of objectives, financing mechanisms and roles of health systems across countries [22, 23]. With many countries adopting HTA processes with different features, the role of pharmacoeconomics in HTA varies. In this section, we consider some of the key defining features in the role of pharmacoeconomics in HTA.

14.3.1 SCOPE

HTA agencies in Europe are generally autonomous bodies with either an advisory or regulatory function. Regulatory function refers to controlling and monitoring quality, safety and efficacy of health technologies. The Italian Medicines Agency, for example, has both advisory and regulatory functions. The results of assessments can inform coverage recommendations in a binding or non-binding way and pricing either directly or indirectly [24]. Non-binding recommendations are used in Germany, where results of clinical or economic evaluations are used to inform the negotiation of price premiums. In England, the outcome of HTA decision-making can have an indirect impact on pricing, as reimbursement status does not affect price, but prices can determine estimates of cost-effectiveness that in turn determine reimbursement status. These characteristics determine the extent to which pharmacoeconomic analyses can directly inform reimbursement decisions.

A distinction should be drawn between assessment, which is the process of evaluation and synthesis of the evidence, and appraisal, which is the production of coverage recommendations based on the results of the assessment and other criteria considered relevant. Some countries have separate agencies to deal with the assessment and appraisal stages. In Germany, for example, the Institute for Quality and Efficiency in Healthcare (IQWiG) is responsible for evaluating the evidence, while the appraisal is carried out by the Federal Joint Committee (G-BA).

HTA can be applied to all health technologies or only pharmaceuticals or medical devices. The majority of the HTA agencies in Europe focuses on pharmaceuticals [25]. In England, NICE appraises a subset of new pharmaceuticals, chosen by the Department of Health and Social Care in consultation with NICE, based on priority criteria. The Scottish Medicine Consortium assesses all new medicines that receive regulatory approval. A topic selection process informs the choice of these technologies based on criteria such as budget impact (see Chapter 8) or uncertainty (see Chapter 13) of the benefits [24].

The geographical scope of HTA can also vary, typically being either national or regional, but it can also be performed in local settings, such as hospitals. In Italy and Spain, for example, some hospitals have experimented with hospital-based HTA to evaluate the clinical, financial and organizational impact of technologies on the hospital unit [22, 26].

14.3.2 MANDATES

With respect to the role of pharmacoeconomics in reimbursement decision-making, HTA agencies can be broadly grouped into three categories: those that mandate the consideration of cost-effectiveness evidence, those that allow it, and those that do not.

All HTA agencies are concerned with estimating the added clinical benefit of a technology. Some countries, such as France, Germany and Italy, focus primarily on the evidence for incremental therapeutic value, as demonstrated by clinical effects from randomised controlled trials compared to the existing standard of care. Other countries, such as England, Sweden and New Zealand, explicitly focus on cost-effectiveness, measured using the incremental cost-effectiveness ratio, where incremental health effects are compared to incremental costs relative to existing treatments. In these countries, QALYs are usually the preferred outcome measure to identify comparable evidence of clinical effectiveness. In countries that don't formally require evidence on economic impact, it may be considered in special cases, such as where there is high expected budget impact and significant incremental therapeutic value (e.g. France), or for use in price negotiations (e.g. Italy).

Most Organisation for Economic Co-operation and Development (OECD) countries mandate the submission of cost-effectiveness evidence as part of the drug reimbursement decision-making process, while others (e.g. France, South Korea) will consider the cost of a new technology and yet others (e.g. Luxembourg, United States) mandate against the consideration of costs [27].

14.3.3 GUIDELINES

In order to support manufacturers' submissions, many agencies provide guidance on the preparation of cost-effectiveness evidence and the use of pharmacoeconomic methods. Such methodological guidelines help to achieve consistency through standardised assessments.

As part of this guidance, some agencies provide a reference case, and some newly established agencies, such as in India, are seeking to do the same [20, 28]. The use of a reference case is also recommended by researchers outside of the decision-making context, including in the United States [29]. Most methods guidance is used such that agencies will consider analyses that deviate from the reference case so long as an analysis that is consistent with the reference case is also provided.

For those agencies that mandate the submission of evidence on costs, most methods guidance recommends cost-effectiveness analysis, with many either exclusively accepting (or, at least, preferring) cost-per-QALY analyses [30]. The Pharmaceutical Management Agency of New Zealand (PHARMAC) is notable for its almost exclusive reliance on cost-per-QALY analyses. In some contexts (e.g. Germany), outcomes are specified but the methods for their analysis are not prescribed.

14.3.4 THRESHOLDS

HTA bodies that mandate the submission of evidence on costs and mandate the use of a particular health outcome could, in principle, establish a threshold level for cost-effectiveness. However, most agencies do not explicitly specify a cost-effectiveness threshold [27], though some do. NICE uses a £20,000–£30,000 cost-per-QALY threshold, while ICER (see Chapters 8 and 15) specify technologies as providing high, intermediate or low value of care according to their cost-per-QALY relative to a 'health-benefit price benchmark' range of $100,000–150,000 [31]. Thailand has become a reference point for new HTA initiatives, as it is the only country in Asia to include an explicit cost-effectiveness threshold as part of the assessment process [32].

Other countries define thresholds with reference to economic indicators. For example, Slovakia specifies a threshold range according to average monthly salary. Where agencies do not specify an explicit threshold, an implicit threshold is often in use and can be identified through research [33]. For instance, depending on severity of disease, technologies assessed in Sweden have been shown to have a 50% chance of approval at either €79,400 or €111,700 per QALY [34].

14.3.5   EQUITY CRITERIA AND MODIFIERS

HTA processes include considerations of wider societal or public health benefits, equity impacts (e.g. disease severity, target population group), innovation and budget impact (see below and Chapter 8). These aspects may enter the appraisal phase rather than being systematically assessed as part of HTA processes or being included in the estimation of cost-effectiveness. As such, they may be considered implicitly or in non-systematic ways. For example, NICE recognises a higher cost-effectiveness threshold for technologies that meet 'end-of-life' criteria. In Italy and Germany, severity is considered implicitly as part of the added benefit assessment.

14.3.6   BUDGET IMPACT

Budget impact has become an increasingly important consideration in HTA, with new treatments that appear to be highly cost-effective while potentially unaffordable (see Chapters 1 and 8 for more information on budget impact). Different countries have varied in their approach considering budget impact, which has given rise to different approaches to reimbursement [35]. Budget impact tends to be presented separately from cost-effectiveness estimates but can be an important decision-making parameter in price negotiations. In England, NICE introduced a budget impact test in 2017, which looks at the net budget impact of new products. Negotiations with NHS England are required for products with an annual net budget impact of £20 million or more, in any of the first 3 years of its use in the NHS. ICER specify an annual budget impact threshold, currently around $820 million based on an algorithm with time-varying market-based factors.

14.4   LESSONS

Recent experience in the spread of HTA has demonstrated that policy solutions can (and should) be context specific. Governments looking to introduce or expand HTA processes need not simply adopt those from any single other country.

Most HTA bodies operate at arms-length from the government and maintain some level of independence. This is particularly important when HTA agencies make recommendations that are controversial and perhaps unfavourable to political goals. Yet, HTA bodies such as NICE, PBAC and CADTH are often perceived as pursuing a payer's agenda despite occasionally making recommendations that are inconvenient to the government.

Independent conduct or validation of pharmacoeconomic analysis is therefore an important part of most HTA processes. Agencies use expert committees, patient representation and stakeholder involvement at various stages and to varying degrees, and these can feed into the conduct or assessment of pharmacoeconomic analyses.

A key feature of publicly funded HTA agencies is that they should be accountable to the public. As a central part of HTA processes, pharmacoeconomic analyses must be conducted with this accountability in mind. Therefore, transparency in the use of pharmacoeconomic analysis is key. This transparency can also be extended to the analyses themselves.

Many HTA agencies provide methodological guidance for pharmacoeconomic analysis, and this is a valuable tool in reimbursement decision-making. By providing guidelines, agencies ensure that internal, external and manufacturer-submitted pharmacoeconomic analyses estimate the value of medicines in a consistent way. Yet, many aspects of HTA methods guidelines remain contentious. A key question in the use of pharmacoeconomic analysis to inform drug reimbursement is the types of outcomes that are to be considered. Most HTA agencies explicitly state the outcomes that will be considered in the decision-making process. Cost-effectiveness thresholds need not be explicitly specified by an agency but can be used implicitly. Explicit thresholds have the advantage of clarity but can create pricing incentives and may restrict a flexible HTA process [36].

A common challenge in low-resource settings, including in South America, Africa, Asia and to some extent Central and Eastern Europe, is that capacity for HTA, in terms of human resources and expertise, is lacking [37]. Arguably, lower income countries face greater opportunity costs from inappropriate decision-making due to the availability of more limited healthcare budgets compared with high-income countries. For this reason and given the lack of sufficient resources to perform HTA, low- and middle-income countries ought to develop clear national roadmaps and increase their involvement in multi-national projects.

While it is important that HTA processes consider the local context, previous experience has demonstrated the value of cross-national collaboration. This may take the form of methodological alignment, shared capacity or collaborative processes to increase the efficiency of HTA.

14.5 CONCLUSIONS

HTA is a truly global phenomenon, and pharmacoeconomic analyses are an increasingly routine input to national decision-making processes. The organisation and authority of HTA bodies, and the nature of the work that they conduct, vary between settings. Policymakers intending to create, formalise or extend the remit of HTA processes can look to other countries for inspiration. Despite the importance of context-specific frameworks, there are several general lessons from international experience to date. These include the need to develop capacity (especially in low-resource settings), establish methodological standards and employ transparent decision-making processes that are protected from undue political bias.

REFERENCES

[1] A. Torbica, G. Fornaro, R. Tarricone, M.F. Drummond, Do social values and institutional context shape the use of economic evaluation in reimbursement decisions? An empirical analysis, *Value in Health* 23(1) (2020) 17–24.

[2] E. Draborg, D. Gyrd-Hansen, P.B. Poulsen, M. Horder, International comparison of the definition and the practical application of health technology assessment, *International Journal of Technology Assessment in Health Care* 21(1) (2005) 89–95.

[3] F. Kristensen, EUnetHTA and health policy-making in Europe, *Eurohealth* 12 (2006) 36–38.

[4] E. Jonsson, Development of health technology assessment in Europe. A personal perspective, *International Journal of Technology Assessment in Health Care* 18(2) (2002) 171–83.

[5] D. Banta, F.B. Kristensen, E. Jonsson, A history of health technology assessment at the European level, *International Journal of Technology Assessment in Health Care* 25(S1) (2009) 68–73.

[6] O. Löblová, Three worlds of health technology assessment: explaining patterns of diffusion of HTA agencies in Europe, *Health Economics, Policy and Law* 11(3) (2016) 253–73.

[7] World Health Organization, *2015 Global Survey on Health Technology Assessment by National Authorities*, World Health Organization, Geneva, Switzerland, 2015.

[8] L. García-Mochón, J.E. Balbino, A.O. de Labry Lima, A.C. Martinez, E.M. Ruiz, R.P. Velasco, HTA and decision-making processes in Central, Eastern and South Eastern Europe: results from a survey, *Health Policy* 123(2) (2019) 182–90.

[9] Z. Kaló, A. Gheorghe, M. Huic, M. Csanádi, F.B. Kristensen, HTA Implementation Roadmap in Central and Eastern European Countries, *Health Economics* 25 (S1) (2016) 179–92.

[10] European Network for Health Technology Assessment, 2020. EUnetHTA Network. [online] EUnetHTA. Available at: https://eunethta.eu/about-eunethta/eunethtanetwork/[Accessed 6 Feb. 2020].

[11] F.B. Kristensen, K. Lampe, C. Wild, M. Cerbo, W. Goettsch, L. Becla, The HTA core model®—10 years of developing an international framework to share multidimensional value assessment, *Value in Health* 20(2) (2017) 244–50.

[12] W. Oortwijn, D. Determann, K. Schiffers, S.S. Tan, J. van der Tuin, Towards integrated health technology assessment for improving decision making in selected countries, *Value in Health* 20(8) (2017) 1121–30.

[13] The Economist Intelligence Unit, Value-based healthcare in Korea: a pioneer in Asia, 2017.

[14] S. Tantivess, Y. Teerawattananon, A. Mills, Strengthening cost-effectiveness analysis in Thailand through the establishment of the health intervention and technology assessment program, *PharmacoEconomics* 27(11) (2009) 931–45.

[15] U. Chaikledkaew, K. Kittrongsiri, Guidelines for health technology assessment in Thailand (second edition)–the development process, *J Med Assoc Thai* 97(Suppl 5) (2014) S4–9.

[16] T. Shiroiwa, T. Fukuda, S. Ikeda, T. Takura, K. Moriwaki, Development of an official guideline for the economic evaluation of drugs/medical devices in Japan, *Value in Health* 20(3) (2017) 372–78.

[17] M. Hasegawa, S. Komoto, T. Shiroiwa, T. Fukuda, Formal implementation of cost-effectiveness evaluations in Japan: A Unique health technology assessment system, *Value in Health* 23(1) (2020) 43–51.

[18] A. Towse, HTA in Japan: Failing to meet international good practice? 2019.

[19] K. MacQuilkan, P. Baker, L. Downey, F. Ruiz, K. Chalkidou, S. Prinja, K. Zhao, T. Wilkinson, A. Glassman, K. Hofman, Strengthening health technology assessment systems in the global south: a comparative analysis of the HTA journeys of China, India and South Africa, *Global Health Action* 11(1) (2018) 1527556.

[20] S. Prinja, L.E. Downey, V.K. Gauba, S. Swaminathan, Health technology assessment for policy making in India: current scenario and way forward, *PharmacoEconomics Open* 2(1) (2018) 1–3.

[21] F. Pearce, L. Lin, E. Teo, K. Ng, D. Khoo, Health technology assessment and its use in drug policies: singapore, *Value in Health Regional Issues* 18 (2019) 176–83.

[22] Health Technology Assessment and Health Policy-Making in Europe: Current Status, Challenges, and Potential, World health organization on behalf of the European observatory on health systems and policies, Copenhagen, 2008.

[23] N. Allen, F. Pichler, T. Wang, S. Patel, S. Salek, Development of archetypes for non-ranking classification and comparison of European national health technology assessment systems, *Health Policy* 113(3) (2013) 305–12.

[24] A. Angelis, A. Lange, P. Kanavos, Using health technology assessment to assess the value of new medicines: results of a systematic review and expert consultation across eight European countries, *Eur J Health Econ* 19(1) (2018) 123–52.

[25] J. Chamova, Mapping of HTA national organisations, programmes and processes in EU and Norway, European Commission, 2017.

[26] L. Sampietro-Colom, M. Soto, C. García, S. Benot, Hospital-Based HTA in three Spanish hospitals, in: L. Sampietro-Colom, J. Martin Eds., *Hospital-Based Health Technology Assessment: The Next Frontier for Health Technology Assessment*, Springer International Publishing, Cham, 2016, pp. 57–69.

[27] L. Barnieh, B. Manns, A. Harris, M. Blom, C. Donaldson, S. Klarenbach, D. Husereau, D. Lorenzetti, F. Clement, A synthesis of drug reimbursement decision-making processes in organisation for economic co-operation and development countries, *Value in Health* 17(1) (2014) 98–108.

[28] S. Swami, T. Srivastava, Role of culture, values, and politics in the implementation of health technology assessment in India: A commentary, *Value in Health* 23(1) (2020) 39–42.

[29] P.J. Neumann, G.D. Sanders, L.B. Russell, J.E. Siegel, T.G. Ganiats, *Cost-Effectiveness in Health and Medicine*, Oxford University Press, New York, 2016.

[30] T. Mathes, E. Jacobs, J.-C. Morfeld, D. Pieper, Methods of international health technology assessment agencies for economic evaluations- a comparative analysis, *BMC Health Services Research* 13(1) (2013) 371.

[31] Institute for Clinical and Economic Review, 2020-2023 Value Assessment Framework, 2020.

[32] R. Schwarzer, U. Rochau, K. Saverno, B. Jahn, B. Bornschein, N. Muehlberger, M. Flatscher-Thoeni, P. Schnell-Inderst, G. Sroczynski, M. Lackner, et al, Systematic overview of cost–effectiveness thresholds in ten countries across four continents, *Journal of Comparative Effectiveness Research* 4(5) (2015) 485–504.

[33] H.-G. Eichler, S.X. Kong, W.C. Gerth, P. Mavros, B. Jönsson, Use of cost-effectiveness analysis in health-care resource allocation decision-making: how are cost-effectiveness thresholds expected to emerge?, *Value Health* 7(5) (2004) 518–28.

[34] M. Svensson, F. Nilsson, K. Arnberg, Reimbursement Decisions for Pharmaceuticals in Sweden: The impact of disease severity and cost effectiveness, *PharmacoEconomics* 33 (2015) 1229–36.

[35] M. Berdud, M. Garau, M. Neri, P. O'Neill, C. Sampson, A. Towse, R&D, Competition and Diffusion of Innovation in the EU: The Case of Hepatitis C, Research Papers, Office of Health Economics, London, 2018.

[36] P. Thokala, J. Ochalek, A.A. Leech, T. Tong, Cost-effectiveness thresholds: the past, the present and the future, *PharmacoEconomics* 36(5) (2018) 509–22.

[37] R. Li, K. Hernandez-Villafuerte, A. Towse, I. Vlad, K. Chalkidou, Mapping priority setting in health in 17 countries across Asia, Latin America, and sub-Saharan Africa, *Health Systems & Reform* 2(1) (2016) 71–83.

15 Value-Based Pricing of Pharmaceuticals in the US and Europe

Renée J.G. Arnold, PharmD, RPh
Icahn School of Medicine at Mount Sinai
Arnold Consultancy & Technology, LLC
New York, NY, USA

Neil X. Hawkins, PhD, MBA, MSc
University of Glasgow
Scotland, UK

TABLE OF CONTENTS

15.1   INTRODUCTION

Value-based pricing (VBP) was first defined as basing the price of a drug on data demonstrating its benefits and harms [1]. This has been broadened to encompass 'any change to traditional payment models for drugs, regardless of the underlying approach to determining the final price of the product' [2]. It was originally developed for a single-payer setting, such as the United Kingdom's National Health Service, to aid in price determinations for novel drugs using a cost per quality-adjusted life year (QALY) threshold of £20,000 to £30,000 and maybe even up to £50,000 per QALY. However, in the United States, where a pluralistic system of insurance providers makes for a great array of coverage options, such a schema is not so straightforward. This chapter will discuss the use of VBP in the US and Europe in terms of cost-effectiveness analyses (CEAs) and negotiating methods.

If one were to follow demand curve economics, there would be no single VBP but instead a distribution of VBPs. One such way of going about this would be to use value-based cost-effectiveness threshold analyses early in drug development to:

- Calculate the minimum changes in clinical effectiveness needed to make a new technology cost-effective for the average patient at various reimbursement levels based on results from pivotal randomized controlled trials (RCTs), the published literature and burden of illness analyses; and,
- Support internal planning by providing thresholds against which to judge cost-effectiveness given expected RCT results.

An example of this last bullet is an analysis to document expected improvements in the clinical effectiveness measures of 1) change in intraocular pressure, 2) medication use and 3) procedure-related costs (including adverse events), – all RCT endpoints expected to be advantageous for a novel injectable for glaucoma. Given assumptions for 2 of these outcomes, the model would then calculate the minimum value of the third outcome needed for the new technology to be cost-effective. In a similar type of analysis, Luttjeboer and colleagues recently published an interesting threshold analysis to validate potential pricing of a therapeutic human papillomavirus (HPV) vaccine in the Netherlands [3] in which scenario testing for €20,000, €50,000 and €80,000/QALY, targeting characteristics of the HPV test being used in screening practice and vaccine efficacy based on RCT results, was performed.

15.2   NEGOTIATION OF TRADE-OFFS

Pauly believes that the 'real alternative [to simple cost-effectiveness thresholds] is to revert to the negotiation model used to develop the UK VBP model' [4]. He states that Medicare is the only US insurer with enough political clout to be able to negotiate prices, although it is currently prohibited by law from doing so. Since CEA is suggested, but not required, in the US for reimbursement decisions, why is it gaining substantial traction in the US now in this regard? There are 2 primary motivations for this:

- The development of value frameworks by prominent groups, including clinician-led organizations; and,
- Publication of new CEA guidelines broadening suggested perspective to include payers [5, 6]

15.2.1   THE DANCE AROUND SUPPLY AND DEMAND IN EUROPE

Pauly [4] discusses the concept of VBP for a 'new break through' technology with no close substitutes in contexts (such as the US) where a single supplier sells its products to various buyers. In this case, the supplier is effectively a monopolist and enjoys corresponding 'market power'. In this section, we look at the context (more commonly found in Europe) where a single supplier sells its products to a single or coordinated buyer. In this case, a bilateral monopoly exists, with the supplier enjoying monopolistic market power and the buyer enjoying monopsonistic market power, implying that whether, and at what price, a technology is reimbursed is subject to negotiation [7]. At a given price, the monopolistic supplier can decide whether they are willing to supply the technology, and the monopsonistic payer can decide whether they are willing to reimburse the technology. If the supplier signals that they are unwilling to supply the technology at a price proffered by a payer, the payer has to decide whether to offer a higher price or threaten not to reimburse the technology. If the payer signals that they are unwilling to reimburse the technology at a price proffered by a supplier, the supplier has to decide whether to lower their price or to threaten not to supply the technology. Although the dynamics of whether it is the supplier or the payer who offers a price may differ between jurisdictions, ultimately the final agreed price will depend on the ability of each party to issue credible threats to either not supply or not reimburse a technology [8–10]. Both parties will typically refer to various measures of value and to support their position within the price negotiation; the credibility of threats not to reimburse or supply will depend on the strength of the incentives and constraints that each party faces.

Payers managing a constrained budget, in general, have a primary incentive to obtain lower prices, as these will leave more money to fund other technologies and services. In some cases, this primary incentive may be tempered by concerns about generating appropriate signals for future technology development and considerations related to national industrial policy [9].

However, a decision not to reimburse a particular technology for an identifiable set of patients may be controversial and lead to political pressure to reverse the decision and, in some cases, judicial review. Conversely, there may be concerns about budget impact (affordability) and the setting of precedents for future reimbursement decisions if a technology is reimbursed [11].

In order to support a credible threat not to reimburse at a given price, a payer may refer to a number of factors, including large budget impact, low magnitude of incremental benefit, price of comparable products, price paid for the technology in other markets, uncertainty in treatment outcomes, overall profitability of the supplier, lack of cost-effectiveness given an established acceptable threshold, and, in extremis, the potential for compulsory licensing. The relative importance given to these factors varies between jurisdictions. Some payers emphasise budget impact, whereas others give greater emphasis to cost-effectiveness and technical efficiency. Some payers emphasise reference pricing and, by implication, the value attached to technologies and strength of credible threats issued by other payers [12].

In contrast, suppliers in general have a primary incentive to maximise revenue. In some cases, this primary incentive may be tempered by concerns about longer term revenues, relationships with payers and the reputational damage of refusing to supply a market. For suppliers, the range of acceptable prices is likely to be constrained at the extreme by the variable cost of goods. In addition, suppliers will be concerned regarding the effect of accepting a given price on the pricing dynamics in other markets, particularly those that employ formal price referencing. In order to support a credible threat not to supply at a given price, a supplier may refer to a number of factors, including small budget impact, large magnitude of incremental benefit, price of comparable products, price paid for the technology on other markets, high cost of technology development and evidence of cost-effectiveness given an established acceptable threshold, and deficiencies in the process of estimation of product value.

Payers can strengthen the credibility of their threats not to reimburse at a given price by establishing an accepted process to estimate the value of a technology. Where the assessment of value is based on a formal assessment of cost-effectiveness, credible threats not to reimburse are strengthened by the research justifying the choice of the acceptable threshold. Credible threats not to reimburse are further strengthened when the assessment of value is conducted by an 'independent' institution. Correspondingly, we have seen many countries set up 'independent' Health Technology Appraisal agencies evaluating the value of technologies using published processes to provide support for reimbursement decisions (see Chapter 14). In this sense, 'value'-based pricing is an integral part of the reimbursement landscape across Europe and increasing beyond [13].

VBP may be based on CEA with the application of an acceptable threshold (e.g., an acceptable cost per QALY threshold) being used to define the maximum effective price. If the threshold represents the opportunity cost of investment in the technology being evaluated, this equates to an objective of promoting technical efficiency (in the generation of QALYs). If this objective is accepted as a [political] priority within the healthcare system, this provides a strong basis to issue credible threats not to pay more than the maximum price that is indicated by the CEA. However, some argue that this approach is 'over-generous,' and that such disclosure of the willingness to pay leads to manufacturers receiving all of the available rent for a technology leaving no consumer surplus [14]. This approach has been taken in the United Kingdom where decisions regarding reimbursement are based predominantly on estimates of cost-effectiveness at a proposed price. Other countries have based their assessment of value, and hence acceptable price, on other, arguably more qualitative, measures of benefit. For example, in France, value of a new technology is assessed by the Haute Autorité de Santé on the five-point Amélioration du Service Médical Rendu [Improvement in Medical Benefit] (ASMR) scale, which runs from 'ASMR V' equating to 'no improvement' to 'ASMR I' equating to major improvement (reserved for an extremely few drugs that have demonstrated effect on mortality in a severe disease). This rating then translates into a determination of the acceptable price. For example, a drug with a rating of ASMR V will only be listed if the price is less than its comparable technologies, whereas drugs with an ASMR I, II or III may achieve maximum allowable prices consistent with the rest of Europe.

Even where the assessment of value is based on CEA and an acceptable threshold, it is not the only determinant of what is ultimately regarded as an acceptable price. Within the United Kingdom, we have seen the introduction of the end-of-life criteria (£50,000 per QALY), Cancer Drug Fund, and the Highly Specialised Technologies process (£100,000–300,000 per QALY) that apply thresholds higher than that which would optimize efficiency in terms of QALYs generated within a fixed budget. These initiatives may be seen as a response to political pressure and an ability to issue credible threats not to pay at prices that would be indicated by an objective of technical efficiency. Once such concessions have been made, they are likely to have a profound impact on the ability to issue future credible threats not to pay as a specific price based on estimated cost-effectiveness [10].

Perhaps one disadvantage of VBP processes based on explicit quantitative assessments of value such as cost per QALY is that any deviation from the accepted threshold creates a strong precedent for future evaluations. In this aspect, there is limited flexibility to respond to acute political pressures and more subjective qualitative assessments of value may, perhaps counterintuitively, lead to more robust VBP processes.

In addition to simple negotiations regarding price, other aspects of pricing may be considered. For example, within the United Kingdom, complex Patient Access Schemes may include individual response-based schemes where, for example, payment is only made for patients who demonstrate a defined response, where treatment for an initial period is free, or treatment after a given period is free. Reimbursement may also be made contingent on future data collection [15]. Examples of both types of schemes have been implemented in the United Kingdom [16, 17].

At a Value Frameworks ISPOR summit held in Washington, DC (October, 2018), McClellan suggested that 'applying value frameworks to systems of care rather than technologies in isolation' could help improve access and outcomes and advance the transition to 'value-based' care systems [18]. Systems of care could include, for example, wireless/remote personal health tools and supportive telemedicine, lower cost methods or sites of care and better coordination of team-based care. The use of open source models, which enhances the ability, transparency and credibility of scenario analyses of cost-effectiveness models in support of VBP, is a concept that has been explored over many years but appears to be gaining some traction in both the US [19–23] and EU (EUnetHTA[24, 25]); it is explored further in Chapter 17 of this book.

15.3 USE OF COST-EFFECTIVENESS THRESHOLDS AS VBP BENCHMARKS

The Institute for Clinical and Economic Review (ICER) in the US has begun to set standards for cost-effectiveness in terms of cost per QALY using benchmarks of <US$100,000/QALY, $100,000 to $150,000/QALY and >$150,000/QALY for high, intermediate and low care value, respectively. Recently, they have modified the cost-effectiveness threshold for ultra-rare diseases (condition/label for fewer than 10,000 patients in the US, which is different from the EU definition) up to $500,000/QALY, although the VBP benchmark remains at $50,000 to $150,000/QALY and incorporates both societal and health system perspectives in many of its deliberations [26]. Regeneron became the first company in the US to publicly adopt a VBP at market entry when it priced its drug dupilumab (Dupixent®) in line with its ICER analysis [2]. Indeed, New York State passed a landmark law in 2017 that allowed, for the first time in the US, New York's Department of Health (DoH) to refer drugs that exceeded the 10-year average inflation rate plus either 5% (2017–2018) or 4% (2018–2019) to a state-wide Drug Utilization Review (DUR) Board created to authorize limits on prescription drug costs based on provided therapeutic value and determination of a target rebate amount [27, 28]. The board may consider drug effectiveness, therapeutic alternatives and the seriousness and prevalence of disease [27].

"If the state and manufacturer fail to agree on a rebate that is at least 75% of the difference between the drug's current price and [the calculated] VBP, the state may waive provisions that currently require managed care plans to cover medically necessary drugs in certain protected classes."

Currently, the basic federal US Medicaid rebate for brand-name medications is greater than 23.1% of the average manufacturer price (AMP) or the AMP minus the best price available to nongovernmental payers. The DUR Board recently recommended that Medicaid pay just under $57 per unit for lumacaftor/ivacaftor (Orkambi®, Vertex Pharmaceuticals), a price that comes to <$150,000/QALY based on the ICER review and which is a medication for cystic fibrosis (CF) [28] that lists for $186 per unit. This $272,000 annual cost of Orkambi has been justified by the manufacturer on the basis of its being the only drug in its class. The class effect limits the state's negotiating power with Vertex because, being the first in its class, New York cannot remove the drug from its formulary, nor waive the prescriber prevails provision of the Medicaid program that affords physicians the final determination over whether a patient requires the drug. Indeed, Vertex has indicated that it does not intend to negotiate further with the state. The DoH is now charged with negotiating with Vertex and, if unsuccessful, the DoH can demand internal information from Vertex about the basis of its pricing. CF is a genetic condition that produces abnormally thick mucus secretions, primarily in the lungs, predisposing to life-threatening infections. It is designated as an orphan disease in the US because it affects <200,000 people (roughly 30,000 people in the US), including 1,660 in New York. New York's Medicaid program covers about 1,000 CF patients; about 1/3 of these are candidates for Orkambi.

Such analyses go towards a drug's affordability. One cannot speak about the VBP or comparative cost-effectiveness of a therapy without discussing its affordability (see Chapter 8 on further discussion about budget impact and affordability). In their review of 3 articles on the topic, Towse and Mauskopf aver that

affordability cannot be separated from the willingness to pay for and/or the opportunity cost of providing a new intervention…Discussion about the affordability of a new health intervention usually means that there is a substantial associated budget impact on a system [29]

15.4 VBP SCHEMA

There are various themes on VBP, including indication-specific pricing, outcomes-based contracts, mortgage pricing and value-based insurance design, among others [2]. Two that are of particular relevance here are indication-specific pricing and outcomes-based contracting. Indication-based pricing sets prices based on the percentage of patients expected to be treated for one of several indications. A form of stratified pricing (reimbursement based on acceptable ICERs in subgroups[30]), although potentially attractive, especially to the manufacturer, may have negative connotations for price and coverage if implemented without negotiation of both [30]. Indeed, from an efficiency standpoint, 'if the price is set according to a higher-value indication, payers may be reluctant to pay that price for lower-value indications, thus restricting the use of the product to fewer indications and patients (static inefficiency)'. Conversely, when prices are based on a lower value indication, industry will be reluctant to invest in research on higher value indications (dynamic inefficiency). Multiple authors have weighed in on the pros (increased transparency leading to rational prices for drugs, potentially lowering prices for lower value indications) and cons (higher prices for patients who benefit the most, higher utilization for patients who benefit the least, higher overall spending and manufacturer profits) of indication-based pricing [29, 31–33].

15.5   EXAMPLES OF VALUE-BASED CONTRACTS

Outcomes-based contracting refunds the cost of a drug when it fails to achieve the promised therapeutic effect in a specific patient. However, as demonstrated by the outcomes-based contract of Amgen with Harvard Pilgrim for evolocumab in heart failure patients, refunding for the approximately 7% of patients who have a myocardial infarction or stroke would only lower the net price from $14,000 per year to $13,620, hardly the cost savings envisioned with such a schema [2, 34]. Clearly, as indicated by many colleagues, insurers and manufacturers need attractive solutions to implement VBP in the US, including reduced restrictions on access, use of VBP benchmarks for initial pricing, facilitated (or nonexistent) prior authorization for drugs priced at their VBP threshold (or varied across multiple thresholds), reduction of or no consumer cost-sharing requirements and placement in preferred formulary tiers without co-insurance if these VBP benchmarks are met by manufacturers [29, 35]. ISPOR has convened a task force to address potential elements of next generation value assessment [36], including those in the following table:

TABLE 15.1

Next-Generation Value Assessment Considerations

- Unmet need
- Rare diseases
- New mechanism/potential for clinical extensions
- Equity for population subgroups with historically worse outcomes

---

(Continued)

TABLE 15.1 (Cont.)

- Labor productivity, e.g. depression treatment for employees
- Better adherence
- Better targeting, e.g. personalized medicine with genetic markers
- Contagion and fear of contagion, e.g. Ebola or Covid-19 vaccine
- Financial protection value for high-cost conditions
- Value of hope/some potential for cure, e.g. Duchenne Muscular Dystrophy treatments
- Option value, i.e. value of opportunity to benefit from future treatment

Other recent examples of new models to pay for costly treatments in the US include (1) Alnylam Pharmaceuticals Inc's calibration of the full $575,000 annual value for its drug givosiran (Givlaari®) to treat acute hepatic porphyria, an inherited liver condition in an estimated 3,000 patients in the US and Europe, based on achieving outcomes similar to clinical trial results and numbers of treated patients; (2) Sanofi's program to provide insulins at a $99/month subscription rate; (3) Novartis' option for insurers to pay over 5 years in equal annual instalments for onasemnogene abeparvovec (Zolgensma®) as a single injection for spinal muscular atrophy and (4) Asegua Therapeutics LLC, a wholly owned subsidiary of Gilead Sciences, Inc., and Abbvie agreeing to provide medications for hepatitis C at a fixed annual cost to the states of Louisiana and Washington regardless of the numbers of patients being treated [37, 38]. In the US, several measures have gone into effect to promote availability of good quality real-world data/evidence (RWD/RWE) to aid in value determination, including passage of the 21st Century Cures Act, which directs the US Food and Drug Administration (FDA) to evaluate the potential use of RWE to support approval of new indications for approved drugs or to support/satisfy post-approval study requirements. In addition, the US Prescription Drug User Fee Act VI requires the FDA to enhance use of RWE in regulatory decision-making. Drafts guidances for both initiatives are expected by the end of 2021 [36, 39]. Moreover, payment reform, such as the framework from the US Healthcare Payment Learning and Action Network, is looking to use such methods as bundled payments (e.g. chronic heart failure episode of care) and specified populations (e.g. accountable care organizations (ACOs)) as alternative payment models to fee-for-service to link healthcare payments to quality and value [36, 40]. Challenges to implementation of VBP payment models include determination of appropriate metrics to establish that outcomes have been met and collection of data to confirm achievement of goals (and trigger contractual terms). A recent study employed a modified Delphi panel construct to establish consensus on indicators for a value-based contract in multiple sclerosis [41]. In terms of data collection, although not a panacea, the near ubiquity of electronic data sources (electronic medical records, claims data, etc.) will help counter the challenge of documenting patient outcomes during negotiations of a VBP.

REFERENCES

[1] P.B. Bach, S.D. Pearson, Payer and policy maker steps to support value-based pricing for drugs, *JAMA* 314(23) (2015) 2503–04.

[2] A. Kaltenboeck, P.B. Bach, Value-based pricing for drugs: Theme and variations, *JAMA* 319(21) (2018) 2165–66.

[3] J. Luttjeboer, D. Setiawan, Q. Cao, T. Cahh Daemen, M.J. Postma, Threshold cost-effectiveness analysis for a therapeutic vaccine against HPV-16/18-positive cervical intraepithelial neoplasia in the Netherlands, *Vaccine* 34(50) (2016) 6381–87.

[4] M.V. Pauly, The questionable economic case for value-based drug pricing in market health systems, *Value in Health* 20(2) (2017) 278–82.

[5] Cost-effectiveness in Health and Medicine, 2nd ed., Oxford University Press, New York, 2016.

[6] P.J. Neumann, G.D. Sanders, Cost-effectiveness analysis 2.0, *N Engl J Med* 376(3) (2017) 203–05.

[7] Management Sciences for Health, Chapter 9: pharmaceutical pricing policy, 2012. www.msh.org/sites/msh.org/files/mds3-ch09-pricing-policy-mar2012.pdf, accessed 22 January 2013.

[8] www.wsj.com/articles/vertex-resolves-yearslong-drug-price-dispute-in-england-11571928563.

[9] M. Vandergrift, P. Kanavos, Health policy versus industrial policy in the pharmaceutical sector: the case of Canada, *Health Policy* 41(3) (1997) 241–60.

[10] S. Grepperud, P. Pedersen, Positioning and negotiations, *The Case of Pharmaceutical Pricing, European Journal of Political Economy* 101853 (2020).

[11] J. Chhatwal, F. Kanwal, M.S. Roberts, M.A. Dunn, Cost-Effectiveness and budget impact of Hepatitis C virus treatment with Sofosbuvir and Ledipasvir in the United States, *Ann Intern Med* 162 (2015) 397.

[12] A.-P. Holtorf, F. Gialama, K.E. Wijaya, Z. Kaló, External reference pricing for pharmaceuticals—A survey and literature review to describe best practices for countries with expanding healthcare coverage., *Value in Health Regional Issues* 19 (2019) 122–31.

[13] M. Drummond, B. Jönsson, F. Rutten, T. Stargardt, Reimbursement of pharmaceuticals: reference pricing versus health technology assessment, *Eur J Health Econ* 12 (2011) 263–71.

[14] K. Claxton, OFT, VBP: QED?, *Health Econ* 16 (2007) 545–58.

[15] L.P. Garrison, A. Towse, A. Briggs, G. de Pouvourville, J. Grueger, P. Mohr, J.L.H. Severens, P. Siviero, M. Sleeper, Performance-Based risk-sharing arrangements—Good practices for design, implementation, and evaluation: Report of the ISPOR Good practices for performance-based risk-sharing arrangements task force, *Value in Health* 16 (2013) 703–19.

[16] M. Duddy, J. Palace, The UK risk-sharing scheme for interferon-beta and glatiramer acetate in multiple sclerosis. Outcome of the year-6 analysis, *Pract Neurol* 16 (2016) 4–6.

[17] www.nice.org.uk/about/what-we-do/patient-access-schemes-liaison-unit.

[18] N. Devlin, Extending the Cope of PROs and QALYs, *ISPOR Summit: New Approaches to Value Assessment: Towards More Informed Pricing in Healthcare*, ISPOR, Washington, DC, 2018.

[19] C.J. Sampson, A call for open-source cost-effectiveness analysis, *Ann Intern Med* 168(7) (2018) 528.

[20] C.J. Sampson, T. Wrightson, Model Registration: A call to action, *PharmacoEconomics - Open* 1(2) (2017) 73–77.

[21] R.J. Arnold, S. Ekins, Time for cooperation in health economics among the modelling community, *Pharmacoeconomics* 28(8) (2010) 609–13.

[22] R.J.G. Arnold, S. Ekins, Ahead of our time: collaboration in modeling then and now, *Pharmacoeconomics* 35(9) (2017) 975–76.

[23] D.M. Eddy, W. Hollingworth, J.J. Caro, J. Tsevat, K.M. McDonald, J.B. Wong, ISPOR-SMDM modeling good research practices task force, Model transparency and validation: a report of the ISPOR-SMDM modeling good research practices task force-7, *Med Decis Making* 32(5) (2012) 733–43.

[24] EUnetHTA, The HTA core model®, 2016.

[25] EUnetHTA, Joint Action 3 Kick-off Meeting, 2018.

[26] R. Chapman, Current Value Frameworks: What's New? *ISPOR Summit: New Approaches to Value Assessment: Towards More Informed Pricing in Healthcare*, ISPOR, Washington, DC, 2018.

[27] T.J. Hwang, A.S. Kesselheim, A. Sarpatwari, Value-based pricing and state reform of prescription drug costs, *JAMA* 318(7) (2017) 609–10.

[28] N. Niedzwiadek, D. Goldberg, State board recommends supplemental rebate for cystic fibrosis drug, 2018. www.politico.com/states/new-york/albany/story/2018/04/26/state-board-recommends-supplemental-rebate-for-cystic-fibrosis-drug-387847. (Accessed January 3 2019).

[29] A. Towse, J.A. Mauskopf, Affordability of new technologies: The next frontier, *Value Health* 21(3) (2018) 249–51.

[30] N. Hawkins, D.A. Scott, Reimbursement and value-based pricing: stratified cost-effectiveness analysis may not be the last word, *Health Econ* 20(6) (2011) 688–98.

[31] P.B. Bach, Indication-specific pricing for cancer drugs, *JAMA* 312(16) (2014) 1629–30.

[32] A. Chandra, C. Garthwaite, The economics of indication-based drug pricing, *N Engl J Med* 377(2) (2017) 103–06.

[33] A. Towse, Indication-based Pricing: A Better Way to Value Drugs? *ISPOR Summit: New Approaches to Value Assessment: Towards More Informed Pricing in Healthcare*, ISPOR, Washington, DC, 2018.

[34] S. Mailankody, P.B. Bach, Money-back guarantees for expensive drugs: Wolf's clothing but a sheep underneath, *Ann Intern Med* 168(12) (2018) 888–89.

[35] J.C. Robinson, S. Howell, S.D. Pearson, Value-based pricing and patient access for specialty drugs, *JAMA* 319(21) (2018) 2169–70.

[36] M. McClellan, Keynote Address, ISPOR Summit: New Approaches to Value Assessment: Towards More Informed Pricing in Healthcare, ISPOR, Washington, DC, 2018.

[37] T. Alcorn, A Plan to Fight Hep C, Volume September 16, 2019, Wall Street J, Dow Jones, New York, 2019, R5.

[38] J. Hopkins, Drugmakers Test New Models to Pay for Costly Treatments, Volume CCLXXV, Wall Street J, Dow Jones, New York, 2020, A1.

[39] A. Ambegaonkar, Recent initiatives in US drug policy to promote innovation, value, access and affordability, Value & Outcomes Spotlight Novemer/December (2018) 28–30.

[40] US Healthcare Payment Learning and action network, about the LAN, 2018. https://hcp-lan.org/. (Accessed January 18 2019).

[41] E.C.S. Swart, L.M. Neilson, C.B. Good, W.H. Shrank, R. Henderson, C. Manolis, N. Parekh, Determination of multiple sclerosis indicators for value-based contracting using the Delphi method, *J Manag Care Spec Pharm* 25(7) (2019) 753–60.

16 Pharmacoeconomics in Disease Management

Practical Applications and Persistent Challenges

Ryung Suh, MD
Georgetown University
Washington, DC, USA

David Atkins, MD, MPH
Department of Veterans Affairs
Washington, DC, USA

TABLE OF CONTENTS

16.1 INTRODUCTION

Disease management (DM) programs refer broadly to programs that seek to improve the care of patients with specific chronic diseases by complementing their usual primary and specialty care with some variety of additional services. Also called care management and care coordination, DM aims to address the common failures of traditional episodic, symptom-based care of chronic diseases like asthma and heart failure by teaching patients to manage their own disease, increasing communication between multiple providers, and emphasizing proactive prevention of exacerbations and complications of chronic disease. DM programs typically target high-risk or high-cost patients; emphasize clinical practice guidelines; employ telephone support to monitor and motivate patients; and aim to be cost-effective by reducing costly complications, hospitalizations, or emergency visits [1].

The promise of DM rests on the observation that many patients with chronic disease do not get all the evidence-based interventions that are indicated [2] and often lack the understanding and skills they need to know how to manage their disease, including how to adhere to their medications, when to seek out care, and how to modify their lifestyles to slow disease progression. The DM industry has grown because various programs have claimed positive financial returns on investment, but the methods to assess the economic returns remain controversial. There have been many initiatives to develop a consensus standard for the economic evaluation of DM programs. Pharmacoeconomic (PE) approaches have been applied to DM programs and to component interventions – largely through observational studies offered by health plans, DM vendors, and academic researchers – but the reliability and validity of many of the studies have been questioned.

16.1.1 EVALUATIONS OF DM PROGRAMS

A number of comprehensive reviews of the literature on the cost implications of DM programs have pointed out frequent flaws in published literature claiming cost-savings. The Congressional Budget Office examined peer-reviewed studies of DM programs for congestive heart failure, coronary artery disease, and diabetes mellitus and determined in 2003 that there was insufficient evidence to conclude that DM programs reduced overall health spending [3]. A systematic review of the literature by Ofman and colleagues [4] in 2004 found that relatively few studies of DM programs evaluated the effects on healthcare utilization and costs and that, among the few studies that demonstrated reductions in utilization or costs, findings were inconsistent, modest, or failed to include program development and implementation costs. A review by Goetzel found that DM programs may reduce direct costs in heart failure and could be cost-saving in depression if productivity gains were included [5]. A RAND Corporation literature review in 2007 examined 317 unique studies and found no evidence of improved cost-savings from DM programs [6].

The introduction of the Medicare Health Support (formerly the Voluntary Chronic Care Improvement) Pilot Program raised hopes that a more rigorous economic evaluation methodology using a randomized design with intervention and comparison groups would lead to a definitive conclusion on the financial benefits of DM. Many programs, however, had difficulty enrolling beneficiaries, and preliminary data indicated that the programs were unlikely to generate sufficient savings to cover the program costs, leading Medicare to end the program earlier than planned and resulting in continued controversy about whether this constituted a good model of economic evaluation principles for DM programs [7].

This chapter outlines how PE principles, discussed in detail elsewhere in this book, have been applied with respect to DM programs. The chapter will begin with an introduction to DM and the characteristics of DM programs that make it unique in the context of economic evaluation. Next, the chapter will examine different approaches and applications of PE principles in the context of DM programs. The final section of the chapter will discuss challenges inherent to integrating these disciplines as the field moves from theory to practice.

16.1.2 DM PROGRAMS

DM programs have been in existence at least since the 1990s and have been proposed as a way to address the failings of the traditional approach to clinical medicine [3]. By providing a standardized, disease-focused approach to patient care, it was envisioned that chronic disease could be managed better through prevention so that acute episodes of illness (usually manifested as hospitalizations and emergency department visits) would be reduced or avoided altogether. Furthermore, DM programs would facilitate knowledge and application of standard of care medicine and improved coordination of care [3].

The term "disease management" has been used to describe a number of component interventions, but the Disease Management Association of America (DMAA) has established a definition that includes a core set of required components [8]. In addition to the use of evidence-based clinical practice guidelines as mentioned above, effective programs must identify the population at risk. Typically, a clinic, health system or health plan uses administrative or clinical databases to identify a target population with a specific disease based on diagnoses, procedures, medication use, lab results, or patient survey data. Commercial DM vendors typically also use administrative data on costs and utilization to target high-risk and high-cost populations who may benefit the most from better management. DM programs also require patient involvement and patient self-management education (to include primary prevention, behavior modification programs, and compliance/surveillance) to equip participants to take a more active role in managing their condition. Beyond the patient-program dynamic, DM authorities generally recognize the need for a collaborative effort among physicians, nurses, technicians, and other members of the care team in order to effectively manage chronic conditions. There must be efforts made to actively evaluate the programs using process and outcomes measurement, evaluation, and management. Finally, there must be routine reporting and feedback loops, including providing feedback to the patient and to the treatment team.

DM programs may be grouped into two general categories: integrated programs (those built into health plans or health systems) and non-integrated programs (stand-alone commercial products) [9]. While many variations exist, the latter programs are designed, marketed, and implemented by third-party vendors with no formal connection to a particular health plan, system, or clinic. This has a significant impact on evaluation strategies, as who is purchasing the DM services, whether patients are embedded within the practice, and whether outreach, recruitment, and coordination costs are included or not have important impacts on the economic costs being measured.

DM programs have been applied to a number of diseases, with diabetes, heart failure, asthma, hypertension, cancer, and depression demonstrating encouraging outcomes data. Other diseases and conditions – for arthritis, pain management, HIV/AIDS, chronic obstructive pulmonary disease, lipid disorders, and others – have been evaluated less frequently but show the potential for benefits as well. With chronic illnesses accounting for nearly 75% of total healthcare expenditures, the expansion of DM programs has accelerated in recent years.

16.2   APPLICATION OF PE PRINCIPLES IN DM PROGRAMS

Despite their intuitive appeal and apparent simplicity, DM programs are highly variable in design, complex in implementation, and have proven difficult to evaluate. PE, in the strictest sense, evaluates cost-effectiveness of drug therapy in terms of the long-term costs and benefits to the patient, to the payer, or to the system. PE principles can be applied to DM programs, inasmuch as the DM program could be viewed like a pharmaceutical treatment and the costs and economic impacts of the treatment can be calculated. Unlike a medication, however, a DM program has multiple targets, including the behavior of patients and multiple providers, each of which have multiple different impacts on healthcare utilization, costs, and health outcomes. This makes a typical PE approach to DM programs difficult. The following section takes a look at different applications of PE principles to DM evaluation.

16.2.1   THE CENTRAL ROLE OF PHARMACEUTICALS

Many DM programs target the appropriate use of evidence-based drug therapy as a way to improve outcomes and reduce costs related to disease exacerbations or progression. For example, heart failure and asthma DM programs all include guidelines that specify the routine use of drugs such as angiotensin-converting enzyme (ACE) inhibitors for congestive heart failure (CHF) or inhaled corticosteroids for asthma, since these have been shown to reduce emergency room visits and hospitalizations. For depression and diabetes, guidelines promote treatments that have been proven to improve symptoms and prevent worsening of the disease and attendant hospitalizations. Effective DM programs assess whether patients are on appropriate therapy and dose, whether they are taking medications as directed, and whether they are responding as hoped.

16.2.2 Cost Analyses of Pharmaceutical Interventions

The crudest justification for DM programs and for pharmaceutical interventions is simple cost of illness (COI) studies (see Chapter 3 for more information on COI). Although COI studies can be useful in identifying candidate conditions with potential for reducing costs, they do not define alternative choices. Using average costs in patients with a given diagnosis (as opposed to marginal costs associated with having the diagnosis on top of other conditions) to assign direct costs of an illness often leads to overestimation of burden attributable to the disease in question and overestimation of the savings from better management of that single condition. Such studies have relatively limited roles in evaluating DM programs themselves, but articulating the burden of illness in financial terms has often been effective in justifying the need for some intervention, especially among healthcare purchasers.

Cost-minimisation analysis (CMA) compares the costs of alternative interventions that are assumed to achieve the same target outcome (see Chapter 6 for more information on CMA). This analysis is most easily applied to pharmaceuticals where there may be evidence that several alternatives are equivalent in relieving symptoms or improving some physiologic endpoint, for example, a specific improvement in blood pressure. A DM program designer or manager may generate a list of all pharmaceuticals approved for use in a particular application within a DM program and identify the least expensive, accounting for direct, indirect, and intangible costs while considering time horizon and discounting to present value (see Chapter 11 on discounting). An example would be to analyze currently approved HMG CoA reductase inhibitors (commonly referred to as statin drugs). While there are distinctions among these drugs in terms of cost, dosing, and evidence on long-term outcomes, if one assumes that there is no clear superiority among available statins (or among a selection of statins) on important outcomes, a simple CMA comparing the various drugs could identify cost-saving strategies for disease managers.

Cost-effectiveness analysis (CEA) calculates both the costs for a series of equivalent treatment or preventive options and the effectiveness expressed as change in a single common dimension of health outcomes, for example, cases avoided, admissions avoided, life-years gained, deaths avoided, cases identified, etc. (see Chapter 7 for more information on CEA). Researchers in the United Kingdom have compared a group of statin medications with regard to the cost to achieve a certain reduction in low-density lipoprotein cholesterol and total cholesterol [10, 11]. In these studies, researchers were able to name a specific drug as being the most cost-effective in the cohort examined. Such information can be useful in choosing among different interventions that may vary in effectiveness (e.g., in formulary decisions). CEA can also be used to decide if a new intervention, such as a DM intervention, provides reasonable "value" relative to other health programs, even if it is not strictly cost-saving.

Cost–benefit analysis is distinct from the previous analytic methods described as it strictly adheres to costs and benefits in monetary terms [12]. These tend to be comprehensive comparisons of all social costs and consequences, taking a societal perspective to maximize social welfare; these are not routinely used in the evaluation of DM programs as they require assigning monetary values to all health outcomes.

Cost–utility analysis (CUA) compares alternative interventions using the health outcome of individual "utility" based on preferences for different states of well-being (see Chapter 7 for more information on CUA). As mentioned previously, the quality-adjusted life year (QALY) is a common unit of measurement in North American studies. Unlike CEA, CUA can account for a variety of disparate outcomes, such as effects on symptoms, mortality, and unanticipated harms of treatment. Several challenges complicate the use of CUAs: utilities must be assigned to a comprehensive set of outcomes; a small change in the disutility assigned to a common outcome (e.g., the inconvenience of monitoring one's blood sugar regularly) can have big effects on overall assessments, and finally, the results can be difficult for lay people to interpret. There is also no consensus about what cost per QALY represents a "reasonable" value. That is, there are generally no hard cut-offs for an acceptable cost to save one QALY. A common cut-off in the U.S. has been $50,000, although these have been changing (see Chapter 15), but different thresholds may be used in the United Kingdom and other European countries [13]. A conference on evaluation of DM sponsored by the Agency for Healthcare Research and Quality (AHRQ) in 2002 recommended the use of natural history models that combine the expected benefits of improvement from multiple outcomes measures into a single composite measure (the QALY), with the need for data validation and appropriate case-mix adjustments [14].

16.2.3   ACTUARIAL ANALYSIS OF DM PROGRAMS

Actuarial approaches to DM evaluation are more common than health economic approaches. Actuarial methods allow for analyses of DM programs that have been applied to an entire target population and where there is no concurrent comparison group. Actuarial analysis, instead, analyzes historical trends and relies on a set of methodological tools and techniques applied to financial risk and uncertainty. Actuarial analysis has a number of features: a financial focus, an interest in long-term outcomes, prediction based on historical experience, sensitivity testing on assumptions, the use of sophisticated statistics, and a marriage of pragmatism and theory [15]. Predictive modeling and assessments of DM interventions in terms of impacts on actuarial trend lines have become the dominant evaluation model. In its simplest form, actuarial analysis measures cost trends before and after a DM intervention and calculates the savings from the project cost trend line. The evaluation strategy is straightforward and unbiased as long as the analysis is applied to all eligible patients but assumes that models can adjust for other secular factors that may affect cost trends. Trends (and estimated savings) can also be influenced by the duration of baseline data.

16.2.4 DEVELOPMENTS IN THE ECONOMIC EVALUATION OF DM PROGRAMS

Although actuarial analysis predominates with commercial programs, a number of other reports have sought economic evaluations with more reliable concurrent controls. The Medicare Prescription Drug, Improvement, and Modernization Act of 2003 instituted a Chronic Care Improvement Plan for traditional fee-for-service Medicare beneficiaries. This is a volunteer program to evaluate the use of DM programs in the Medicare population. The name for this initiative was later changed to the Medicare Health Support (MHS) program. Briefly, this program called for DM vendors – selected vendors are henceforth referred to as Medicare Health Support Organizations (MHSOs) – to target enrollees with the selected conditions of heart failure and/or diabetes and to provide services incorporating those already in use in commercial DM and case management programs. Thirty thousand participants were identified and randomized into either the intervention group (enrolled in an MHSO program) or the control group.

The first of four Reports to Congress was released in 2007 and presented preliminary findings from the first six months of the trial [16]. There were no significant differences between the intervention and the control groups in processes of care, acute care utilization (outcomes), or changes in Hierarchical Condition Code. Additionally, the authors of the first report did note as key findings that the cost per beneficiary in the intervention and comparison groups drifted apart between randomization and the start dates of the pilot; the intervention group (those that volunteered to participate) tended to be healthier and less expensive than the intervention group as a whole; and that the programs have generally not been cost-effective for Medicare. While this initial report did not offer promising information for supporters of DM programs, additional data are needed to draw firm conclusions. The 18-month interim report on MHS again failed to identify financial cost-savings and continues to create controversy. The MHS experience illustrates a fundamental challenge of non-integrated DM programs in effectively engaging the sickest patients.

The RAND Corporation conducted a literature review on the available evidence for the impacts of DM programs [6]. The authors reviewed three evaluations of large population-based programs, ten meta-analyses, and sixteen systematic reviews. In total, 317 unique studies were included in the review. The report concluded that there is no evidence for improved cost-savings by using DM programs despite improvements in processes of care and, in a very limited number of circumstances, reduced utilization. The overarching theme of the review was that scientific evidence had not kept pace with the growth of the DM industry. The report also contained a useful perspective on how to classify DM programs as the authors recommended analyzing a DM program by both the severity of illness and by the intensity of the intervention. This perspective may prove useful for future work using economic evaluation applied to DM programs as programs can be grouped and compared more easily if they are classified according to what they have in common.

AHRQ's report on Patient Self Management Support Programs also addressed evaluation issues in DM [17]. As discussed above, DM programs depend on patient education as a key component of their approach to managing disease. Many of the observations here are applicable not only to patient self-management efforts but also to DM programs as a whole in that both focus on changes in behavior. These observations also provide opportunities for inclusion of PE techniques into the development, implementation, and evaluation of DM programs. The most specific example of how PE analysis may play a role in promoting positive behavior change pertains to medication compliance. This in turn belongs to a broader set of evaluation measures that help program managers determine the success of their program as well as areas for improvement. The authors emphasized the importance of aligning program objectives with measured objectives so that the results are meaningful. This is an area where PE analysis may be particularly useful. For example, when planning what to measure, managers may desire to perform a CEA specifically related to medication use within the DM program. Program managers working closely with PE experts in the development process will ensure that their program is generating appropriate data easily analyzed in future work, hence, opening the door for meaningful program evaluation and improvement.

DMAA has also made significant contributions to developing practical approaches to the economic evaluation of DM programs. Their Outcomes Guideline Report (Volumes I and II) outlined recommended practices for measuring outcomes in DM and other population-based programs to include key clinical measures, applications to wellness programs, and approaches to small populations. Volume III expanded on the clinical and financial measures from the preceding volumes, validated an identification methodology, recommended a measure of medication possession ratio (a metric of patient adherence to medications), and outlined principles for evaluating programs for more than one chronic medical condition [18].

16.2.5 Effective Use of PE Data

DM programs depend on the selection of best medications, their use in a correct regimen, and patient and provider compliance. Patient compliance alone may directly tie to the patient's ability to pay for the medication, an important area for PE if patient cost sharing is a factor. There are recent examples of direct application of PE data to disease processes that are also managed under DM programs. All of the examples below demonstrate the role that PE can play in guiding DM programs, potentially at more than one stage of the program life cycle.

For example, clopidogrel is an antiplatelet agent used to treat a variety of vascular diseases, including the U. S. Food and Drug Administration -approved indications of acute coronary syndrome, stroke, and peripheral artery disease, all within specified time frames with respect to hospitalization or diagnosis. A study by Choudhry found that as much as 40% of a 5,000-person Medicare population was prescribed the drug despite it having no clear advantage over alternate or no therapy [19]. Many of the patients in this cohort would have been equally well treated by using aspirin. In this particular example, there is abundant literature on use of clopidogrel to include good scientific understanding of which specific patients benefit from its use versus aspirin alone. This information is important from an economic perspective as there is a great difference in price between clopidogrel and aspirin, with clopidogrel costing as much as several hundred times that of aspirin per tablet [20]. Choudhry estimated that potentially inappropriate use of clopidogrel cost the state of Pennsylvania as much as $2.87 million in one year (using FDA indications for clopidogrel use). It is then reasonable to suppose that were PE data such as these applied to DM programs, real and substantial cost-savings could be achieved in a short time. Operationally, it would not be difficult to assign DM program participants into categories based on the clinical indicators for particular treatments, as risk stratification is already a part of some DM programs.

Seen from a different angle, the ability of a DM program to support medication compliance may be significantly enhanced by provision of payment for medications where there is strong evidence for their use in treating specific conditions. Choudhry also examined how providing full coverage for drugs enhanced compliance with treatment regimens for post-myocardial infarction patients [21]. He found that among Medicare beneficiaries, eliminating patient responsibility for paying for essential drugs such as aspirin, beta-blockers, ACE inhibitors or angiotensin receptor blockers, and statins, there was an improvement in cost-utility of $7,182 per QALY saved despite the program not being strictly cost-saving. Choudhry made the macroeconomic argument that, from a societal perspective, this is beneficial. An application to DM programs might be offering enrollees full or partial drug coverage for those medications included within the DM program requirements.

In addition to these two examples of PE analysis playing an important role in DM programs, there has been work in gathering similar data from the treatment of illnesses less commonly thought of in the context of a DM program. In 2005, Dubinsky examined the cost-effectiveness of various strategies for treating Crohn's disease, including a comparison of traditional methods with those more tailored to individual patients based on individual variance in metabolism of the main therapeutic drug. She concluded that costs were significantly greater for non-tailored care and that time to reach a response to treatment was longer [22]. Treatment of Alzheimer's disease with a new drug was the topic of a PE review by Lamb [23] who showed that a specific acetylcholinesterase inhibitor, rivastigmine, was associated with cost-savings (not including the cost of the drug itself), which became more significant over time and when initiated early in the progression of the disease. Both of these examples demonstrate situations where cost-effectiveness of a pharmaceutical intervention will be greatest if the drug is prescribed in a controlled environment, such as within a DM program, where patients and their use of particular medications are closely monitored and where changes in therapeutic regimens are potentially simpler to institute, monitor, and modify.

16.3   FROM THEORY TO PRACTICE

The application of PE theory into DM evaluation practice is beset by a number of challenges. Interventions and the components of DM programs that one strives to evaluate take place within complex health systems, and our PE techniques tend to be rather crude, with fundamental biases when applied to DM programs.

16.3.1   EVALUATION STRATEGIES

The purpose of any evaluation is to demonstrate value in terms of cost-savings, clinical improvements, or increased quality of care. Effective evaluations allow one to improve how the program is designed or delivered and help to sustain support for the program within the limitations of time, data, and resources. Good evaluation strategies aim to accurately reflect the impact of programs, avoid measures that conceal or mislead, and use resources for efficient measurement. Hence, the selection of measures and evaluation strategies must balance process and outcomes measures, consider the feasibility of data collection, and the importance of the measure in promoting actual improvements in the program.

Measuring the financial or economic impact of DM programs requires one to recognize the inherent challenges (e.g., allowing a sufficient time horizon for improvements, the turnover of subjects within the program, defining the population and the denominator). One must have realistic expectations about how much evaluation can be achieved in a given DM program and the value of longer, more contentious, and more expensive evaluations. Estimates of costs must be sure to include the costs of the DM program itself and the costs of increased medical care and pharmaceutical interventions. Accurate estimations of cost-savings require a reliable comparison group, and certain comparisons are likely to be biased. For example, pre–post comparisons in high-cost patients are subject to regression to the mean. Likewise, unadjusted comparisons between patients who remain in a given DM program and those who do not are subject to selection bias.

Practical evaluation strategies call for the development of a standardized methodology, but this is beset by a number of conflicting dichotomies. Simplicity in practice comes at the price of accuracy and practicality is at odds with evaluation granularity. The search for comparability makes it difficult to achieve customizability.

16.3.2   PERSISTENT CHALLENGES

Data availability varies considerably from DM program to DM program, and evaluations are often limited to administrative claims data. Beyond actuarial models that focus on financial risk, it is difficult to access data that relate to the broad definitions of economic value. For example, patient quality of life, worker productivity, and patient satisfaction are important, but these data are often unavailable. Case-mix adjustments are required, and one needs to identify all vendor fees and administrative costs associated with a given DM intervention, but data to support these evaluations are also not always available.

The perspectives of different payers (e.g., Medicare, Medicaid, employers, health plans, etc.) may differ substantially and may have conflicting objectives: who captures the savings and when have important implications. Patients and clinicians often view impacts over an entire lifetime, while purchasers and health plans may prefer shorter time horizons that relate to turnover rates. Also, given that significant cost shifting (delays in cost burden) may occur across time, different purchasers are concerned with different analytical approaches that capture this perspective.

Measurement challenges are common and well established in DM evaluation. Regression to the mean resulting from the targeted evaluation of high-risk or enrolled subpopulations only and selection bias resulting from selective enrollment or turnover remain critical challenges. Pre/post study designs without a control group are most practical, although evaluations with whole populations or probability sampling with case-mix adjustment and a comparison group would likely be more valid. Secular trends, technology changes, medical inflation, differential program ages, local pricing or accounting differences, enrollee turnover, treatment interference, and other factors may be significant confounders.

The generalizability of results from economic evaluations remains limited. It is difficult to attribute conclusions and results from specific interventions given that diseases, populations, and settings vary considerably. Multiple comorbidities add complexity, although most chronic diseases have significant comorbidities that must be managed concurrently. In addition, different diseases may have varying timelines for long-term economic returns.

16.4 CONCLUSIONS

The economic evaluation of DM programs depends largely on the structure of the DM programs and the objective of the evaluation. DM programs target multiple levels – patient behaviors, provider behaviors, and health system change – and each level must be appropriately incentivized. Patient self-management practices only work on those willing to be engaged. Moreover, incentives to change provider behavior depend on the model or embedded system of care within which providers operate. Systems integration and measurement depend on whether DM programs are stand-alone or integrated, and all DM interventions take place in complex health systems.

The practical application of PE principles often relies on over-idealistic assumptions about DM. It is important to recognize that economic evaluations are not simple and that they are not inexpensive. The analytic strategies that one chooses must recognize the fundamental limitations of traditional PE approaches and the need to select appropriate approaches and models in evaluating DM. Actuarial analysis and predictive modeling are likely to remain the dominant analytical strategy, both for their reliance on relatively easily accessible data and their relative simplicity, but one must also recognize that the challenge of evaluating practice change at multiple levels within complex healthcare systems requires the use of different analytical tools and approaches as needed.

REFERENCES

[1] S.L. Norris, R.E. Glasgow, M.M. Engelgau, P.J. O'Connor, D. McCulloch, Chronic disease management, *Disease Management & Health Outcomes* 11(8) (2003) 477–488.
[2] E.A. McGlynn, S.M. Asch, J. Adams, J. Keesey, J. Hicks, A. DeCristofaro, E.A. Kerr, The quality of health care delivered to adults in the United States, *New England Journal of Medicine* 348(26) (2003) 2635–2645.
[3] Congressional Budget Office, *Congress A to Z*, CQ Press, Washington, DC, 2008.
[4] J.J. Ofman, E. Badamgarav, J.M. Henning, K. Knight, A.D. Gano, R.K. Levan, S. Gur-Arie, M.S. Richards, V. Hasselblad, S.R. Weingarten, Does disease management improve clinical and economic outcomes in patients with chronic diseases? A systematic review, *The American Journal of Medicine* 117(3) (2004) 182–192.
[5] R.Z. Goetzel, R.J. Ozminkowski, V.G. Villagra, J. Duffy, Return on investment in disease management: A review, *Health Care Financ Rev* 26(4) (2005) 1–19.
[6] S. Mattke, M. Seid, S. Ma, Evidence for the effect of disease management: Is $1 billion a year a good investment?, *Am J Manag Care* 13(12) (2007) 670–676.
[7] D. Peikes, A. Chen, J. Schore, R. Brown, Effects of care coordination on hospitalization, quality of care, and health care expenditures among medicare beneficiaries, *JAMA* 301(6) (2009) 603.
[8] D.M.A.o. America, 2008. www.dmaa.org/dm_definition.asp. (Accessed December 29 2008).
[9] J.P. Geyman, Disease management: Panacea, another false hope, or something in between?, *The Annals of Family Medicine* 5(3) (2007) 257–260.
[10] S. Palmer, A.J. Brady, A. Ratcliffe, PCV19 A probabilistic model to assess the cost-effectiveness of a new statin (rosuvastatin) in the UK, *Value in Health* 6(6) (2003) 649–650.
[11] K. Wilson, J. Marriott, S. Fuller, L. Lacey, D. Gillen, A model to assess the cost effectiveness of statins in achieving the UK National Service Framework target cholesterol levels, *PharmacoEconomics* 21(Supplement 1) (2003) 1–11.
[12] R. Lee, *Economics for Healthcare Managers*, Health Administration Press, Chicago, IL, 2000.
[13] K.L. Rascati, The $64,000 question – What is a quality-adjusted life-year worth?, *Clinical Therapeutics* 28(7) (2006) 1042–1043.
[14] J.V. Selby, D. Scanlon, J.E. Lafata, V. Villagra, J. Beich, P.R. Salber, Determining the value of disease management programs, *The Joint Commission Journal on Quality and Safety* 29(9) (2003) 491–499.
[15] J. Adler, Actuarial forecasting for health, September 12, 2007. www.sepho.org.uk/download.aspx?urlid=10963&amp:urlt=1. (Accessed December 29 2008).
[16] Centers for Medicare and Medicaid Services, Report to Congress. Evaluation of Phase I of Medicare Health Support (Formerly Voluntary Chronic Care Improvement) Pilot Program Under Traditional Fee-for-Service Medicare, June 2007.
[17] R. Health, *Patient Self-Management Support Programs: An Evaluation. Final Contract Report to the Agency for Healthcare Research and Quality*, AHRQ, Rockvville, MD, November 2007.

[18] Disease Management Association of America, *Outcomes Guidelines Reports*, Volumes I–III, Disease Management Association of America, Washington, DC, 2008.
[19] N.K. Choudhry, R. Levin, J. Avorn, The economic consequences of non–evidence-based clopidogrel use, *American Heart Journal* 155(5) (2008) 904–909.
[20] Drugstore.com. www.drugstore.com. (Accessed December 28 2008).
[21] N.K. Choudhry, A.R. Patrick, E.M. Antman, J. Avorn, W.H. Shrank, Cost-effectiveness of providing full drug coverage to increase medication adherence in post–myocardial infarction medicare beneficiaries, *Circulation* 117(10) (2008) 1261–1268.
[22] M.C. Dubinsky, E. Reyes, J. Ofman, C.-F. Chiou, S. Wade, W.J. Sandborn, A cost-effectiveness analysis of alternative disease management strategies in patients with Crohn's disease treated with azathioprine or 6-mercaptopurine, *The American Journal of Gastroenterology* 100(10) (2005) 2239–2247.
[23] H.M. Lamb, K.L. Goa, Rivastigmine, *PharmacoEconomics* 19(3) (2001) 303–318.

17 From Machine Learning in Drug Discovery to Pharmacoeconomics

Sean Ekins, PhD
Collaborations Pharmaceuticals, Inc.
Raleigh, NC, USA

Renée J.G. Arnold, PharmD, RPh
Icahn School of Medicine at Mount Sinai
Arnold Consultancy & Technology, LLC
New York, NY, USA

TABLE OF CONTENTS

17.1 INTRODUCTION

The area of artificial intelligence is gathering increasing visibility, with self-driving cars and voice assistants coming to the market. In the pharmaceutical industry, we have seen pockets of use for computers and machine learning for aspects of drug discovery for several decades [1]. At its core, machine learning is just "using patterns in data to label things" [2]. Recent developments in deep learning exemplified by deep neural networks (DNNs) that have become more accessible [3–6] have accelerated the interest such that this has become a hot trend in the industry [7–10]. These technologies can assist us in mining complex data, learning from images, and perhaps in identifying future important drugs. Beyond the hype, the reality always sets in [11]; what we are seeing are discrete pockets where this technology excels. Otherwise, algorithms developed decades ago are still holding their own in the many recent comparisons for drug discovery applications [12–14], with DNN occasionally outperforming the other methods marginally for drug discovery applications [15]. We can learn from the decades of use and development of computational and machine learning models in the pharmaceutical industry and apply them elsewhere in areas like pharmacoeconomics, for example.

As stated in the American College of Physicians position paper,

> given the as-yet uncontrolled explosion of health care costs... and the limited resources of our society, the time has come for patients, physicians, insurers, and health care policymakers to explicitly and transparently factor the comparative effectiveness, comparative cost, and cost-effectiveness of both new and existing health care interventions into their decisions. [1]

Attempts to provide that computational evidence have sometimes been disastrous. For example, a computational (decision analysis) model that was used to compare the expected health outcomes and resource requirements for mammography screening caused a furor by calling for limited screening below the age of 50 and increasing the screening interval to every other year for all but high-risk breast cancer candidates [16]. The model interpretation was debated in journal articles, published and further debated in online newspaper stories, blogs, and various other scattered information sources without a centrally located source not only for making the model available for examination but also for discussion surrounding the model once published. It was rumored that insurance companies would stop paying for annual mammograms. As mentioned in the online Health Care Blog, "What a golden opportunity has been missed to educate Americans about the implications of their health care choices" [17]. Fortunately, practitioner societies, such as the American Society of Clinical Oncology and the American Heart Association in conjunction with the American College of Cardiology, independent associations, such as the Institute for Clinical and Economic Review (ICER), academicians, managed care organizations and other healthcare institutions, have all recently established or proposed the so-called "value frameworks" (see Chapter 15) that encompass measures of cost (affordability) and/or cost-effectiveness of drugs and other initiatives [18–20].

The International Society for Pharmacoeconomics and Outcomes Research (ISPOR), Health Technology Assessment International (HTAi), Academy for Managed Care Pharmacy (AMCP), and Society for Medical Decision Making (SMDM) have called for transparency and availability of models so that they can be examined and vetted (e.g., by journal reviewers and policy makers), "reused" with different data, further validated, and continually revised as new information becomes available [21–24]. The difficulty with these requirements is illustrated by the following:

1. Models are often created for a single purpose and then languish in journal archives, health authority databases, or various proprietary settings, often reinvented when the need arises for a new evaluation to inform health policy decisions or drug reimbursement guidelines;

2. Rather than using/updating a pre-existing model, new models are often created for new medications or new indications at considerable time (up to a year) [25] and expense;

3. Because of lack of a platform and standards for easily sharing such computer-based models, very few are ever made available to peer reviewers, let alone expert readers, public health officials, and decision makers other than in the form of a paper print-out of the model or certain of its generated reports; and,

4. Currently, the medical specialty journals remain the primary medium for communicating the content and results of decision models to the healthcare research community.

There are an increasing number of online tools that are viable for storing science-related content, e.g. FigShare (Digital Science), SlideShare (Microsoft), Mendeley (Elsevier), Dropbox, etc. and consortia to coordinate and make data accessible like OpenPhacts [26, 27], ATOM [28], as well as a myriad of other initiatives to free up data [29–31]. In addition, there are several efforts that have enabled the sharing of machine learning models for drug discovery [32–34].

We envisage a future in which there is a massive growth in open science and we see the urgent need for a model exchange (ModEx). This represents a knowledgebase for real-time management of data and models fully supporting the FAIR (Findable, Accessible, Interoperable, Reusable) principle for research data [35] and updates an earlier idea we published in 2010 that many groups [22, 23, 25, 27, 36] are now embracing, namely, to build a web-based platform for the exchange and enhancement of healthcare models that determine comparative effectiveness (CE) and/or cost-effectiveness of different healthcare strategies (Figure 17.1). Bertagnolli and colleagues [37] have discussed data sharing of clinical trial results—a feat more than 60 years in coming—and hampered largely by similar forces to those facing the sharing of pharmacoeconomic models, namely, lack of "access to enabling data systems technology, bioinformatics expertise and legal agreements that facilitate sharing." Some of these barriers to data sharing of clinical trial results are slowly being overcome via gatekeeper models (a central repository overseen by an independent expert committee and subject to review of a research proposal), active open source data-sharing models (upload and download of publicly-available patient-level datasets, incorporating templates of legal agreements and other documentation to facilitate data-sharing), and federated data models (the data requester's analytical programs are copied into the data owner's computer, the programs are run and the aggregated results are sent back to the requester) [37]. We have published the concept in a peer-reviewed journal [25, 36] and have been contacted by researchers from around the globe who are eager to participate. A secondary effect of ModEx will be to have a positive global impact on the pace, usage, scholarship, cost, and relevance of computational model development for pharmaceutical/device company customers (Pharma), policy makers, and the researchers who generate these models. We will build on our recent work to develop software for sharing machine learning models including Assay Central [13, 14, 38], which

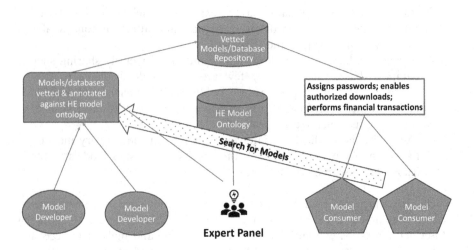

FIGURE 17.1 Creation of an interactive model exchange/marketplace prototype. The figure represents the web processes transactional system components. ModEx will store all data in a database backend and provide an administrative interface for users. It will be comprised of several major subsystems and a number of connected services.

provides a considerable foundation for ModEx and will improve data sharing and collaboration.

The following sections illustrate some of the algorithms and approaches that have been applied successfully in drug discovery. In addition, we will describe some applications of software in pharmacoeconomics and ultimately suggest how we could use such approaches to create a decision-making algorithm for pharmaceutical research and development.

17.2   QUANTITATIVE STRUCTURE–ACTIVITY RELATIONSHIPS

Quantitative Structure–Activity Relationships (QSARs) are mathematical models relating a molecular structure to a chemical property or biological effect using statistical techniques. When a significant correlation is achieved for a set of training molecules with available biological data, the model can then be used to predict the biological effect for other molecules, although there may be some limitations to model applicability [39]. QSAR is a key component of modern medicinal chemistry and pharmacology, with much of the early work in the field published by Hansch and co-workers in the 1960s onwards [40]; since this time, there have been thousands of models generated [41, 42]. QSAR uses a wide array of molecular descriptors (one dimensional, two dimensional, and three dimensional [3D]) as numerical representations of chemical structures [43, 44] and methods to select those that are most relevant [45]. 3D-QSAR methods, including comparative molecular field analysis [46] and comparative molecular similarity indices analysis [47], are perhaps the most widely used. Of course, the real value of these QSAR methods is in using them to make predictions for new molecules or as frequently used in the process of scoring and ranking molecules in large chemical libraries for their likelihood of possessing affinity for a target of interest (also known as virtual screening) [38]. The pharmaceutical industry has learnt to accept that virtual screening methods represent an efficient complement to high throughput screening [48–50]. Virtual screening requires either a ligand-based model of the protein of interest, a QSAR or pharmacophore, or the target itself (target-based virtual screening) [51, 52].

A diverse range of ligand-based virtual screening methods is available [53] (for more details, see recent reviews [39, 54]). Perhaps the most widely employed methods requiring 3D structure representations of molecules are those exploiting the concept of pharmacophore similarity [55], where a pharmacophore is the 3D arrangement of molecular features necessary for bioactivity [56–60]. Pharmacophore approaches have subsequently been applied to many therapeutic targets for the virtual screening of compound databases [61–63]. Successful pharmacophore applications include the identification of hits for a variety of targets [64, 65], such as absorption, distribution, metabolism, excretion, and toxicity (ADME/Tox)-related proteins, using database searching protocols [66–69]. Hence, pharmacophore-based approaches have considerable versatility and applicability.

17.3   MACHINE LEARNING METHODS

Machine learning approaches have been widely used for several decades for ADME/Tox and drug discovery, and they have enabled the prioritization of compounds prior to testing *in vitro* (Figure 17.2). The large volumes of available *in vitro* data have motivated the field to initially focus on computational models to predict properties such as aqueous solubility and metabolic stability. Some of the machine learning models, e.g. solubility, human liver microsomes, or mouse liver microsomes [70, 71], have proven relatively useful. Drug discovery is about making better decisions. Every day, drug discovery teams in large Pharma must decide which hits to take forward from a high throughput screen, which compounds to synthesize, which compounds to take into a pharmacokinetic study, and ultimately, which compounds to take into development and subsequently the clinic.

Collaborations Pharmaceuticals Inc. has been involved in making available as open source software various machine learning technologies, such as algorithms and descriptors [72–74], which have recently eliminated the barrier of expensive proprietary software for cheminformatics [75]. One product we are developing is Assay Central (Figure 17.3), a cheminformatics tool for building and validating machine learning models for high throughput and other datasets in drug discovery [12, 76, 77]. The Assay Central project has been previously described [12, 76, 77]. It uses the source code management system Git to gather and store structure–activity datasets from diverse sources in addition to storing scripts for thorough curation. These scripts employ a series of rules for the

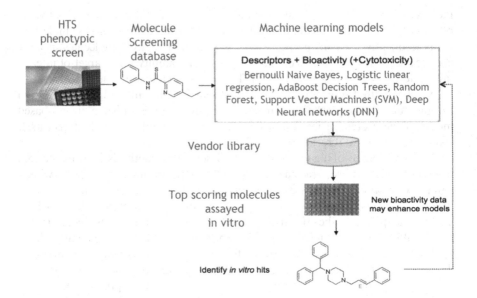

FIGURE 17.2 Machine learning process schematic.

detection of problem data that are corrected by a combination of automated structure standardization (including removing salts, neutralizing unbalanced charges, and merging duplicate structures with finite activities) and human re-curation. The output is a high-quality dataset and a Bayesian model that can be conveniently used to predict activities for proposed compounds. We utilize Assay Central to prepare and merge datasets collated in Molecular Notebook [76], as well as generate Bayesian models of training data. These models utilize extended connectivity fingerprints maximum diameter 6 (ECFP6) descriptors [78, 79], which are circular topological fingerprints generated by applying the Morgan algorithm that have widely been noted for their ability to map structure–activity relationships [77]. Each model in Assay Central includes common statistics to evaluate predictive performance. Assay Central allows us to wrap up models as an app and share them with collaborators (model 17.1). This achieves one of our goals to make the models accessible to collaborators and they can be shared privately or publicly (e.g., as supplemental data for publications).

We have also compared various machine learning models across multiple drug discovery and toxicity end points [12]. We use the RDKit open source cheminformatics software [78] to generate Extended-Connectivity Fingerprints (ECFP6) [79] for the training set compounds that serve as the chemical features for QSAR modeling training. Then, a variety of machine learning algorithms are used to learn the relationship between the chemical features and the target activity within the training compounds. These include "classic" machine learning algorithms Bernoulli Naive Bayes [80], AdaBoost Decision Trees [81], Random Forest (RF) [82], Support Vector Classification [83], and k-Nearest Neighbors [84] as implemented through the software package scikit-learn (http://scikit-learn.

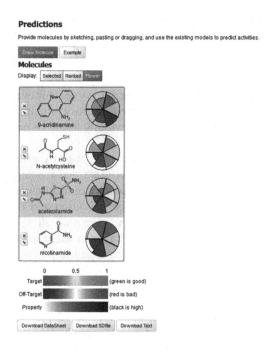

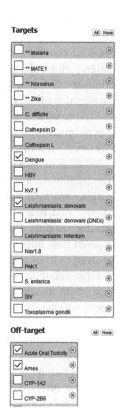

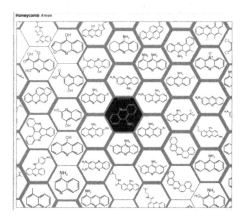

FIGURE 17.3 Assay Central interface and inset showing test set molecule (black) surrounded by training set actives (green) and inactives (no shading).

org/) [85]. Additionally, DNN [86] using multiple hidden layers and implemented using Keras [87] is included in our comparisons. We frequently use a stratified five-fold cross validation technique that maintains similar ratios of active and inactive molecules amongst the splits. This five-fold cross validation is performed exhaustively for each combination of hyper-parameters to identify the best set as measured by the area under the receiver operating characteristic curve. However, due to the increased training times needed for DNN, the five-fold cross validation is performed on a single set of hyper-parameters that we previously found to perform well on a variety of diverse datasets [12].

What is a success for us as modelers may not be seen that way by other scientists/investors, etc. How we pick the endpoint to demonstrate that machine learning works is therefore critical. In order to succeed, the pharmaceutical industry and pharmaceutical researchers must promote internal collaboration and the sharing of data that can be mined efficiently rather than generating silos of impenetrable information. Drug discovery and development has been suggested to be composed of distinct decision gates [88, 89], where key questions can be asked of a candidate molecule and answers may be provided using experimental studies. One could imagine that these decision gates could represent individual computational models which ultimately lead to the development of decision analytic methods, which will be useful to determine whether a molecule should progress through additional steps of the drug discovery and development process. The decisions suggested in such an approach could be based on one of a number of algorithms such as a decision tree approach that has been used widely in health economic analysis [90] and drug innovation assessment algorithm analysis [91], and that incorporates probability models and weights at each step. This may represent an opportunity for the industry to consider predictions from many computational simulations in different areas of research alongside experimental data.

17.4   SHARING PHARMACOECONOMIC MODELS

Healthcare rationing, that is, deciding who gets what healthcare service, is influenced in the United States and, indeed, around the world, by computer models that compare available treatments, so-called CE models, to see which works and costs the least based on research findings. The US Institute of Medicine defines CE research as the study of methods to "prevent, diagnose, treat, and monitor a clinical condition or to improve the delivery of care," including alternative approaches to healthcare delivery, to assist "consumers, clinicians, purchasers, and policy makers to make informed decisions that will improve health care at both the individual and the population levels." Computerized models help to objectify the complexities of CE and cost-effectiveness of different therapeutic options to aid in decision-making by pharmaceutical/device manufacturers, health authorities, and healthcare practitioners regarding therapeutic guidelines, reimbursement/coverage, and overall patient health. Many of these models are created annually. However, these models are often static versions published in journals, not transparent, open to public scrutiny, or updated in a timely fashion.

We believe that the time has come to embrace development of the registry of CE models which we proposed 10 years ago and that the technology available to do this is even more robust now. This effort will include classic machine learning methods such as Bayesian, RF, and SVM, as well as cutting edge machine learning methods such as DNNs, which have been used to advance many other fields [8]. Algorithms could also highlight potential problems with the model(s), and similar methods would provide the quality check, followed up by an Advisory Panel evaluating the model for basic validity according to AdViSHE recommendations, including validation of the conceptual model, input data, computerized model calculations, and accurate model outcomes [92]. Sharing of CE models goes far beyond the company-level collaboration [93]. It is long overdue for a consortium to be formed which might consist of the major stakeholders such as societies (e.g., ISPOR, HTAi, SMDM, and AMCP), academic centers of excellence (e.g., University of York, Tufts Medical Center), health technology assessment bodies (e.g., National Institute for Health and Care Excellence, ICER, Canadian Agency for Drugs and Technologies in Health), and the pharmaceutical industry, who could break down their CE model silos and cooperate for the good of patients. The proposed ModEx offers a platform for the sharing of models, allows for a network of model creators/potential to meet, and has a much broader base of user types. It is also a central forum for discussion and peer-review around the models and their implications. The project is also intended to bring together open and pre-publication data and models, facilitating research around this data. By connecting focused groups of disparate individuals and organizations scattered about the country or globe, the ample opportunity exists to both gather and disseminate important information to a highly relevant target audience. Team members will be able to borrow and reuse a growing collection of existing data and/or models.

A large number of such models are created and published annually. Indeed, a Medline search for "cost-effectiveness analysis" (one of the model types that will be supported in ModEx [Figure 17.1]) yielded 22,681 abstracts over the past 5 years. Therefore, there are many researchers in the field creating and publishing their models in journals. These models are expensive to create.

Although gaining traction in the health economic press lately, as noted above, the concept of an exchange for CE and cost-effectiveness models is innovative, has never been accomplished for this purpose, and will have a positive impact in the modeling community, and, ultimately, in healthcare research. Although there is a precedent for collaborative modeling, the Global Diabetes Model [94–96], ModEx, will catalyze a level of collaboration and peer-to-peer networking that does not currently normally occur in the modeling community— amongst modelers, potential "customers" for the models, public health officials, and members of the public. Indeed, the germ for this idea was the request of one of the others by two very different entities—an academic institution and a large, public, CRO—that she donate a working copy of a decision tree model that she had previously published so that they could further modify it for their needs [90]. ModEx will assist model developers not only by increasing their visibility but also by increasing the return on their development efforts by selling the models to multiple customers or through contracts to customize their models for other applications. Model development and validation would likely become more rapid and cost-effective because many models have common bases, and a modeler could build on that base rather than starting from scratch. In some cases, simply using a different data set (e.g., a managed care vs. Medicaid database) for a new client would result in novel conclusions. Furthermore, collaborations between modeling experts from industry, academia, and government may result in more and better ideas. ModEx will be a centralized marketplace for the exchange of pre-existing models, new models, and collaboration amongst various stakeholders in the CE debate. The ModEx platform aims to serve modelers in the CE, decision analysis, and health economics communities, which are currently without a platform for sharing models. These users will have secure accounts from which they can share models they desire (when published, for example) or keep them private by default if they are only using ModEx for collaboration amongst a small group. In addition, the ModEx platform would include a search as well as networking component, enabling users to post queries and collaborate with colleagues and others working on modeling projects. Ensuring authenticity and integrity of models and data generated is possible by implementing a DataLedger [97, 98], which represents an open source framework based on the approach and technology used in Blockchain [99] and Hyperledger [100].

17.5   CONCLUSION

Computational tools and algorithms can have an impact when used alongside other types of data in drug discovery and development [1]. In recent years, we have seen more data sharing by big Pharma and considerable efforts at open innovation [31, 101–106]. The machine learning tools and models are, however, usually used in isolation to make discrete decisions and rarely shared. Part of this may derive from commercial tools limiting the sharing of models to those with licenses for the software used. Open source software has changed the dynamic in cheminformatics to some degree [72, 74, 107–113]. We propose that pharmacoeconomics could also benefit from the sharing of models, and enabling this will require the development of a new database and software tools. Challenges ahead include the funding of such initiatives and the willingness of the community to both contribute and share their models while using those developed by others. While we describe just 2 discrete areas of drug discovery that utilize computational approaches, one could imagine many more that could learn from these initiatives.

ACKNOWLEDGMENTS

S.E. kindly acknowledges Dr. Alex Clark, Mr. Daniel Russo, Mr. Valery Tkachenko and colleagues at Collaborations Pharmaceuticals. This work is supported by NIH/NIGMS R43GM122196, R44GM122196-02A1.

REFERENCES

[1] S. Ekins, *Computer Applications in Pharmaceutical Research and Development*, John Wiley & Sons, Inc., Hoboken, NJ, 2006.

[2] C. Kozyrkov, Machine learning—Is the emperor wearing clothes? https://medium. com/@kozyrkov/machine-learning-is-the-emperor-wearing-clothes-928fe406fe09., (2018).

[3] Anon, Deepchem. https://deepchem.io/.

[4] Anon, Tensorflow. www.tensorflow.org (2018).

[5] Anon, Amazon Sagemaker. https://aws.amazon.com/sagemaker/.

[6] Anon, Cloud AutoML. https://cloud.google.com/automl/docs/.

[7] H. Chen, O. Engkvist, Y. Wang, M. Olivecrona, T. Blaschke, The rise of deep learning in drug discovery, *Drug Discov Today* 23(6) (2018) 1241–1250.

[8] S. Ekins, The next era: Deep learning in pharmaceutical research, *Pharm Res* 33(11) (2016) 2594–2603.

[9] E. Gawehn, J.A. Hiss, G. Schneider, Deep learning in drug discovery, *Mol Inform* 35(1) (2015) 3–14.

[10] T. Unterthiner, A. Mayr, G. Klambauer, S. Hochreiter, Toxicity prediction using deep learning, 2015.

[11] A.M. Jordan, Artificial intelligence in drug design-the storm before the calm?, *ACS Med Chem Lett* 9(12) (2018) 1150–1152.

[12] A. Korotcov, V. Tkachenko, D.P. Russo, S. Ekins, Comparison of deep learning with multiple machine learning methods and metrics using diverse drug discovery data sets, *Mol Pharm* 14(12) (2017) 4462–4475.

[13] T. Lane, D.P. Russo, K.M. Zorn, A.M. Clark, A. Korotcov, V. Tkachenko, R.C. Reynolds, A.L. Perryman, J.S. Freundlich, S. Ekins, Comparing and validating machine learning models for mycobacterium tuberculosis drug discovery, *Mol Pharm* 15(10) (2018) 4346–4360.

[14] D.P. Russo, K.M. Zorn, A.M. Clark, H. Zhu, S. Ekins, Comparing multiple machine learning algorithms and metrics for estrogen receptor binding prediction, *Mol Pharm* 15(10) (2018) 4361–4370.

[15] K. Liu, X. Sun, L. Jia, J. Ma, H. Xing, J. Wu, H. Gao, Y. Sun, F. Boulnois, J. Fan, Chemi-Net: A molecular graph convolutional network for accurate drug property prediction, *Int J Mol Sci* 20(14) (2019) 3389.

[16] H.D. Nelson, K. Tyne, A. Naik, C. Bougatsos, B.K. Chan, L. Humphrey, U.S.P.S.T. Force, Screening for breast cancer: An update for the U.S. Preventive Services Task Force, *Ann Intern Med* 151(10) (2009) 727–37, W237-42.

[17] M. Goozner, The Health Care Blog: So much for comparative effectiveness. http://thehealthcareblog.com/blog/2009/11/20/so-much-for-comparative-effectiveness/#more-15032, (2010).

[18] P.B. Bach, New math on drug cost-effectiveness, *N Engl J Med* 373(19) (2015) 1797–1799.

[19] P.J. Neumann, J.T. Cohen, Measuring the value of prescription drugs, *N Engl J Med* 373(27) (2015) 2595–2597.

[20] P.J. Neumann, G.D. Sanders, Cost-effectiveness analysis 2.0, *N Engl J Med* 376(3) (2017) 203–205.

[21] SMDM, *ISPOR- SMDM Joint Modeling Good Research Practices Task Force*, ISPOR, Princeton, NJ, 2010.

[22] ISPOR, *Model Transparency and Validation Working Group*, ISPOR, Princeton, NJ, 2011.

[23] AMCP Partnership Forum, Principles for sound pharmacy and therapeutics (P&T) committee practices: What's next?, *J Manag Care Spec Pharm* 26(1) (2020) 48–53.

[24] C.J. Sampson, R. Arnold, S. Bryan, P. Clarke, S. Ekins, A. Hatswell, N. Hawkins, S. Langham, D. Marshall, M. Sadatsafavi, W. Sullivan, E.C.F. Wilson, T. Wrightson, Transparency in decision modelling: What, why, who and how?, *Pharmacoeconomics* 37 (2019) 1355–1369.

[25] R.J.G. Arnold, S. Ekins, Time for cooperation in health economics among the modelling community, *PharmacoEconomics* 28(8) (2010) 609–613.

[26] www.openphacts.org/, OpenPHACTS.

[27] K. Azzaoui, E. Jacoby, S. Senger, E.C. Rodriguez, M. Loza, B. Zdrazil, M. Pinto, A.J. Williams, V. de la Torre, J. Mestres, M. Pastor, O. Taboureau, M. Rarey, C. Chichester, S. Pettifer, N. Blomberg, L. Harland, B. Williams-Jones, G.F. Ecker, Scientific competency questions as the basis for semantically enriched open pharmacological space development, *Drug Discov Today* 18(17–18) (2013) 843–852.

[28] Anon, ATOM. https://atomscience.org/, (2018).

[29] A.J. Hunter, The innovative medicines initiative: A pre-competitive initiative to enhance the biomedical science base of Europe to expedite the development of new medicines for patients, *Drug Discovery Today* 13(9–10) (2008) 371–373.

[30] J. Hunter, Precompetitive collaboration in the pharmaceutical industry, in: S. Ekins, M. Hupcey, A.J. Williams (Eds.), *Collaborative Computational Technologies for Biomedical Research*, Wiley and Sons, Hoboken, NJ, 2011, pp. 55–84.

[31] J. Hunter, S. Stephens, Is open innovation the way forward for big pharma?, *Nat Rev Drug Disc* 9(2) (2010) 87–88.

[32] S.J. Capuzzi, I.S. Kim, W.I. Lam, T.E. Thornton, E.N. Muratov, D. Pozefsky, A. Tropsha, Chembench: A publicly accessible, integrated cheminformatics portal, *J Chem Inform Model* 57(2) (2017) 105–108.

[33] I. Sushko, S. Novotarskyi, R. Korner, A.K. Pandey, M. Rupp, W. Teetz, S. Brandmaier, A. Abdelaziz, V.V. Prokopenko, V.Y. Tanchuk, R. Todeschini, A. Varnek, G. Marcou, P. Ertl, V. Potemkin, M. Grishina, J. Gasteiger, C. Schwab, Baskin, II, V.A. Palyulin, E.V. Radchenko, W.J. Welsh, V. Kholodovych, D. Chekmarev, A. Cherkasov, J. Aires-de-Sousa, Q.Y. Zhang, A. Bender, F. Nigsch, L. Patiny, A. Williams, V. Tkachenko, I.V. Tetko, Online chemical modeling environment (OCHEM): Web platform for data storage, model development and publishing of chemical information, *J Comput Aided Mol Design* 25(6) (2011) 533–554.

[34] Anon, NCATS Predictor. https://predictor.ncats.io/, (2018).

[35] P.C. Matthews, Fairness in scientific publishing, *F1000Research* 5 (2016) 2816.

[36] R.J.G. Arnold, S. Ekins, Ahead of our time: Collaboration in modeling then and now, *PharmacoEconomics* 35(9) (2017) 975–976.

[37] M.M. Bertagnolli, O. Sartor, B.A. Chabner, M.L. Rothenberg, S. Khozin, C. Hugh-Jones, D.M. Reese, M.J. Murphy, Advantages of a truly open-access data-sharing model, *N Engl J Med* 376(12) (2017) 1178–1181.

[38] T.I. Oprea, H. Matter, Integrating virtual screening in lead discovery, *Currnt Opin Chem Biol* 8(4) (2004) 349–358.

[39] S. Ekins, J. Mestres, B. Testa, In silico pharmacology for drug discovery: Applications to targets and beyond, *Br J Pharmacol* 152 (2007) 21–37.

[40] C. Hansch, T. Fujita, p-σ-π Analysis. A method for the correlation of biological activity and chemical structure, *J Am Chem Soc* 86(8) (1964) 1616–1626.

[41] C. Hansch, D. Hoekman, A. Leo, D. Weininger, C.D. Selassie, Chem-bioinformatics: Comparative QSAR at the interface between chemistry and biology, *Chem Rev* 102(3) (2002) 783–812.

[42] A. Kurup, C-QSAR: A database of 18,000 QSARs and associated biological and physical data, *J Comput Aided Mol Design* 17(2/4) (2003) 187–196.

[43] M. Karelson, *Molecular Descriptors in QSAR/QSPR*, Wiley-VCH, New York, 2000.

[44] R. Todeschini, V. Consonni, *Handbook of Molecular Descriptors*, Wiley-VCH, Weinheim, 2000.

[45] W.P. Walters, B.B. Goldman, Feature selection in quantitative structure-activity relationships, *Curr Opin Drug Discov Dev* 8(3) (2005) 329–333.

[46] R.D. Cramer, D.E. Patterson, J.D. Bunce, Comparative Molecular Field Analysis (CoMFA). 1. Effect of shape on binding of steroids to carrier proteins, *J Am Chem Soc* 110 (1988) 5959–5967.

[47] G. Klebe, Comparative molecular similarity indices analysis: CoMSIA, *Persp Drug Disc Design* 12-14 (1998) 87–104.

[48] J. Bajorath, Integration of virtual and high-throughput screening, *Nat Rev Drug Discov* 1(11) (2002) 882–894.

[49] K.H. Bleicher, H.-J. Böhm, K. Müller, A.I. Alanine, Hit and lead generation: Beyond high-throughput screening, *Nat Rev Drug Discov* 2(5) (2003) 369–378.

[50] F. Stahura, J. Bajorath, Virtual screening methods that complement HTS, *Combinat Chem High Throughput Screen* 7(4) (2004) 259–269.

[51] A. Evers, G. Hessler, H. Matter, T. Klabunde, Virtual screening of biogenic amine-binding G-protein coupled receptors: Comparative evaluation of protein- and ligand-based virtual screening protocols, *J Med Chem* 48(17) (2005) 5448–5465.

[52] Q. Zhang, I. Muegge, Scaffold hopping through virtual screening using 2D and 3D similarity descriptors: Ranking, voting, and consensus scoring, *J Med Chem* 49(5) (2006) 1536–1548.

[53] T. Lengauer, C. Lemmen, M. Rarey, M. Zimmermann, Novel technologies for virtual screening, *Drug Discov Today* 9(1) (2004) 27–34.

[54] S. Ekins, J. Mestres, B. Testa, In silico pharmacology for drug discovery: Methods for virtual ligand screening and profiling, *Br J Pharmacol* 152 (2007) 9–20.

[55] J.S. Mason, A.C. Good, E.J. Martin, 3D pharmacophores in drug discovery, *Curr Pharm Des* 7 (2001) 567–597.

[56] O. Guner, *Pharmacophore, Perception, Development, and Use in Drug Design*, University International Line, San Diego, 2000.

[57] T. Langer, R.D. Hoffman, *Pharmacophores and Pharmacophore Searches*, Wiley-VCH, Weinheim, 2006.

[58] Y.C. Martin, 3D database searching in drug design, *J Med Chem* 35(12) (1992) 2145–2154.

[59] Y.C. Martin, M.G. Bures, E.A. Danaher, J. DeLazzer, I. Lico, P.A. Pavlik, A fast new approach to pharmacophore mapping and its application to dopaminergic and benzodiazepine agonists, *J Comput Aided Mol Design* 7(1) (1993) 83–102.

[60] C.-G. Wermuth, C. Robin Ganellin, P. Lindberg, L.A. Mitscher, *Glossary of Terms Used in Medicinal Chemistry (IUPAC Recommendations 1997)*, Annual Reports in Medicinal Chemistry, Elsevier, New York, 1998, pp. 385–395.

[61] D. Barnum, J. Greene, A. Smellie, P. Sprague, Identification of common functional configurations among molecules, *J Chem Inf Comput Sci* 36 (1996) 563–571.

[62] P.W. Sprague, Automated chemical hypothesis generation and database searching with Catalyst, *Perspect Drug Disc Design* 3 (1995) 1–20.

[63] P.W. Sprague, R. Hoffman, CATALYST pharmacophore models and their utility as queries for searching 3D databases, in: H. van de Waterbeemd, B. Testa, G. Folkers (Eds.), *Computer-assisted Lead Finding and Optimization*, Verlag Helvetica Chimica Acta, Basel, 1997, pp. 225–240.

[64] S. Ekins, V. Kholodovych, N. Ai, M. Sinz, J. Gal, L. Gera, W.J. Welsh, K. Bachmann, S. Mani, Computational discovery of novel low micromolar human pregnane X receptor antagonists, *Mol Pharmacol* 74(3) (2008) 662–672.

[65] O. Guner, O. Clement, Y. Kurogi, Pharmacophore modeling and three dimensional database searching for drug design using catalyst: Recent advances, *Curr Med Chem* 11(22) (2004) 2991–3005.

[66] C. Chang, P.M. Bahadduri, J.E. Polli, P.W. Swaan, S. Ekins, Rapid identification of P-glycoprotein substrates and inhibitors, *Drug Metab Dispos* 34(12) (2006) 1976–1984.

[67] C. Chang, S. Ekins, P. Bahadduri, P.W. Swaan, Pharmacophore-based discovery of ligands for drug transporters, *Adv Drug Deliv Rev* 58(12–13) (2006) 1431–1450.

[68] S. Ekins, J.S. Johnston, P. Bahadduri, V.M. D'Souza, A. Ray, C. Chang, P.W. Swaan, In vitro and pharmacophore-based discovery of novel hPEPT1 inhibitors, *Pharmaceut Res* 22(4) (2005) 512–517.

[69] S. Ekins, P.W. Swaan, Development of computational models for enzymes, transporters, channels, and receptors relevant to ADME/Tox, in: K.B. Lipkowitz, R. Larter, T.R. Cundari (Eds.), *Reviews in Computational Chemistry*, John Wiley & Sons, Inc., New York, 2004, pp. 333–415.

[70] T.P. Stratton, A.L. Perryman, C. Vilcheze, R. Russo, S.G. Li, J.S. Patel, E. Singleton, S. Ekins, N. Connell, W.R. Jacobs, Jr., J.S. Freundlich, Addressing the metabolic stability of antituberculars through machine learning, *ACS Med Chem Lett* 8(10) (2017) 1099–1104.

[71] A.L. Perryman, T.P. Stratton, S. Ekins, J.S. Freundlich, Predicting mouse liver microsomal stability with "pruned" machine learning models and public data, *Pharmaceut Res* 33(2) (2016) 433–449.

[72] A.M. Clark, K. Dole, A. Coulon-Spektor, A. McNutt, G. Grass, J.S. Freundlich, R.C. Reynolds, S. Ekins, Open source bayesian models. 1. Application to ADME/Tox and drug discovery datasets, *J Chem Inform Model* 55(6) (2015) 1231–1245.

[73] A.M. Clark, K. Dole, S. Ekins, Open source bayesian models. 3. Composite models for prediction of binned responses, *J Chem Inform Model* 56(2) (2016) 275–285.

[74] A.M. Clark, S. Ekins, Open source bayesian models. 2. Mining a "Big Dataset" to create and validate models with ChEMBL, *J Chem Inform Model* 55(6) (2015) 1246–1260.

[75] S. Ekins, R.R. Gupta, E. Gifford, B.A. Bunin, C.L. Waller, Chemical space: Missing pieces in cheminformatics, *Pharm Res* 27(10) (2010) 2035–2039.

[76] A. Clark, Molecular Notebook, 2018. http://molmatinf.com/MolNote/, (2018).

[77] J. Hert, P. Willett, D.J. Wilton, P. Acklin, K. Azzaoui, E. Jacoby, A. Schuffenhauer, Comparison of topological descriptors for similarity-based virtual screening using multiple bioactive reference structures, *Organ Biomol Chem* 2 (22) (2004) 3256.

[78] Anon, RDKit: Open-Source Cheminformatics Software. www.rdkit.org.

[79] D. Rogers, M. Hahn, Extended-connectivity fingerprints, *J Chem Inform Model* 50 (5) (2010) 742–754.

[80] N. Friedman, D. Geiger, M. Goldszmidt, Bayesian network classifiers, *Mach Learn*, 29(2/3) (1997) 131–163.

[81] H. Drucker, Improving regressors using boosting techniques. https://pdfs.semanticscholar.org/8d49/e2dedb817f2c3330e74b63c5fc86d2399ce3.pdf., (1997).

[82] L. Breiman, Random Forests, *Mach Learn* 45 (2001) 5–32.

[83] C. Cortes, V. Vapnik, Support vector networks, *Mach Learn* 20 (1995) 273–293.

[84] N.S. Altman, An introduction to kernel and nearest-neighbor nonparametric regression, *Am Stat* 46 (1992) 175–185.

[85] F. Pedregosa, G. Varoquaux, A. Gramfort, V. Michel, B. Thirion, O. Grisel, M. Blondel, P. Prettenhofer, R. Weiss, V. Dubourg, J. Vanderplas, A. Passos,

D. Cournapeau, M. Brucher, M. Perrot, E. Duchesnay, Scikit-learn: Machine learning in python, *J Mach Learn Res* 12 (2011) 2825–2830.

[86] Y. LeCun, Y. Bengio, G. Hinton, Deep learning, *Nature* 521(7553) (2015) 436–444.

[87] Anon, Keras. https://keras.io/, 2018.

[88] S. Nwaka, R.G. Ridley, Virtual drug discovery and development for neglected diseases through public-private partnerships, *Nat Rev Drug Discov* 2(11) (2003) 919–928.

[89] J.F. Pritchard, M. Jurima-Romet, M.L.J. Reimer, E. Mortimer, B. Rolfe, M.N. Cayen, Making better drugs: Decision gates in non-clinical drug development, *Nat Rev Drug Discov* 2(7) (2003) 542–553.

[90] R.J. Arnold, R. Kim, B. Tang, The cost-effectiveness of argatroban treatment in heparin-induced thrombocytopenia: The effect of early versus delayed treatment, *Cardiol Rev* 14(1) (2006) 7–13.

[91] L. Caprino, P. Russo, Developing a paradigm of drug innovation: An evaluation algorithm, *Drug Discov Today* 11(21–22) (2006) 999–1006.

[92] P. Vemer, I. Corro Ramos, G.A.K. van Voorn, M.J. Al, T.L. Feenstra, AdViSHE: A validation-assessment tool of health-economic models for decision makers and model users, *PharmacoEconomics* 34(4) (2016) 349–361.

[93] A.J. Hatswell, F. Chandler, Sharing is caring: The case for company-level collaboration in pharmacoeconomic modelling, *PharmacoEconomics* 35(8) (2017) 755–757.

[94] Mount Hood 4 Modeling Group, Computer modeling of diabetes and its complications: A report on the Fourth Mount Hood Challenge Meeting, *Diabetes Care* 30(6) (2007) 1638–1646.

[95] J.B. Brown, A. Russell, W. Chan, K. Pedula, M. Aickin, The global diabetes model: User friendly version 3.0, *Diab Res Clin Pract* 50 (2000) S15–S46.

[96] A.J. Palmer, Computer modeling of diabetes and its complications: A report on the fifth Mount Hood Challenge Meeting, *Value Health* 16(4) (2013) 670–685.

[97] J. Brogan, I. Baskaran, N. Ramachandran, Authenticating health activity data using distributed ledger technologies, *Comput Struct Biotechnol J* 16 (2018) 257–266.

[98] T.T. Kuo, H.E. Kim, L. Ohno-Machado, Blockchain distributed ledger technologies for biomedical and health care applications, *J Am Med Inform Assoc* 24(6) (2017) 1211–1220.

[99] Anon, Blockchain. https://en.wikipedia.org/wiki/Blockchain_(database).

[100] Anon, Hyperledger. www.hyperledger.org/.

[101] M. Allarakhia, Exploring open innovation with a patient focus in drug discovery: an evolving paradigm of patient engagement, *Exp Opin Drug Discov* 10(6) (2015) 571–578.

[102] H. Dorsch, A.E. Jurock, S. Schoepe, M. Lessl, K. Asadullah, Grants4Targets: An open innovation initiative to foster drug discovery collaborations, *Nat Rev Drug Discov* 14(1) (2014) 74–76.

[103] T. Melese, S.M. Lin, J.L. Chang, N.H. Cohen, Open innovation networks between academia and industry: An imperative for breakthrough therapies, *Nat Med* 15(5) (2009) 502–507.

[104] N. Nilsson, J. Felding, Open innovation platforms to boost pharmaceutical collaborations: Evaluating external compounds for desired biological activity, *Fut Med Chem* 7(14) (2015) 1853–1859.

[105] A. Roy, P.R. McDonald, S. Sittampalam, R. Chaguturu, Open access high throughput drug discovery in the public domain: A mount everest in the making, *Curr Pharm Biotechnol* 11(7) (2010) 764–778.

[106] P. Talaga, Open innovation: Share or die ..., *Drug Discovery Today* 14(21–22) (2009) 1003–1005.

[107] R.R. Gupta, E.M. Gifford, T. Liston, C.L. Waller, M. Hohman, B.A. Bunin, S. Ekins, Using open source computational tools for predicting human metabolic stability and additional absorption, distribution, metabolism, excretion, and toxicity properties, *Drug Metab Dispos* 38(11) (2010) 2083–2090.

[108] O. Spjuth, J. Alvarsson, A. Berg, M. Eklund, S. Kuhn, C. Mäsak, G. Torrance, J. Wagener, E.L. Willighagen, C. Steinbeck, J.E.S. Wikberg, Bioclipse 2: A scriptable integration platform for the life sciences, *BMC Bioinform* 10 (2009) 397.

[109] O. Spjuth, L. Carlsson, J. Alvarsson, V. Georgiev, E. Willighagen, M. Eklund, Open source drug discovery with bioclipse, *Curr Topics Med Chem* 12(18) (2012) 1980–1986.

[110] O. Spjuth, T. Helmus, E.L. Willighagen, S. Kuhn, M. Eklund, J. Wagener, P. Murray-Rust, C. Steinbeck, J.E.S. Wikberg, Bioclipse: An open source workbench for chemo- and bioinformatics, *BMC Bioinform* 8 (2007) 59.

[111] J.C. Stålring, L.A. Carlsson, P. Almeida, S. Boyer, AZOrange—High performance open source machine learning for QSAR modeling in a graphical programming environment, *J Cheminform* 3 (2011) 28.

[112] V.J. Sykora, D.E. Leahy, Chemical Descriptors Library (CDL): A generic, open source software library for chemical informatics, *J Chem Inform Model* 48(10) (2008) 1931–1942.

[113] Z. Wu, B. Ramsundar, E.N. Feinberg, J. Gomes, C. Geniesse, A.S. Pappu, K. Leswing, V. Pande, MoleculeNet: A benchmark for molecular machine learning, *Chem Sci* 9(2) (2017) 513–530.

18 Speculations on the Future Challenges and Value of Pharmacoeconomics

J. Jaime Caro, MDCD, FRCPC, FACP
McGill University
Montreal, Canada
Evidera, Boston, USA

TABLE OF CONTENTS

18.1 HOW BADLY DID WE DO?

Before launching into further speculations on the future, it is worth revisiting those that we made a decade ago for the first edition of this book. At that time, we worried about pharmacoeconomics sinking into irrelevance, weighted down by burdensome theory that led to methods that were not aligned with the concerns of decision makers and failed to provide substantive, defensible guidance. We were concerned that the preoccupation with QALYs and their use in cost-per-QALY comparisons with evidence-free thresholds would prompt many stakeholders to jettison our field and look for alternatives that better addressed their needs. We, rather optimistically, called for the field to move beyond the QALY and incremental cost-effectiveness ratios to embrace more relevant, fit-for-purpose approaches and offered some thoughts on alternatives that were already available.

Well, the QALY is still with us, but calls for its replacement, or at least extensive modification, have grown more strident. Recognition that it is not a good measure of therapeutic benefits, nor a solid basis for their valuation, is now widespread but the field clings stubbornly to the QALY, alleging a variation of the old saw, "but it's the best we have". Now, the claim is that we have invested so much effort on this measure and there are such extensive data on its use that we cannot possibly abandon it at this juncture. Instead, it is said that it can be modified—with little clarity on how—to address the main concerns. I very much doubt it can be saved because the flaws are so fundamental, and the required modifications so profound that any resulting new version, if it is to be truly useful, would no longer be a QALY. Indeed, there are already various proposed new approaches that forego the QALY and related "incremental cost-effectiveness analysis" entirely; more on this below.

Another prediction we made was that decision-analytic models would be forced to become increasingly sophisticated to better accord with reality and provide a solid basis for considering the complex issues that attend to appraisal of new interventions. Although the basic, oversimplified cohort Markov approach continues to be the most prevalent, it has lost its monopoly. Our field has finally recognized that better methods are needed to realistically model the course of chronic diseases over time; the many therapeutic alternatives and sequences; increasing knowledge of the determinants—particularly biomarkers; and newer mechanisms of action. Most well-regarded models today are individual patient simulations that can properly reflect the required intricacy. Indeed, novel methods, such as discretely integrated condition event (DICE) simulation discussed in Chapter 10, have made significant inroads, and I expect that in the near future we will consign the cohort Markov approach to the very limited role it deserves (finally!).

Along with our prediction that modeling would need to grow in sophistication was our sense that we would need to vastly improve the validation of the models that underpin appraisals of new technologies. We worried that impossibly short timelines, a penchant for one-time use models, and software restrictions that led to very obscure implementations would further erode any trust that decision makers might have in the results of model-based analyses. There has been some progress in this regard. Although predictive validation—the most persuasive kind —remains rare, most model reports now include some sort of validation and methods to facilitate it and improve transparency have become more prevalent. Similarly, there are increasing examples of models designed for repeated use over many years, increasing the impetus for validation. In parallel, we are seeing calls for models to join the open source movement, allowing many eyes to view the structure, inputs, calculations, and results, thus helping ensure that errors are caught earlier, and the models continually improve. Some national HTA agencies have even started pursuing construction of their own core models aimed at standardizing simulation in those therapeutic areas and reducing structural uncertainty, or at least rendering it plainly visible.

Apart from speculations on the maturation of the field methodologically, we also ventured the idea that clinical trials would become market oriented rather than remaining focused on producing the highly artificial "efficacy" estimates necessary to get past the regulatory hurdles. This has decidedly not happened. Despite some innovation in designs and use of wearables to collect data, development of new medicines remains entrenched in the traditional three phases, with the randomized clinical trial the gold standard. Nevertheless, there are some signs of recognition that the needs of the markets require loosening the strictures and leveraging novel methods, particularly those that can validly extract useful information from the very large datasets that are now becoming ubiquitous. Further thoughts on this are discussed below.

18.2 RENEWED SPECULATIONS

Mindful of our much less than perfect record so far, I will nevertheless venture thoughts on some of the most active areas in our field, and their implications for further developments.

18.2.1 CONCERNS WITH COST, AFFORDABILITY AND PURSUIT OF VALUE

Although pharmacoeconomics is by no means concerned solely, or even primarily, with therapeutic costs, this is by far the aspect that causes the most ado and draws in clinicians, patients, politicians, the press and others who would not otherwise show much interest. This is not a new phenomenon—in many ways it was the stimulus that gave origin to our field—but the proliferation of highly effective therapies for previously incurable diseases at very high prices has propelled concerns with costs and questions of value to the forefront.

One consequence of these heightened concerns is the rise of the so-called value-frameworks in the United States. The idea behind these frameworks is seductive: fully assess the value of a new intervention in order to appraise whether it is sufficient to justify the proposed price. The items incorporated on each list and the manner of assessing them differs but the focus is on ensuring the catalog is comprehensive. Unfortunately, this misses the core methodological challenge: what is the reasonable amount to pay for a given set of benefits? Answering this vital question remains elusive because assigning monetary value to health and other less tangible effects is very problematic without actively trading them in a market.

The prevailing approach supported by many economists is the idea of opportunity cost: if for the amount to be paid, you are obtaining more benefit elsewhere, then the price is too high. While this appears to be sensible, it turns out to be extremely difficult to apply in practice. Determining how much benefit is obtained for a given healthcare expenditure requires data that are rarely available; benefits are not always evident, particularly if one insists on using the QALY; and the few studies that have attempted it, have found enormous variability across therapeutic areas. Thus, the threshold price to pay remains an arbitrary choice in all jurisdictions. This is unlikely to be remedied any time soon.

In part to avoid these issues, many countries (e.g., France, Germany, Japan) had refused to pursue this avenue, preferring instead to embark on negotiations without theoretical foundations. The much greater pressures generated by enormous therapeutic advances coupled with vastly higher prices are forcing everyone to wade into these treacherous waters. It is unclear where this will lead. Though fraught with difficulties, one option is to modify the opportunity cost yardstick from one based on estimates of what we pay to one that considers explicitly what we would give up in order to fund the new intervention. This is already being done at the hospital level in some countries and would clarify for everyone the trade-offs required if implemented more broadly. Of course, it is one thing to talk about what one might give up and another thing altogether to actually disinvest in those activities. So far, there has been very little progress in this regard and people are very reluctant to withdraw established funding. Nevertheless, it seems inevitable that formal processes will be established to assess existing expenditures (possibly extending beyond the healthcare system) for reassignment.

Another option is to directly intervene, without a theoretical basis, to limit the prices paid. Even those who do not accede to the threshold-based approach must recognize that it does provide an effective club with which to beat back high prices. More draconian tools will become increasingly attractive if better solutions are not found—and industry does itself no favors by raising prices, with little justification, after products achieve market access.

The concern with costs will not abate in the near future. Instead, pressure will mount to make novel interventions available at more affordable prices, and this will motivate many new actors to take a stab at new ways to measure benefits and establish their value.

18.2.2   THE RISE OF MECHANISM OF ACTION PRODUCTS
ACROSS INDICATIONS

As we learn more about the underlying abnormalities that lead to disease, it is becoming clear that many conditions that were considered distinct illnesses are simply different manifestations of the same problem. This has led to development of interventions that attack a particular underlying defect that may result in various diseases. These mechanism of action (MoA) products are, therefore, not limited to one indication—they may be of benefit in several conditions, with the specific clinical effects differing.

The applicability of a single product to many conditions poses a new set of challenges for our field. A big one has to do with what price should be set. Given the differences across indications in manifestations; management practices; alternative treatments; prognosis; the clinical effects of the treatment; and other major components of the pharmacoeconomic assessment, it is unclear which ones should drive pricing considerations and how any given price should be assessed. A seemingly obvious solution may be to set a different price in each indication, but it is not evident why the same product should not have the same cost regardless of the indication. Moreover, there are many practical challenges to implementing differential pricing. For manufacturers, there are many immediate concerns, including which indication to prioritize and how to position their asset. MoA products will become increasingly common, and this will force our field to grapple with these issues. Perhaps economic models will expand to consider the broader range of indications, and the specific indications will be deemphasized. This may even lead to modifying the specialties that clinicians pursue, focusing on a MoA rather than an organ or physiological system.

18.2.3   The Impact of "Personalized" Medicine

Along with deeper understanding of the mechanisms of disease, there is increasingly detailed elucidation of the factors that determine prognosis and the response to treatment. This enables developers of interventions to tailor them more specifically to individuals and opens the door for highly personalized approaches to treating disease. While it is hard to view these advances negatively, they do confront us with important new problems.

To recoup the large investments in research and development, firms must be able to generate substantial revenues with those products that are successful in reaching market. As treatments become more individualized, the potential volume of users necessarily drops, shrinking the market substantially. This leaves pricing as the only way to achieve the desired revenue, with the resulting numbers reaching stratospheric heights that further challenge efforts to balance costs and benefits. Bespoke products in any area are always much more expensive than mass-market ones, but these are typically considered luxuries, and the decision to spend money on them is left to the wealthy consumer. This is not (at least not yet) an option for medicines with much higher, potentially curative, efficacy coupled with fewer side-effects. Dealing with the inexorable progress in precision medicine will require substantial innovations across pharmacoeconomics, insurance, health technology appraisal, funding mechanisms, legal, regulatory, and other areas. There is little time for these to take place, yet efforts remain disparate, poorly funded, and tentative.

18.2.4   New Approaches to Valuation

The conflicting demands resulting from the promising scientific advances and funding imperatives are, fortunately, breaking the hold of the entrenched cost-per-QALY dogma and fostering interest in alternatives. One major area has to do with the failure of the QALY to capture many of the effects of interventions. Some researchers have tried to retain the familiar measure by somehow broadening it to encompass other aspects of value. This has not yet produced a usable, widely accepted variant. It is doubtful that these efforts will result in a better QALY because they fail to address its fundamental problems.

A more radical approach is to abandon the QALY altogether and leverage other methodologies. One that has stirred much interest is multi-criteria decision analysis (MCDA), see Chapter 9. In an MCDA, any number of criteria can be considered, and the appraisal can weight their importance in whatever way is judged appropriate. Thus, there is no inherent limitation to what the analysis covers, and the theoretical failings of the QALY are avoided. Still, important and difficult challenges remain. MCDA was not intended for recurrent decisions across many and diverse areas. If criteria and weights are standardized and fixed, the method will lose its flexibility, but without that, it is unclear how it can be validly applied to our problems. The scores produced, even with standardized criteria and weights, have no inherent meaning and their value in monetary terms is not established. Whether costs should be incorporated in the MCDA or be kept separate is a matter of controversy. Of course, MCDA is subject to the more general problem of getting humans to coherently value consequences in the abstract.

Another alternative that departs from the QALY is to desist from forcing its two dimensions into a single index. The originators of the QALY and other researchers at the time felt strongly that a single measure would ease difficult decision-making, but much of the QALY's weaknesses stem from that choice. If the dimensions are kept distinct, then the effects of disease and of interventions on mortality can be appraised separately from those on quality of life, even if dependencies remain (e.g., hair loss is relatively inconsequential with a life-saving treatment but would scarcely be tolerated to alleviate minor pain). Recently, this idea has been advanced further by proposing a two-dimensional measure of value that considers the deadliness of the illness and its non-fatal impact relative to the inexorable consequences of senescence. This measure— the "BADI"—properly assigns the (0, 0) point to absence of disease and provides unbounded scales to assess whatever condition affects health adversely. The effect of an intervention can then be represented as a decrease in deadliness, or in non-fatal impact, or both, and its value can be gauged conditional on the severity of the illness. Whether this new measure, which can provide for more valid assessment, is adopted and leads to more acceptable decisions remains to be seen.

18.2.5   LEVERAGING VAST DATA SETS

It is evident that vast quantities of information on individuals' characteristics, behaviors, clinical status, and even their genomes are being rapidly assembled and linked to other enormous datasets. The challenge medicine faces is turning this massive information into knowledge that can enhance assessments, support better decisions, and, ultimately, improve outcomes. For better or worse, this challenge has attracted the attention of the large corporations whose business is, to a great extent, in dealing with huge datasets and who have, thus, acquired substantial expertise in wringing the most value from their collections. For now, their target seems to be largely clinical medicine and related research, but it won't be long before they sniff out the possibilities in pharmacoeconomics. Hopefully, our field can successfully surf that tsunami, but there is substantial risk that our methods will be swept away into irrelevance or just not implemented appropriately.

The methods applied by those corporations, variously grouped under "machine learning" and "artificial intelligence," are being applied in efforts to discern patterns that would otherwise have gone unnoticed and there have been some successes. Their application to pharmacoeconomics remains a work in progress, however. We are unsure how to incorporate the stochastic outputs of those analyses into our economic models, and the distrust of "black boxes" will only grow as we try to make use of these much less transparent frameworks. Major efforts to render them comprehensible will be essential if they are to be considered by health technology assessment agencies in their appraisals.

One area where knowledge gained from large datasets can be readily leveraged is the identification of subgroups where an intervention is more efficient. This efficiency can be gained simply by reserving the intervention for individuals who manifest characteristics that have been identified as markers of higher mortality or, worse, non-fatal impacts. Pursuing these risk factors is not new, and our field has done well applying equations derived with standard statistical methods, but harnessing vast datasets with the newer approaches offers the tantalizing possibility of taking this to a much more refined level.

It is much more difficult, however, to move beyond identifying patterns of risk factors to understanding causal relationships that make it possible to predict the impact of altering the individual's conditions, behaviors, or environment. Nevertheless, such models would allow much better forecasting of effects and this enhanced precision could take us from the rather sketchy and difficult to validate estimates made today in highly artificial simulated contexts to actual predictions of what will happen to actual patients in the conditions of the real world. Whether we ultimately want to head into that messy sphere may not be entirely in our control—it will be extremely difficult to stop that "progress."

One very fertile ground for machine learning is improvement of the randomized clinical trial (RCT). Today, we still have to enroll large numbers of participants because the majority of them will not manifest the outcomes of interest, thus making it much harder to detect any signal. If knowledge derived via machine learning can improve admissibility criteria so that we target the experiment to those who are very likely to experience the outcomes, the trials will become much more efficient. These better targeted criteria will also reduce heterogeneity, ultimately perhaps approaching the levels attained in the lab, where cloned organisms can be ethically studied.

Though still very much a pipe dream, these developments in machine-learning-derived knowledge, coupled with genomics and much more precise understanding of the mechanisms of disease and the actions of interventions, may one day lead to fully *in silico* trials that can accurately predict the expected effects in precisely defined types of patients. This would, of course, simultaneously achieve a major goal of "personalized" medicine.

18.2.6   WILL HTA AND REGULATORY APPROVAL COME TOGETHER?

In today's world, the process of evaluating the evidence regarding a product's intended and united effects remains distinct from that of assessing the economic implications of these effects; this separateness is underscored in all jurisdictions by assigning these responsibilities to different agencies. This has led to the increasingly common, yet very awkward, situation where the evidence that a product is beneficial is judged sufficient for it to be given market authorization, but market access is withheld or restricted because its price is not appraised as efficient enough. This is particularly uncomfortable when there is unanimity on the former across jurisdictions, yet the citizens of some countries are allowed to benefit while those of others are forbidden. This might be viewed as reasonable when the countries' economies are vastly different, but it is much more difficult to justify when they are quite similar.

One hope has been to minimize this by harmonizing processes, even to the extent of bringing them into one agency or closely related entities. This would also achieve substantial efficiencies by reducing repetition of tasks with similar objectives. After all, the underlying evidence is the same, even if the manner of processing it may differ. Initiatives in this regard are ongoing, but, so far, there has been little tangible progress. Getting from the lab to the patient still requires a product to pass through a complex set of distinct hurdles that do not necessarily cohere.

One of the justifications given for this inefficiency and incoherence is the differences in actual practices, costs, and preferences across borders. Undoubtedly, these exist, but their impact can be handled by improving the way we approach the evidence and the appraisal of value. The regulatory process must leave behind the hypothesis-testing focus and move towards detailed quantification of a product's effects over time, conditional on patient characteristics, and against relevant comparators. This should include consideration of all relevant data, not just from the development-phase trials, and bring to bear techniques such as meta-analysis, simulated treatment comparisons, and quantitative benefit-risk modeling. The goal should be as full a quantitative understanding of the product's intended and unintended effects as possible, relative to those of its therapeutic alternatives. The regulatory decision, presumably, would rest on whether these effects are judged to be sufficiently beneficial.

The assessment of the economic implications can then take the detailed estimates of effects and incorporate them directly into the appropriate model. Indeed, if properly coordinated, this model would simply be an extension of the one used to support the regulatory decision. It should not be difficult to add to this model those aspects that pertain to value, ensuring that they are readily adaptable locally as needed. This adaptability is already a feature of many of the economic models constructed today. If a common model is used, ideally open source and endorsed by the agency, we will greatly improve the efficiency of the process and the consistency of the estimates, though the decisions themselves may still turn out differently because of local considerations not incorporated in the model.

18.3 CONCLUSIONS

Despite its on-the-go development, borrowed methodologies, and seat-of-the-pants experts, pharmacoeconomics is still here—indeed, it is thriving. Our congresses now number participants in the thousands; many formal educational graduate-level programs have been established and there is no shortage of eager students; and mainstream media increasingly take notice. Perhaps the most conspicuous sign of relevance is the formal involvement of clinicians and their professional societies together with the increasing attention paid by patient groups. Even politicians in countries without a national healthcare system have realized that pharmacoeconomics offers tools to address the costs increasingly perceived to be unsustainable.

We now have the opportunity to play a major role in the shaping of health care, the development of new products, and the leveraging of novel methods and tools. Achieving these enticing aspirations will require a new generation of leaders willing to take the field into unexplored areas, to break with the dogma we have depended on and focus on doing the very best we can to ensure that our efforts properly support the difficult decisions looming in the near future.

19 Pharmacoeconomics in the Era of the Novel Coronavirus

Renée J.G. Arnold, PharmD, RPh
Icahn School of Medicine at Mount Sinai
Arnold Consultancy & Technology, LLC
New York, NY, USA

As mentioned previously throughout this book, it is important to assess the trade-offs between the economic costs of a strategy and the benefit derived from that strategy to determine comparative cost-effectiveness of competing approaches. Multiple journal editorials and letters to the editor have referenced the many SARS-CoV-2 (novel coronavirus or COVID-19) forecasting models (see Table 19.1), sometimes with wildly diverging predictions [1]. The problem is that the code and inputs are unavailable to understand how these results were derived. Some have weighed in that

> it would be much simpler to require publicly funded academics to publish data and code as a matter of course; the possibility of competing teams checking their work might encourage development of the quality-control culture that seems lacking within the academy. It would also mean that in a crisis, when traditional academic peer review would move too slowly to be useful, a crowdsourced review process could take place. [1]

The use of open source models (OSMs), those for which all data and programming associated with the model are made openly available to enhance transparency and, perhaps, facilitate replication and ongoing modifications of the model, have the potential to allow for faster access to critical knowledge [2–5]. Use of OSMs, perhaps in an easily accessible database, could allow for the aforementioned "crowdsourced" model review and more accurate/timely models, at least as far as the existing data allow. Although there have been relatively few articles published on the cost-effectiveness of methods, for example, partial or full quarantine/isolation, masking, screening, and testing, of dealing with the novel coronavirus to date because of the newness of the situation, inclusion of cost-effectiveness in these epidemiological models would "help to inform decisions about the most efficient, comprehensive and feasible strategies" [6] to employ in any pandemic situation.

Cost-utility analysis (CUA), as discussed in Chapter 1 and other chapters about modeling, is a subtype of cost-effectiveness analysis (CEA) wherein the effectiveness component of the equation is "adjusted" by the impact of a

TABLE 19.1

Sample of COVID-19 Forecast and Projection Models

Model and Organization(s) Responsible	Primary Approach	Outcomes Estimated and Timeframe	Selected Model Findings/ Notes
Imperial College "Non-Pharmaceutical Intervention" (NP) Model	SEIR	Projected US cases, deaths across a range of different mitigation and suppression scenarios, over the next year (to April 2021)	Projected 2.2 million US deaths might occur in an "unmitigated" scenario
Institute for Health Metrics and Evaluation (IHME) COVID-19 Model	Curve-fitting /extrapolation	Forecasts number of hospitalizations and deaths in the United States and by state, along with the timing of in the peak of hospitalizations and deaths, through August 2020	Initially, the model forecast 81,000 deaths in the United States by July. Results are updated daily, and as of April 12, 2020, that death estimate has been revised downward, to 61,545 by August 4, 2020.
COVID-19 Model from Northeastern University. Fogarty International Center, Fred Hutchison Cancer Center, University of Florida and others	Agent-based	Projects cases and deaths in the United States and by state, under no mitigation vs. "stay-at-home" scenario, through April 30, 2020	As of April 4, 2020, the model projected US deaths would peak on April 8, 2020, and there would be approximately 52,575 COVID-19 deaths (range: 35,381 to 88,269) by April 30, 2020.
Columbia University Severe COVID-19 Risk Model (& Mapping Tool)	SEIR	Provides projections on number of severe cases, hospitalizations, critical care, ICU uses, and deaths under different social distancing scenarios, for 3-week and 6-week periods starting April 2, 2020	In different regions of the United States anywhere from 33,986 and 185,192 deaths could be averted through social distancing.
Los Alamos National Laboratory Confirmed and Forecasted Case Data Model	Curve-fitting /extrapolation	Forecasts cases and deaths by US state using assumptions about the growth rate in cases and deaths and the presence of social distancing interventions through May 20, 2020	As an example, the model best guess forecast for California as of April 8, 2020, is that there would be 138,100 cases and 4,082 deaths.

(Continued)

TABLE 19.1 (Cont.)

Model and Organization(s) Responsible	Primary Approach	Outcomes Estimated and Timeframe	Selected Model Findings/ Notes
University of Pennsylvania COVID-19 Hospital Impact Model for Epidemics (CHIME)	SIR	Model allows users to set inputs and assumptions and then provides forecasts on the expected number of hospitalizations, ICU bed demand, ventilator demand, and number of days these demands would exceed capacity at hospitals in a given area based on those inputs, over the next three months.	Using inputs for three University of Pennsylvania Health System hospitals, the model projected best- and worst-case scenarios for total hospital bed capacity needed would reach 3,131–12,650, including 338–1,608 ICU beds and 118 to 599 ventilators.

therapeutic pathway on a patient's quality of life. As discussed in Chapter 12, a common metric used in CUA is the quality-adjusted life year (QALY), which considers the modification of mortality (years of life saved) by the quality impact on those life-years. CUAs are typically reported as incremental cost-effectiveness ratios (ICERs), calculated as $(Cost_1 - Cost_2)/(QALYs_1 - QALYs_2)$; see Chapters 1, 4, and 7. One of the major advantages of using cost per QALY is that it is a metric that can be examined in League tables (see Chapter 1) in comparison to other analyses that use cost per QALY as their primary outcomes metric. It is for this reason that many health technology authorities require CUA to use cost per QALY as the major indicator of the ICER threshold or value framework (see Chapters 13, 14, and 15).

In an attempt to quantify cost-effectiveness of pandemic strategies, in general, a blog on the Tufts Medical Center (Center for the Evaluation of Value and Risk in Health [CEVR]) website reported on the frequency with which the cost-effectiveness of disease outbreak control and/or prevention strategies had been published in peer-reviewed literature as entered into the Tufts-CEVR CEA Registry (https://cevr.tuftsmedicalcenter.org/databases/cea-registry) [6]. Out of the more than 8,000 cost per QALY studies with >20,000 ICERs, the researchers found only 38 published articles (0.5%) that met the desired criteria. Of the 143 intervention-specific ICERs reported, approximately 70% evaluated vaccine or pharmaceutical strategies, with the remainder focused on screening/testing and other strategies. The ICERs ranged from US$440 / QALY (intravenous antiviral agents to treat hospitalized patients with influenza-like (H1N1) illness) to US$15,000,000/QALY (universal meningococcal serotype B vaccination), with a median of US$49,000/QALY, which would be considered quite cost-effective in major nations around the globe (see Chapter 15).

Thirty-seven interventions (e.g., one-dose varicella vaccination) were considered cost-saving (see Chapters 1 and 7).

Three primary modeling methods of epidemiologic forecasting and projections for COVID-19 include Susceptible, Exposed, Infectious, Removed/Recovered (SEIR)/Susceptible, Infectious, Recovered (SIR) models; agent-based models; and curve-fitting/extrapolation models; examples of some of the most often-discussed models are shown in Table 19.1 [7].

One of the few available cost-effectiveness articles on COVID-19 strategies, in a medRxiv preprint (non-peer-reviewed as of this book's printing), examined the comparative cost-effectiveness of global versus focused isolation of people at high risk of exposure with extensive polymerase chain reaction (PCR) testing in Israel during the SARS-CoV-2 pandemic over a 200-day time frame [8]. They used a modified SEIR, six-compartment simulation model (Susceptible, Exposed, Exposed asymptomatic, Infected, Recovered, Death) to compare the two strategies in controlling the spread of COVID-19 and evaluated two outcomes: cost per one avoided death and cost per QALY. Results of the base case analysis are seen in Table 19.2.[1]

A sensitivity analysis demonstrated that the virus transmission rate and daily mortality rate were the two most influential variables. The authors suggested that to "transform" their cost per avoided death to cost per QALY, one could equate loss of one life to loss of 10 QALYs (a rather unusual method), suggesting a cost per QALY of $74,690,035/10 = $7,469,004 per QALY, a very cost-ineffective number.

A preliminary CEA (CUA) of remdesivir, an agent that has shown promise in reducing the length of hospitalization for patients with advanced COVID-19 illness and lung involvement, used a short-term decision tree with a long-term Markov model (see Chapter 4), the health system perspective and a lifetime time horizon to calculate a reasonable price for remdesivir [9]. The Institute for Clinical and Economic Review took the unusual approach of framing the analysis as a "cost recovery" evaluation, that is, framing it as one that compensates the manufacturer for the costs of production without additional profit. Costs and outcomes (cost per QALY) were discounted at a rate of 3%. Value-based

TABLE 19.2

Comparative Cost-effectiveness of Global versus Focused Isolation of High-Risk Populations

	Deaths	Cost (USD)	ICER (Cost/death avoided)
Global isolation	322	10,694,000,000	$74,690,035
Focused isolation	464	88,015,000	

1 N.B. that the manuscript reports a rounded ICER of $75,110,000 per death avoided.

TABLE 19.3
Value-Based Prices Using Various CEA Thresholds

Threshold ($)	Base-Case Model (Assuming Mortality Benefit) ($)	Scenario Analysis (Assuming No Mortality Benefit) ($)
50,000/QALY	4,460	390
100,000/QALY	28,670	780
150,000/QALY	52,880	1,170

prices were calculated assuming a mortality *benefit* with remdesivir, although evidence from the Adaptive COVID-19 Treatment Trial did not demonstrate a statistically significant benefit for the drug. As a result, a scenario (sensitivity) analysis assuming no mortality benefit was also conducted (see Table 19.3).

Therefore, assuming the minimum threshold of $50,000/QALY, remdesivir should be priced no higher than $4,460 if the mortality benefit holds or $390 for a 5- or 10-day course if there is no mortality benefit.

While both of these are unpublished studies and subject to change based on peer review, the goal of performing CEAs to determine appropriate allocation of healthcare resources and, ultimately, providing a practical tool for decision-makers faced with making reimbursement decisions across widely different healthcare technologies and strategies is laudable and necessary. Future analyses will surely be conducted for this and other drugs/vaccines for the novel coronavirus.

Interestingly, the first edition of this book focused on a public-private partnership to develop comparative CEAs that would help in allocation of resources and determine global pricing and availability of a vaccine to bring another deadly virus under control—human papillomavirus (HPV) —which in 2018 caused approximately 570,000 cases of cervical cancer (the fourth most common cancer in women) and 311,000 deaths from the disease [10]. Even with the licensing of the HPV vaccine in over 100 countries since 2006, this disease remains deadly, more so in low-income countries [11]. This second edition of our book now coincides with the arrival of a global virus, SARS-CoV-2, that is the deadliest in a century, with similar requirements for public-private partnerships. Indeed, in this time of constrained resources and need to determine the most cost-effective strategies to address the horrendous loss of life, socioeconomic disparity, mental anguish, and inadequate planning that have been associated with the novel coronavirus, pharmacoeconomic analyses are an objective way to determine likely budget impact of various strategies and how to most efficiently invest in future healthcare.

REFERENCES

[1] B. Peiser, A. Montford, Coronavirus lessons from the asteroid that didn't hit earth, *Wall Street Journal*, Dow Jones, June 1, 2020.
[2] R. Arnold, S. Ekins, Ahead of our time: collaboration in modeling then and now, *Pharmacoeconomics*, 35(9) (2017) 975–976.

[3] R.J. Arnold, S. Ekins, Time for cooperation in health economics among the model-
     ling community, *Pharmacoeconomics*, 28(8) (2010) 609–613.

[4] A.J. Hatswell, F. Chandler, Sharing is caring: the case for company-level collabor-
     ation in pharmacoeconomic modelling, *Pharmacoeconomics* 35 (2017) 755–757.

[5] C.J. Sampson, R. Arnold, S. Bryan, P. Clarke, S. Ekins, A. Hatswell, N. Hawkins,
     S. Langham, D. Marshall, M. Sadatsafavi, W. Sullivan, E.C.F. Wilson, T. Wrightson,
     Transparency in decision modelling: what, why, who and how?, *Pharmacoeconomics*
     37 (2019) 1355–1369.

[6] D. Ollendorf, L. Do, D. Kim, J. Cohen, P. Neumann, The cost-effectiveness of out-
     break responses: considerations in the COVID-19 era, Tufts Medical Center for the
     Evaluation of Value and Risk in Health (CEVR), April 6, 2020.

[7] J. Michaud, J. Kates, L. Levitt, COVID-19 models: can they tell us what we want to
     know?, 2020. www.kff.org/coronavirus-policy-watch/covid-19-models/. (Accessed
     June 4 2020).

[8] A. Shlomai, A. Leshno, E. Sklan, M. Leshno, Global versus focused isolation
     during the SARS-CoV-2 pandemic-A cost-effectiveness analysis, medRxiv preprint.
     (2020). doi: https://doi.org/10.1101/2020.03.30.20047860 posted April 5, 2020.

[9] M. Whittington, J. Campbell, Alternative pricing models for remdesivir and other
     potential treatments for COVID-19, Institute for Clinical and Economic Review,
     2020, pp. 1–7.

[10] M. Arbyn, E. Weiderpass, L. Bruni, S. de Sanjose, M. Saraiya, J. Ferlay, F. Bray,
     Estimates of incidence and mortality of cervical cancer in 2018: a worldwide analysis,
     Lancet Glob Health, 8(2) (2020) e191–e203.

[11] L.E. Markowitz, V. Tsu, S.L. Deeks, H. Cubie, S.A. Wang, A.S. Vicari, J.
     M. Brotherton, Human papillomavirus vaccine introduction-the first five years,
     Vaccine, 30(Suppl 5) (2012) F139–F148.

Index

Printed in the United States
by Baker & Taylor Publisher Services